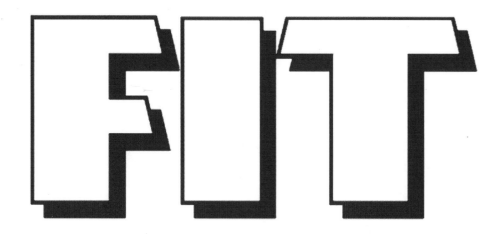

FIT

Lon Kilgore
Michael Hartman
Justin Lascek

ISBN-10 0615497063
ISBN-13 9780615497068

Killustrated Books - Iowa Park - Texas
www.killustrated.com

CONTENTS

Be authentic to your dreams, be authentic to your own ideas about yourself. Grind away at your own minds and bodies until you become your own invention. Be mad scientists.

Doktor Sleepless
in Doktor Sleepless #5 by Warren Ellis

THE AUTHORS

Lon Kilgore currently holds a post at the University of the West of Scotland. He has taught fitness physiology and exercise anatomy in undergraduate pre-physical therapy, exercise physiology, and graduate exercise physiology programs for nearly two decades. He has developed a unique perspective and approach relative to the application of science to sport and exercise that he passes on to his students - or anyone else who will listen. He graduated from Lincoln University with a Bachelor of Science in Biology, earned a Masters in Kinesiology, and a Doctorate from the Department of Anatomy and Physiology from Kansas State University. He has competed in weightlifting to the national level since 1972 and coached his first athletes to national championship event medals in 1974. He has also competed(s) in powerlifting, wrestling, rowing, and golf. He has worked in the trenches as a coach, as a sports science consultant with athletes from rank novices to professionals and the Olympic elite, and as a head university strength coach. His interest in developing better weightlifting coaches, strength coaches, and fitness professionals have driven much of his academic and professional efforts. He spent a decade as a certifying instructor for USA Weightlifting and was a frequent lecturer and researcher at the US Olympic Training Center in Colorado Springs. His authorship and co-authorship efforts include Starting Strength (1st & 2nd editions), Practical Programming, Anatomy Without a Scalpel, magazine columns, and numerous research journal publications. His illustration efforts have similarly appeared in many books, journals, and online. His former students have assumed elite coaching and scientific positions across the USA and internationally.

Michael Hartman is an Assistant Professor of Exercise & Rehabilitative Science at Texas Wesleyan University. He earned his Doctorate in Neuromuscular Physiology from the University of Oklahoma and also holds degrees in Exercise Science (Bachelor of Science) and Kinesiology (Master of Science). As a Research Sport Scientist, he specializes in the neuromuscular adaptations associated with strength training and conditioning. His research efforts have been published in scientific journals and presented extensively at national conferences. He has previously worked at the US Olympic Training Center, where he was a member of the inaugural USA Weightlifting Performance Enhancement Team, he is an Olympic Weightlifting coach and also has experience as a Collegiate Strength and Conditioning Coach.

Justin Lascek is a professional coach, trainer, and owner of the strength and conditioning website 70sBig.com. He has a Bachelor of Science degree in Kinesiology with an emphasis in Exercise Science from Georgia Southern University. He has experience as a strength & conditioning coach at the high school and collegiate levels, has coached athletes in powerlifting and weightlifting, has coached many CrossFit trainees (he is a CrossFit Level II certified trainer), and has worked with many general fitness trainees. He has a broad background in sport and exercise to include playing collegiate football and competing in the 2010 USA Weightlifting Senior National Championships. His specialties are coaching and programming of strength and combined fitness element training.

ACKNOWLEDGEMENTS

We would like to thank our many and diverse personal and professional influences. To list them all would be a chapter in and of itself. We would, however, like to specifically thank Shelley Hancock and Tiffany Stewart for their in-front-of-the-camera work. We would also like to commend Shelley for her research and organizational assistance with this project, we could not have asked for a better project assistant.

Lon
Michael
Justin

FITNESS: WHAT IT IS

Have you ever thought about what fitness really means? Everyone has a rough idea about what fitness ***means to them***, lean and rock hard abs, finishing a marathon, benching double bodyweight, being able to play their favorite recreational sport, the ability to do 15 minutes in the octagon, or maybe just the habit of training. But what does the word fitness really mean? If we harken back to the days of old, science tells us that fitness is essentially survivability. This may not be an especially relevant definition for modern times, or is it?

Every day people use the term "fitness" when they talk about exercise, sport, health, disease, and rehabilitation. Every exercise or health profession has their own preferred terms like "physical fitness," "health-related fitness," "muscular fitness," and there are many more such terms present in the exercise lexicon. Are any of them talking about the same thing? The short answer is "No", and this poses a large problem for those of us that actually want to get fit or study fitness.

The US government, every major health, medical, and exercise professional organization, and most people in the USA will claim a link between fitness and health so one would assume that there must be a universally accepted definition of fitness in support of this assertion. We would also assume that the definition is time tested and precise. Most professionals would agree that this assumption is true. BUT when pressed to define, in absolute terms, what fitness is, 100 professionals would likely provide 100 different definitions. And the definitions provided would be nebulous in form and content. You would not expect this, but "fitness" is a poorly defined term across all professions and occupations who propose to improve it.

In the 1920s through the 50s, fitness had a fairly specific meaning in the exercise literature. "Fitness" was synonymous with the term physical fitness and with the term physical work capacity. The western definition of physical fitness as late as the mid-sixties (1) referred to the possession of:

Strength	Endurance	Body control
Speed	Coordination	Flexibility
Power	Balance	Agility

Having a degree of development in the above elements was assumed to have a direct affect on ones performance or work capacity.

When one examines the independently developing Soviet sports science literature from the same era, it is interesting to note that they had derived the important basic physical qualities of fitness for sport to be strength, speed, endurance, and flexibility (2).

Work capacity was a very simple concept. The more work you can do, the more fit you are. During the American fitness boom of the 60s and 70s, work capacity, in the research laboratory and medicine, mutated in definition from referring to the maximal level of metabolism (work) of which an individual is capable (3) to focusing only on work accomplished with the support of the cardiorespiratory system. Essentially fitness went from having nine elements to having only one - endurance.

With the dissolution and disregard of previous definitions, in the early days of the American fitness boom (1960s and 70s) an alternative definition of "physical fitness" was developed:

> "The ability to carry out daily tasks with vigor and alertness, without undue fatigue, and with ample energy to enjoy leisure time pursuits and meet unforeseen emergencies" (4).

This short definition was very easy to remember in the college classroom setting. It was also very inclusive so that even peripheral issues could be related to fitness in some vague manner. But this generality rendered fitness, in respect to the definition, difficult to measure and use in practice. Fatigue in physical structures is hugely different from emotional fatigue and are all types of fatigue included? "Vigor" can be measured in plants but it is a difficult thing to measure, quantify, and employ in sport and exercise. "Alertness" is a behavioral concept and is not really something trained or generally measured in fitness practice. And then there is the idea of "energy" contained in the definition. Energy is a very well defined term and has a extremely specific physical/chemical/biological meaning. This early definition of fitness used the word in such a lax fashion the definition became meaningless.

Further dissolution and weakening of the definition occurred at the hands of one of the US's greatest proponents of exercise, Kenneth Cooper MD. In a 1987 NY Times interview he stated that he had "broadened the fitness concept to make it one of moderation and balance". In his new concept, bodyweight control, diet, smoking, alcohol consumption, stress management, and periodic physician examinations were now included. A fairly significant deviation from what is considered "fit", as personal habits and disease processes (historically the realm of "health") were now part of the fitness definition.

Although it was obvious to many that the previous modified definitions were irrelevant, it took more than twenty five years for a revision of the 1970s definition to appear in the literature. In 1996 the United States Department of Health and Human Services (USDHHS), and then in 2000 the American College of Sports Medicine (ACSM), modified the definition of fitness in their standards of practice doctrine. One might expect it to have been refined and improved. What occurred was that it was trimmed down to an even more cursory definition:

> "A set of attributes that people have or achieve relating to their ability to perform physical activity" (5,6).

The best thing that can be said about this definition was that it implied that fitness is trainable and focused on physical abilities. But it remained a nebulous and immeasurable concept.

It is apparent to most that a more precise and functional definition of fitness should have been developed since there was a great deal of data being produced relative to exercise in science laboratories around the world. The fact that some exercise professional groups, such as the National Strength and Conditioning Association (NSCA), did not and do not even define fitness in their standards of practice resources is chilling (7). How can an organization produce "authoritative standards" about an entity, fitness, which they do not or cannot define?

The specific "attributes" of fitness to which the USDHHS and ACSM referred in 1996 were later elaborated on in their 2006 exercise guidelines documents:

> "A multidimensional concept that has been defined as a set of attributes that people possess or achieve that relates to the ability to perform physical activity and is comprised of skill-related, health related, and physiologic components. Skill related components of physical fitness includes agility, balance, coordination, speed, power, and reaction time, and are mostly associated with sport and motor skills performance. Health related physical fitness is associated with the ability to perform daily activities with vigor, and the possession of traits and capacities that are associated with a low risk of premature development of hypokinetic diseases. Health related components of fitness include cardiovascular endurance, muscular strength and endurance, flexibility, and body composition. Physiologic fitness differs from health-related fitness in that in includes nonperformance components that relate to biological systems influenced by habitual activity. Physiologic fitness includes - (a) Metabolic Fitness: The status of metabolic systems and variables predictive of the risk for diabetes and cardiovascular disease. (b) Morphologic fitness: The status of body compositional factors such as body circumference, body fat content, and regional body fat distribution. (c) Bone integrity; The status of bone mineral density." (8)

This is a simple laundry list of things that the authors of the definition proposed might be in some way correlated to fitness. This is not a definition, as a mere listing of attributes cannot serve as a coherent definition.

If the "authoritative" definitions of fitness are inadequate, or flat out wrong, how should fitness be defined?

DECONSTRUCTING FITNESS

The human body is an integrated living system, one that must follow the laws and theories of biology, chemistry, and physics. These fields are structured upon foundations of definition and measurement. Any definition of fitness must be quantifiable. If we focus our definition of fitness on the many decades old works of Darwin, Nietzche, Bernard, Selye, and many more, we will create a definition rooted in the science of physical abilities, adaptation, and survival (9,10,11,12). But what physical abilities are related to survival? If we consider the physical abilities that help us function and conquer the spectrum of physical stresses and life tasks with which have historically and presently encountered, we can categorize them into three basic physical abilities:

Strength   Endurance   Mobility

Strength is the ability to move the body under load and is expressed as an ability to generate muscular force across a spectrum of movement speeds. Strength is a physical entity driven by the biological need to overcome the force of gravity acting on the body or on environmental entities with which the body interacts. It is easily measured using apparati commonly found in gyms (barbells) or laboratories (force platforms, dynamometers, and other force measurement devices). Strength can be further subdivided into muscular force generated with no body movement - isometric strength; muscular force generated at slow speeds - low velocity strength; and muscular force generated at high speeds - high velocity strength.

Endurance is the ability to sustain a task over time. Standing and sitting are the two most sustained things humans do in modern life. Neither require any type of physical effort as the body is anatomically structured to minimize exertion and caloric expenditure when seated or standing. Endurance is a characteristic of movement, physical activity, exercise, and sport. Many things we do require a level of endurance - walking across campus, carrying groceries up to a fourth story walk up, jogging a couple miles, and playing a hard half of football for example. Endurance is primarily a bioenergetic entity, related to the ability to deliver oxygen and energetic nutrients to the working muscles at adequate rates and for long enough durations to accomplish the task at hand. As endurance is time dependent, it is easily measured with a watch and measuring tape or any number of other common or laboratory measurement devices. Endurance can be subdivided into continuous endurance, where the activity is sustained, as in jogging - and intermittent endurance, where work-recovery cycles are repeated for long durations, as in digging post holes for a fence row.

Mobility is the ability to move the body and its constituent parts in a variety of directions and carry out both simple and complex motor tasks. Mobility is an important - but under attended - element of fitness. Stable, controlled, and coordinated movement within our occasionally unstable and frequently unpredictable home, work, and play environments facilitates adequate function and survival. Mobility is likely the most complicated element of fitness as it is comprised of range of motion, agility, balance, and coordination. Each of these entities is measurable in the gym or in the laboratory using simple instruments.

A VIABLE DEFINITION

Once we know what fitness is comprised of, we can create a functional definition. The definition for physical fitness used in this book is simple, functional, and measurable:

> Possession of adequate levels of strength, endurance, and mobility to provide for successful participation in occupational effort, recreational pursuits, familial obligation, and that is consistent with a functional phenotypic expression of the human genotype (13).

This definition applies to the general population but it can be extended to occupational and sporting populations. We can also abbreviate it to make it precisely applicable and measurable by the average coach, trainer, or trainee through omission of the clause about genotype - an assessment of ones genetic make-up and function which is measurable only in the laboratory. This will be our approach throughout this text. Various occupations require more (or less) of one of the elements of fitness, and sport has goals and specializations that merely emphasize or de-emphasize pre-determined components of physical fitness to varying degrees - a weightlifter has focused on strength, a marathoner on endurance. Each has accelerated fitness in one area and has an average ability or potential weakness in the others. As we progress though this book you will find out how to develop each component of fitness individually and also how to develop all three elements simultaneously - enabling the tailoring of training to any purpose or goal.

One would hope that it is a logical concept that knowing what fitness is and what it is not is essential knowledge before it can be manipulated and improved. The definition here clearly states that physical fitness is functional and that the elements of fitness are strength, endurance, and mobility. It follows that improvements in physical fitness are dependent on progressive strength, endurance, and mobility training that force our bodies to adapt. It should also be apparent that physical fitness is not a set of variables that cannot be directly measured or do not manifest as outward physical performance. Further, physical fitness should not be considered an abstract concept or set of intangible feelings. These things are by-products of fitness - as a trainee becomes more physically fit, their ability to function within their own circumstances improves, making them feel better about themselves. This change is not "fitness" but rather a change in self-perception driven by their awareness of the tangible increases in performance produced by training and of becoming more fit. The perception of wellbeing is directly attributable to systematic and progressive exercise training delivering something of substance and value to the trainee, fitness.

Fitness is defined as the possession of adequate levels of strength, endurance and mobility to provide for successful participation in any given occupational effort, recreational pursuit, or familial obligation.

Strength is the ability to move the body under load and is expressed as an ability to generate force across a spectrum of movement speeds.

Endurance is the ability to sustain a task over time.

Mobility is the ability to move in a variety of directions and carry out both simple and complex motor tasks.

Exercise is planned movement that is intended to produce an improvement in one or more components of fitness (i.e., lifting weights, running, swimming, etc).

Training is a longer duration (weeks, months, and years), planned, and systematic application of exercise or exercises toward achievement of a fitness goal.

Physical activity is unplanned and spontaneous movement that has no specific intent other than recreation or as an occupational requirement (mowing the yard, movement in the workplace, etc).

REFERENCES

1. de Vries, H.A. Physiology of Exercise for Physical Education and Athletics. W.C. Brown Company, Dubuque, IA, 1966.

2. Matveyev, L. Fundamentals of Sport Training. Progress Publishers, Moscow, USSR, 1977 (1981 translation by A. Shafransky).

3. Wahlund, H. Determination of the physical working capacity. Acta Medica Scandinavica 131(s215):51-70, 1948.

4. Clarke, H.H. (ed). Basic understanding of physical fitness. Physical Fitness Research Digest 1(1), 1971. Presidents Council on Physical Fitness and Sport. Washington, DC.

5. US Department of Health and Human Services. Physical activity and health; A report of the Surgeon General. U.S. Department of Health and Human Services. Atlanta, GA, 1996.

6. American College of Sports Medicine. ACSM's guidelines for exercise testing and prescription. Lippincott, Williams, and Wilkins, Baltimore, MD, 2000

7. Baechle, T.R. and R.W. Earle (eds.). Essentials of Strength and Conditioning. Human Kinetics. Champaign, IL, 2000.

8. American College of Sports Medicine. ACSM's guidelines for exercise testing and prescription. Lippincott, Williams, and Wilkins, Baltimore, MD, 2006.

9. Darwin, C.R. On the origin of species. John Murray, London, 1859.

10. Nietzche, F.W. Götzen-Dämmerung, 1889. Cited in Twilight of the Idols: Or How to Philosophize with a Hammer (Introduction by M. Tanner, Translation by R.J. Hollingdale), Penquin Books, New York, NY, 1998.

11. Bernard, C. La fixité du milieu intérieur est la condition de la vie libre; Oevures xvi, 113 Phénomènes de la vie, tome i, 1865. Cited in J.M.D. Olmstead. Claude Bernard, Physiologist. Harper & Brothers, New York, NY, 1938.

12. Selye, H. A Syndrome produced by Diverse Nocuous Agents. Nature, 138:32, 1936.

13. Kilgore, J.L. and C.M. Rippetoe. Redefining fitness for health and fitness professionals. Journal of Exercise Physiology, 10(2):34-39, 2007.

Any workout which does not involve a certain minimum of danger or responsibility does not improve the body - it just wears it out.

Norman Mailer

FITNESS ADAPTATION - HOW WE BECOME FIT

Now that we understand what it is we want to change, we now are faced with a problem. The problem needing solving is that we - trainees and trainers alike - are not as physically fit as we could be. The solution we need is a defined means of improving fitness levels. And the improvements produced by those means must be predictable. We can begin that quest with a look at the works of one individual, Hans Selye, M.D.

Who Is Hans and Why Do I Care?

Adaptation is not a new concept. Friedrich Nietzsche's attributed quote, "That which does not kill us makes us stronger," is a famous adage used in reference to the many challenges we face in life. The fact that it's from the 1800s means we have known for hundreds of years that the human body, when presented with a sub-lethal physical, psychological or chemical stress, can adapt to the source of stress, allowing the body to tolerate incrementally larger similar stresses.

Numerous and earlier historical writings in science and medicine provide observations that mirror Nietzsche's. But none of these writings provided us with anything other than anecdotes - nice observations of the end results of adaptation. It was not until the 1936 synthesis of the general adaptation syndrome by Seyle that we had our first understanding of how the adaptation occurred. Selye, an endocrinologist and professor at McGill University in Montreal, Quebec, spent a lifetime pursuing a goal of understanding how humans responded and adapted to all types of stress. His work in this area forms the essential foundation of exercise physiology. The entirety of the discipline exists as extensions of Selye's theory of biological adaptation.

Through Selye's own works and his analysis of other scientists' discoveries, he was able to develop a generalized pattern of organismic responses and adaptations to a variety of stressors. The general adaptation syndrome outlines a series of stages through which the body passes as it successfully adapts, or the stages that lead to a failure to adapt.

Selye's 1936 paper was titled *A Syndrome Produced by Diverse Nocuous Agents* and examined structural and functional changes in organisms, single cell to human, after exposure to "nocuous" (harmful) stresses such as injury, cold exposure, intoxication, drugs and - most important for our purposes - exercise (1).

Seyle proposed that all organisms mount an acute response, then a chronic adaptation after surviving exposure to stress. The final adaptation enables the organism to tolerate a subsequent and more intensely stressful exposure to the same type of stress - a physiological expression of Nietzsche's popular quote.

The general adaptation syndrome has three basic stages: alarm, resistance and exhaustion. The former two are quite useful and represent a positive adaptation leading to survival. The latter stage represents a failure to adapt to an overwhelming stress and might result in death of the organism. Let's look at each stage individually and examine what occurs and why.

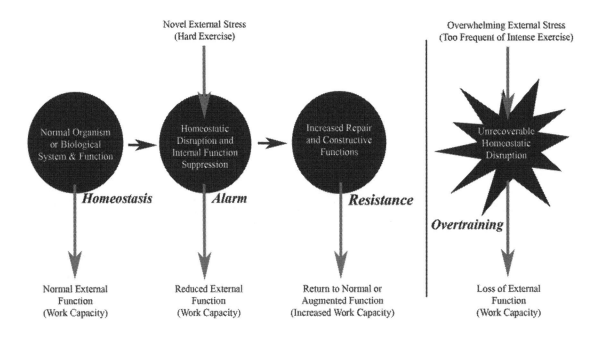

Figure 1. A representation of the stages of Selye's General Adaptation Syndrome. A positive outcome is depicted in the left three images and a negative outcome in the right image.

Setting off the Alarm

In the alarm stage, the body experiences a novel stress or novel level of magnitude or frequency of a previously experienced stress. That the magnitude or frequency of stress application exceeds the levels previously experienced is very important. It takes such a level of stress to disrupt the internal equilibrium of the cell, tissue or organism and induce the alarm stage.

Once the cascade of events is triggered, we see the physiologic intent of this stage is survival at all costs. The stressed cell or tissue diverts all available resources - energy, metabolic resources and architectural substrates - from carrying out normal functions to the maintenance of cell-structure integrity. Making new and replacing normal cellular chemicals and structures slows to a crawl while creation of cell-stabilizing stress proteins, acute-phase proteins, and beneficial inflammatory mediators increases. This selective increase in production acts like basic life support, keeping the cell from being damaged further in the presence of the stress.

Once the stress is removed, there is a fairly rapid return of homeostasis, within six to 48 hours (Selye's proposition). It must be understood that the alarm stage is the stimulus for adaptation, and for us it is the stimulus for improved fitness. If this is understood, it should also be understood that if exercise is to drive adaptation (fitness gain), the work done in training must continually progress in load. No increased stress leads to no improvement in fitness.

The idea of progression, just like the concept of adaptation, is not new. Its origin is often credited to the Greek Olympian Milo of Croton (circa 400 B.C.), who became the strongest of all the original Olympians by reputedly lifting a bull each day of its life, from calf to full-grown bull. So the idea of progression as a training reality has been accepted for a couple millennia. Selye simply provided us with a lucid physiological explanation for how and why it occurred - no increased exercise load leads to no improvement in fitness.

Resistance Is Not Futile

The second phase of the syndrome is the resistance stage. During this stage, the organism starts producing more metabolic and structural elements that are required to enhance its ability to withstand another exposure to the damaging stress. That makes sense: resistance to stress is developed. While the alarm stage is absolutely crucial to initiating fitness gains, the resistance stage is where fitness gains actually occur. A better name for this stage would be the adaptation phase.

The duration of this phase is greatly variable from days to months, depending on a number of issues including the magnitude of homeostatic disruption. Was the workload a little or a lot more than normal? Was it a single or cumulative overload? Is the trainee fit or unfit? The end result is always the same: an enhanced physiological ability to tolerate a specific stress.

Here is a good place to introduce the basic premise of specificity. While the stages of the general adaptation syndrome follow the same pattern regardless of stress type, a specific stress such as running 10 kilometers for the first time will produce a set of physiologic adaptations intended to make the trainee able to run the distance again with a lower degree of perceived stress as well as less, if any, homeostatic disruption. Running 10 kilometers generally will not improve sprint speed or squat strength to any appreciable extent because long, slow distance running cannot induce the specific set of adaptations required to do so effectively.

Exhaustion on a Cellular Level

The third stage is known as the exhaustion stage. Selye envisioned it as a stage where the organism's adaptive capacity was overwhelmed, or "exhausted." Homeostasis has been disrupted, and the magnitude of disruption is so profound that recovery is impossible. The repercussions of this stage can be quite dire, with death being among the possibilities.

We all know exercise can kill you - Selye considered it a nocuous stress - but deaths among healthy exercising individuals are rare. This means the third stage, relative to exercise, is usually manifested as something less dire. We will call it "overtraining."

We will look at stage three, or overtraining, as being induced by excessive volume (exercise duration, frequency, or both) or intensity (level of exertion relative to maximal ability) of exercise - or a combination of all of the variants. The physiological results of overtraining are quite diverse, individual, and destructive, but in general they are marked by an inability to compete or train at expected levels. Fitness has decayed.

The Flow of Adaptive Information

When we disrupt homeostasis, a series of events affects our physiology at the most molecular of levels. Exercise, when programmed appropriately, affects the operation of our genes, little segments of DNA (deoxyribonucleic acid) sequestered in the nuclei of our cells. Our genes control pretty much everything about our anatomy and our physiology through a handy-dandy little informational flow: DNA makes RNA (ribonucleic acid) makes protein makes function.

Initially a novel exercise stress shuts down, represses or down-regulates the activity of many normally active genes in favor of activating, promoting or up-regulating the activity of other survival genes. This is Selye's first stage. The up-regulation of survival genes and down-regulation of normally active genes leads to a different profile of proteins produced by the cell and changes the nature of the functions of the cell, tissue or organism. In this instance normal cell metabolism and function is repressed in favor of producing transient architectural proteins and other emergency proteins that aid in cellular survival.

After the exercise stress has been removed, the survival status of the cell is not immediately altered. Many of the emergency proteins and their related functions remain present and function for some time. But over the hours and days following a single exercise stress, during the resistance stage, the normally active genes become un-repressed and begin amping up their production and function again. But this time either more copies of them will be activated, or they will experience an increased efficiency in function. We can also see previously inactive genes become active in order to augment function.

As survival-gene activity and their product's activities abate, the new and enhanced set of genes now active will produce new architectural proteins (things like actin and myosin) and metabolic proteins (such as enzymes controlling energy production) that set up improved performance. The magnitude of change following a single exercise bout is not truly large and may in fact be immeasurable in practice, but the cumulative result of a series of homeostatically disruptive training sessions will be measurable in terms of strength or endurance depending on the type of training done.

Realize here that the body will arm itself for survival by activating specific genes that contribute to its ability to survive (physical fitness in our example), a further demonstration the relevance of the concept of specificity.

Making Fitness Gain out of Performance Loss

During stage one of the general adaptation syndrome, we commonly see a depression in physical capacity: our performances in training or competition are less than our best. We feel tired, a little sore, or maybe sluggish. This is normal, expected and even desired as these sensory phenoma tell us that we have indeed disrupted homeostasis, our training goal at this point.

But how do we turn a homeostatic disruption and reduction in physical ability into a positive, fitness-enhancing result? It's fairly simple but also extremely complex. The idea of super-compensation is fairly well known and elementary. When we train, we become fatigued. Fatigue exists not just as the feeling of tiredness we get after training hard but also as a set of biochemical and architectural phenomena occurring in cells, tissues and systems. We can consider it the opposite of fitness, the ability to do work. In fact, fatigue is defined as a reduction in the ability to do work. The balance and timing of the physiological processes of both fitness and fatigue can produce fitness gains through "super-compensation. Think of it as the disruption of homeostasis and the occurrence of stage one of the general adaptation syndrome events that induce fatigue, metabolically and structurally.

Also occurring during Stage 1 is the reduction of normal function. Fitness, or the ability to do work, will have been compromised as a protective device to prevent further damage. Over time, the results of Stage 1 will diminish, or fatigue will diminish and the emergency proteins and processes will return to their low baseline: "normal" or absent levels of production or activity.

Right after the withdrawal of stress (the end of the training session or series of cumulative sessions), anabolic processes kick in to restore function (fitness) to the system as rapidly as possible. The magnitude of activity is very large in the time shortly after the end of training but decays in the hours and days following cessation of training. The decay will at some point return back to the original level of function existing prior to the training stimulus. The return of fatigue or the return of fitness back to baseline is not remarkable and does not lead to fitness gain. It is the timing of decay in both that leads to fitness gain.

If the rate of fatigue reduction (recovery) is slower than the rate of fitness restoration, then the net effect is either no fitness gain or a reduced performance ability - a loss of fitness. If however, the rate of fatigue reduction is faster than the decay of fitness restoration processes, we will experience "super-compensation" and enhanced fitness, an increased ability to do work (Figure 2). Super-compensation represents the successful entry and completion of Stage 2 of the general adaptation syndrome.

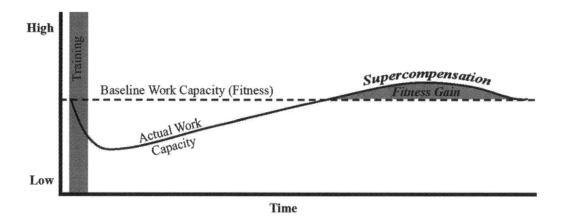

Figure 2. The simple concept of supercompensation. The difference between baseline work capacity (previous best maximum) and the peak reduction in work capacity in an appropriately designed program will generally range from five to eight percent. Larger reductions are suggestive of overtraining.

At this point, recovery methodologies become relevant. Adequate nutritional support and sleep provide the body with the elements necessary for maximizing the magnitude of fitness restoration processes while also facilitating more rapid fatigue reduction. Not only can poor nutritional habits, such as low protein and low energy diets, and inadequate sleep duration reduce the degree of super-compensation produced by a training session or program, but such neglect can also move a trainee toward our application of Selye's third stage: overtraining.

The general adaptation syndrome and the concept of super-compensation are important to researchers and practitioners alike. They are important to the former as these two entities provide a conceptual basis for the study of the human during exercise intended to improve physical fitness. They are important to the latter because the practitioner must, through the delivery of training, elicit these physiological phenomena in a controllable, reliable and repeatable manner.

Unfortunately, the practitioner is largely left to his own devices in this task as relevant experimental scientific literature regarding such programming is sparse and often questionable in content. It is advisable for aspiring coaches and trainers to not only become knowledgeable about anatomy and physiology of the human body and how its structure and function dictate exercise programming, but also to apprentice under successful professionals in order to learn how to apply that knowledge toward effective professional exercise practice.

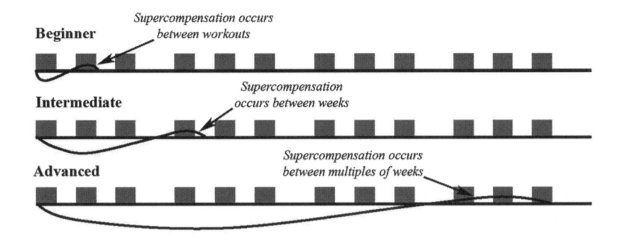

Figure 3. As one continues to train progressively, the length of time required to adapt to new and higher workloads increases. A beginner can adapt between workouts, an intermediate in about a week, and advanced trainees require approximately a month to adapt.

PROGRESSION OF SINGLE AND MULTIPLE FITNESS ELEMENTS

When we train we do so for a specific purpose unique to us. If we have fitness goals that isolate one fitness element we need to understand how to train to enhance performance in that single element. If we have more broadly scoping goals that involve all three elements, we need to understand how to improve performance in strength, endurance, and mobility and how this differs from specialization.

The development of strength as a single fitness component requires some consideration. How do you build strength? The approach taken should be dependent on the training status of the individual. The beginning exerciser needs to develop a base of strength using just a few multi-joint exercises organized into a basic progressive schema. Exercises like theSquat, Bench Press, Deadlift, Press, and Power clean are strongly suggested as beginner appropriate. These movements develop the foundations of strength - static, low velocity, and high velocity - around virtually every mobile joint in the body. After a beginner has trained for sufficient time to develop some functional strength, there will be a transition to the intermediate stage of training. The intermediate trainee will have enough developed strength to benefit from adding a variety of other exercises: different weighted exercises, bodyweight exercises addressing mobility, and even endurance exercises. They will also benefit from some added variation in periodicity of training loads and in exercises included. Modifications such as these provide a continued adaptive stimulus, although the rate of fitness gain will be slower in intermediates than in beginners. Most people will use weight training as an ancillary activity, contributing to fitness for another work or sporting purpose. This means that the majority of the population will never progress past the level of an intermediate strength trainee. Progress past this level of training to the advanced and elite stages of strength training will be associated with some type of sport or performance goals requiring great deals of strength and those programming methods are described in great detail in the references at the end of the chapter (2,3).

Endurance training for fitness also merits careful consideration. This particular fitness component has enjoyed the attention of virtually every expert, self proclaimed or legitimate, for the past 50 years and is the first component people work on when they attempt to "get fit" - think about it when people decide they want to get fit, the first thing they usually do is go out and jog. But that attention has not created any kind of useful information. Midgely and coworkers (4) examined the scientific literature regarding methods of improving aerobic fitness and concluded there was not enough hard data, despite nearly a century of experimentation, to provide a definitive methodology for improving it. Despite the dearth of real guidance, creating the ability to "endure" a mixture of volume (time or distance) and intensities (how hard the work) of sustained effort is desirable. The term "aerobic" is frequently used in respect to endurance. The term "aerobic exercise" describes essentially any continuous activity that lasts longer than 90 seconds. That means that it is not just running a mile or a marathon that is aerobic; any activity sustained through the function of primarily oxidative metabolic pathways can be considered "aerobic". The beginner who is aerobically unfit can initially use walking as an entry level exercise, then progress with added distance, and then increase the intensity to jogging in order to develop a baseline of continuous endurance before adding interval type training to develop intermittent endurance. The intermediate aerobic trainee, as with the intermediate strength trainee, will benefit from a variety of aerobic exercise modalities (running, cycling, rowing, etc.) and will also be ready to reap the endurance benefits of more extensive interval training. It is important to have interval training strongly represented in the training of the intermediate in order to assist in driving and maximizing the aerobic adaptations made possible by longer duration and continuous activities, and should be incorporated in a variety of distances and speeds of movement. Variation in distances and speeds (A) represents the varied aerobic demands of life and (B) their use in training promotes the development of the body's ability to extract, transport, and utilize oxygen during exercise in a variety of conditions. Running or riding the same route at the same speed every training session cannot improve endurance in anyone except the beginner. The basic tenets of biology strongly support this concept (1). And as with strength, most endurance trainees will never progress, or need to progress, past the intermediate level of training organization.

Mobility and the methods needed to improve it have not received any significant attention in the fitness community or laboratory. As it is a bit of an obscure topic with very little scientific literature available about its improvement through training, it has become an easy target for hucksters and marketeers selling the uninformed public (and scientist) gimmicks. What is known, scientifically, is primarily drawn from military motor control research and has been known for nearly a century. Most coaches understand that mobility can be developed through the intelligent selection of both strength and endurance activities but they do not know why. What is known in practice tells us that the Squat, Bench press, Deadlift, Press, and Power Clean strongly develop balance, coordination, and range of motion around most joints of the body in the beginner, IF these exercises are taught correctly and correct technique is enforced in all training sessions. Similarly, mobility in beginners can be enhanced initially by simply moving over a variety of terrains during endurance training. For intermediates, introducing exercises that challenge proprioception - the sense of balance and position relative to the environment - are needed to enhance mobility. For strength, this could be different barbell exercises, bodyweight exercises with gymnastic elements, the Olympic lifts, or work with kettlebells and dumbbells. During endurance training, inclusion of work in unstable environments like swimming, rowing, or biking is appropriate to enhance mobility. Contrary to contemporary trends and exercise fashion, there is no need to spend significant time on "agility" and "balance" drills using interesting toys UNLESS they have been shown to make a specific contribution towards achieving a specific strength or endurance performance goal. Will juggling 3 little sand bags while balancing on one foot on an under-inflated half ball at the same time dodging tennis balls thrown at you help make progress towards a strength goal, endurance goal, improve the ability to make a tackle, or hit a ball?

Single Element Progression

When we decide we want to focus on one single fitness element, all of our body's resources are available to assist in recovery and adaptation. This allows the rate of performance gain in this one fitness element to occur as rapidly as biologically possible. Most people understand the law of diminishing returns is active in fitness - a beginner will get fit fast and then will plateau. At this point he becomes an intermediate who will not only progress at a slower rate of gain but who will also require different training methods. This pattern is repeated as the trainee plateaus as an intermediate, marking the transition to advanced. Let's look at the basic concept we use to explain the changing program requirements of an individual trainee over a training career. Figure 4 represents the relationship between performance improvement (or fitness), the rate of adaptation, and the need for training complexity. The most important of these relationships is that as an individual's fitness/performance increases and approaches genetic potential, so does the need for complexity in his or her training program.

The following diagram suggests that the best program for a beginner would be simple linear progression (i.e., increasing the load each workout) and then, once the gains from that programming are maximized, switching to increasing the load on a weekly basis, and then, eventually, to increasing the load on a monthly basis. Each segment of the training progression line is associated with a progressively more complex training organization. This is a fairly simple concept and it works well to explain maximal progress toward any fitness component, whether it be strength, endurance, or mobility.

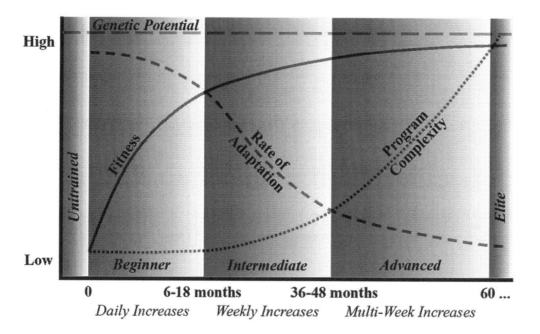

Figure 4. Every time we train and disrupt homeostasis and then recover from it, we make progress toward our genetic potential. The rate of fitness gain and the need for increasingly complex training are inversely associated (2,3,5). This graphic depicts the first five years of progressive and regular training however the diagram can be extended to the right for up to thirteen years of fitness gain (6).

Multiple Element Progression

When multiple fitness elements are trained as part of a program the rate of gain of an individual element will be slower than if it was the only element trained. It should be intuitive that if we want to improve any one of the constituent elements of fitness *as fast as possible*, more time needs to be spent training just that particular element.

To understand this simply think of each element of fitness having its own independent plot on the diagram in figure 5. You can be at an advanced level in your strength progression and thus require complex strength training while at the same time be at a beginning level of endurance progression and require a simple training program for that and also be at an intermediate level of gymnastic or mobility development and thus require moderate-complexity gymnastics training. Every individual will have their own unique profile, and the fitness element that is least developed will always improve fastest under an even-handed approach to fitness where all three elements receive equivalent attention. At some point, the elements reach similar levels of progression relative to the individual's genetic potential and the gains in each of the elements will even out and occur at similar rates.

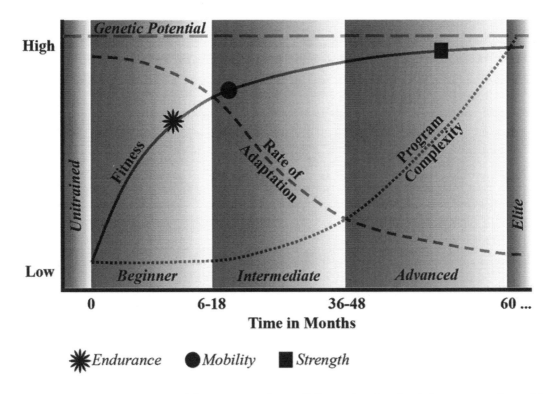

Figure 5. Different components of fitness can exist at different levels of training progression. This means that the programming needed to maximize gains in one area may be different from that for another. In this example endurance is least developed, mobility is moderately developed, and strength is well developed (5).

Fitness as we define it here fits nicely on the figure 4 if we consider overall fitness as a single entity. Overall fitness itself - not just one of its components - is the entity that general fitness training develops; all other elemental considerations are derivative. We use combined strength, endurance, and mobility training to develop the single entity of fitness. This means that the line labeled "performance improvement" on the diagram actually represents fitness as a whole, not merely a derived element.

Still, we are left to think about how to resolve the problem of different rates of fitness gains in different elements of fitness. If you train more with weights, won't the other components suffer? Yes, they will, but look at it this way: your body can recover effectively from only a finite amount of training stress. Let's say I'm a beginner and my body can tolerate and recover from 100 work units in 72 hours. If 80 percent of those work units takes the form of weight training, 20 percent is done in the form of endurance work, and 0 percent is mobility type work (gymnastic exercises for example), obviously the fastest gain is going to come in strength. Consistently using this same organization will develop endurance at a tremendously slower rate than strength. Gymnastic ability would not be directly affected except, of course, in terms of the roles that strength and endurance play in it, and not accounting for the increases in body control and awareness, active flexibility, and other qualities that necessarily come with improvements in strength and endurance. When combined, the total gain from all three elements represents "fitness" gain (figure 6).

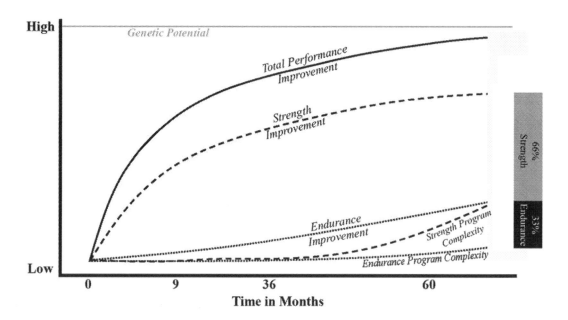

Figure 6. In diagram of progression, the solid line (top) represents the total fitness improvement possible from training at an individual's maximal and recoverable work tolerance. This absolute quantity of possible fitness gain is unaffected by the bias of training among the three elements of strength, endurance, and mobility. However, the magnitude of gain for those individual elements is affected by bias toward any one of them. For example, splitting training effort into 66 percent strength and 33 percent endurance yields a faster gain in strength compared to endurance. Summing the gains in both elements represents total fitness improvement. If we were to split training effort and duration evenly in thirds among strength, endurance, and mobility, fitness gain in all three elements would be slower than if either a single- or dual-element program were used. However the cumulative gain in each fitness element sums to the same overall absolute fitness gain. It is informative to note that every time a fitness element is added in, the complexity line for each individual element flattens. As elemental complexity is increased, the complexity of the program required to improve fitness is reduced (in other words, the more elements you train, the simpler program organization you can use). This is why general fitness training (all three elements included) can sustain steady increases in fitness longer and use simpler programming than any model of single-element training (5).

A general fitness program should include roughly equal numbers of fitness element stresses within the training week, such that the composition of the training might be 33 units of strength work, 33 units of endurance work, and 33 units of mobility work. This means that although the distribution of work and the resulting magnitude of individual element progress are different from the previous example - in this case, there is less strength gain but greater endurance and mobility gains - the total "fitness" gain through adaptation is about the same, but with a differing profile bias.

This also means that some training programs are more right for certain fitness goals and stages of progression - novice through elite - than others. Using an advanced endurance focused program on a beginning trainee with strength as a goal will obviously yield less than stellar progress towards the goal. If any strength gains result, they will occur at a rate slower than if the right program - one intended to improved strength - was used. This should be a logical conclusion to all, but situations like this occur in practice more frequently than not.

LOSING FITNESS OR STANDING STILL

The door to fitness swings both ways. There are conditions that make fitness gain move forward and there are conditions that slow, stop, or even make fitness regress. Understanding something about those conditions can help you select the right training program for you at the right time to use it.

Wrong Training

Using a training program that does not address, at its core, the trainee's fitness goal will assuredly not help them reach their goal. It is imperative that the goal for training be carefully articulated and understood by the trainee, be it improving one of the three elements of fitness, an even handed improvement in all three elements, or something more vanity associated - getting six-pack abs, losing weight, etc. With a clearly identified fitness goal, or even with a vanity goal, a program of training can be created that precisely matches the goal and will deliver positive results. Realize that if your goal is strength, a good program will make you significantly stronger but it likely will not make you the world's strongest man or woman UNLESS you inherited a killer set of genes from your parents. If you have a vanity driven goal, a good program will deliver results that will sate your vanity appetite but the likelihood the program will make you look like a Hollywood star is remote. One of the authors here could look like a Hollywood star. Unfortunately it is Gimli from the Peter Jackson's Lord of the Rings. No amount of training can change that.

Another type of wrong training is where the program used is inconsistent with the trainee's level of training progression. As discussed earlier, a beginner is best served by using simple linear progression, where a little more of an exercise load is added in every workout (the specifics of this are detailed later). If we use an advanced program, one where the load is increased on a monthly basis and that includes higher volumes and intensity of work, the trainee will not progress as quickly and in fact may become over-trained. The lack of progress can come because the load is only added monthly, the supercompensation wave is repeatedly missed, or over-training can cause regression of fitness as it is a catabolic (destructive) condition.

The final type of wrong training is the use of inappropriate training tools. Be cautious of any modern exercise gimmick or apparatus promising easy fitness in a hurry. In general those three easy credit card payments will provide you no fitness benefit but will add weight to the marketers wallet while losing weight in your own. Try to remember that tried and true, time-tested, and widely used training methods are probably a better investment of time and resources.

Stop Training

If you stop training, obviously soon after there will be a loss of fitness. This is a given. However, fitness is relatively persistent with its performance benefits lasting many weeks and months or more after cessation of training. The rate of loss is rather dependent on the fitness element. Endurance decays fairly quickly and a few weeks of inactivity can reduce performance to a point where it is physically noticeable. Strength has a less steep slope of performance decay and although you may have lost significant strength over a year's layoff, you will still be stronger than you were before you started training. Mobility is a bit of a mixed bag. The motor pathways developed during training are persistent - you don't unlearn how to ride a bike. But as strength and endurance decay so does mobility. The good news is that fitness lost is regained more quickly than when it was developed for the first time. If you progressed to a 300 pound squat over a years training then you stop training for a year, it might only take three months of progressive training to regain that level of strength.

WHAT IT ALL MEANS

Hopefully it is now understood that fitness is always some combination of strength, endurance, and mobility and that the combination is represented by an individual's training goal. We can isolate our training efforts on developing a single fitness element and it will progress faster than if we distribute our training efforts across all three elements - and this is not a bad thing.

It should also be apparent that progressively harder work is always required for fitness to improve. Basic biological imperatives make this so. Using the same training routine all the time and never increasing time, distance, speed, weight, or whatever is the source of exercise stress, will not make you more fit. Progression is key. And this means getting fit will become harder over time BUT as you get more fit you adapt to being able to do harder work and recover from it.

And finally, choosing an exercise program organization that is appropriate to the trainees level of advancement - novice, intermediate, advanced, or elite - is essential to capitalize on the body's ability to adapt and create fitness gain. Learning to make those choices is where we are heading for the rest of this book.

REFERENCES

1. Selye, H. A Syndrome produced by Diverse Nocuous Agents. Nature, 138: 32, 1936.

2. Rippetoe, C.M. and J.L. Kilgore. Starting Strength: A Simple and Practical Guide to Coaching Beginners. Aasgaard Company, Wichita Falls, TX, 2005.

3. Rippetoe, C.M. and J.L. Kilgore. Practical Programming for Strength Training. Aasgaard Company, Wichita Falls, TX, 2007

4. Midgley, A.W., L.R. McNaughton, and A.M. Jones. Training to enhance the physiological determinants of long-distance running performance: can valid recommendations be given to runners and coaches based on current scientific knowledge? Sports Medicine 37(10):857-880, 2007.

5. Kilgore, L. Dissecting the Fish: Plotting Progress in Multi-Mode Training. CrossFit Journal 69: 33-37, 2008.

6. Wells, J.R. Rate of strength gain in competitive weightlifters. Masters thesis, Midwestern State University, Wichita Falls, TX, 2009.

FIT

Nearly all the things I do that are of any merit at all start off just being good fun.

Brian Eno

STRENGTH

Strength does not come from winning. Your struggles develop your strengths.
When you go through hardships and decide not to surrender, that is strength.

Arnold Schwarzenegger

Strength is probably the most useful, most respected, and most feared element of fitness. Every culture (and subculture) either directly or indirectly places a value upon it. Today, virtually every media presents strength as an entity that helps us achieve success in the physical world. But there are so many historical misconceptions about getting and being strong that many many people are afraid to train to be strong. The myths that getting huge like a Mr. or Ms. America is inevitable, that if you are strong you are muscle-bound and slow, the stereotypes of physical strength coupled to mental feebleness do not paint an attractive picture. But these fallacies are baseless as strength is simply the ability to move the body under load and is expressed as an ability to generate force across a spectrum of movement speeds. Strength is a physical entity driven by the biological need to overcome the force of gravity acting on the body or on environmental entities with which the body interacts. Everyone is strong to some degree.

Why strength is a good thing

Normally when people talk about the value of strength, it is usually in a context of sport. Stronger is always better as when two equally matched athletes face off, the advantage is on the side of the stronger. This concept is not too difficult to accept as we see it over and over again in professional sports like football, MMA, and many others. But it is also very relevant to endurance sports where it has been repeatedly shown that making endurance athletes stronger increases time to exhaustion (they can run farther) and decreases running event time (they can run faster). But strength has also long been known as a strong contributor to improving quality of life. When someone gets stronger they feel better about their ability to participate in life and its challenges - it's because they can do more and they engage in life's activities more aggressively. Whether it is something seemingly as meaningless as being able to open a jar of pickles or something as significant as shouldering a soldier wounded in an ongoing firefight and doing a series of roof top sprints and six foot gap jumps to return him to cover and safety, strength can keep you fed and strength can save your life.

In fact, a study in the British Medical Journal suggests that if you are in the top third of the population in terms of strength, you are less likely to die from all causes (disease, accident, etc.)(1). These researchers found, as one would expect, that those in the lowest third of strength died faster than the other two thirds. This sets up a fairly interesting dose response - the stronger you are the more likely you are to survive. There are several other studies in print with similar findings. It is important to note that even though the data driving this "fact" is science based, the data is correlational in nature (A is associated to B) it does not establish causality (A causes B). As there is no causality data available, we will proceed assuming that increasing strength likely causes improved survival.

Strength is the "tone" people want

Lots of people have a seemingly simple goal of "toning up" when they start to exercise. Strength training is the best way to accomplish this. Let's actually identify what the desired tone is. Essentially people are envisioning it as being able to poke their abs or their pecs and that the muscles are going to be taught and hard not doughy. This particular phenomenon, changing the texture of muscle is a function of how much baseline electrical activity is going on in the muscles at rest. Physiologically this is called "muscle tonus". Many of us know someone who has suffered a stroke. When that person lost part of their neural bed what happened? The muscles in affected area began to droop. It no longer was receiving nervous input at rest and the muscle was no longer maintaining a baseline of tension. The same thing, although to a lesser extent, occurs when we get out of shape. The amount of baseline electrical activity decreases and the muscles become more flaccid - sort of soft and doughy.

When you train with weights, especially heavier ones, you are conditioning your muscles to produce tremendous amounts of electrical activity. The baseline amount produced at rest increases and baseline muscle tension increases as an adaptation thus producing the desired "tone" - firm and athletic. Endurance exercise does not produce a significant amount of tone improvement as it does not produce the same large magnitude electrical impulses required in weight training.

An alternative concept of "tone" used by the public has nothing to do with tone at all - its about fat. Sometimes when someone says they want to "tone up" they actually mean they want to reduce fat enough for the muscle underneath to have some shape. Regardless of the definition or intent, strength training moves the trainee forward in gaining tone faster than other modes of training.

Why strength facilitates endurance and mobility

Joggers and academics with an aerobic exercise bias don't like to hear this BUT having a foundation of strength enhances your ability to improve endurance. People will argue that strength training is not specific, metabolically or in movement pattern, to endurance and endurance activities so it cannot contribute in such a manner. Guess what? The science data is already in the literature that it does (2,3,4). The joggers have just never been told its there and the academics ignore it.

If I have a baseline strength of 100 units and running at a comfortable speed requires 40 units of strength, there exists a ratio of strength to desired endurance performance. If I increase my baseline strength to 200 the ratio of strength to desired performance is improved. This means that maintaining the comfortable running speed still requires 40 units of strength, but since that now represents a lower level of strength exertion there is less chance for a disruption of homeostasis and fatigue. In fact, the lower relative stress level means I should be able to run a little farther and a little faster than before, just by becoming stronger. Obviously there will be a law of diminishing returns in operation here. Going from untrained to novice levels of strength would provide the largest benefit here. Reaching the intermediate strength level would still provide significant endurance performance benefit. But reaching the advanced and elite levels of strength would likely produce little if any additional benefit to endurance performance. Being strong is also very relevant to the rate at which endurance can be developed. Essentially a stronger trainee can work at a higher absolute work rate than can a weaker trainee, able to produce through exercise a higher adaptive stress that leads to faster fitness gain. The weaker trainee also cannot handle as much accumulated work load; their weaker, less dense structures will break down quicker than stronger structures. A training program that includes more work produces better disruption of homeostasis and induces adaptation efficiently. It is often the case with weak trainees that they cannot do enough work fast enough to disrupt homeostasis and drive fitness adaptation effectively. This is very relevant to developing intermittent endurance - the time domain and the nature of most of life's activities. For this reason, strength training should be the first element of fitness developed.

Strength is also relevant to enhancing mobility. Strength holds your body in a desired position. Strength moves your body in a specific manner. Strength decelerates your body and re-accelerates it in a change of direction. Strength enables you to hold and move an implement with motor stability. If a trainee is weak, mobility and the rate of mobility improvement with training will be less than if they were strong.

Strength training does not automatically make you huge

If it did there would be sixty three million he and she hulks stomping the terra in the US. That's how many people train, at least a couple times a week for a few weeks a year, with weights. There seems to be a misconception, especially among women, that lifting weights will cause you to "bulk up". Actually, if done correctly you initially get smaller by lifting weights. In general a women's dress size will go down with weight training (and no dieting). This is because (A) it is exercise and it burns calories and (B) as muscle tone increases, the space the body takes up decreases.

Once this initial size loss occurs, more size loss can occur by weight training induced fat loss. If the muscles produce more baseline tension, expending more calories at rest, then we consume more calories and if diet is held constant (no dieting) then fat loss will follow. Also the muscles will increase SLIGHTLY in mass and more mass burns more fat calories at rest and during exercise. All in all a continuous loss of dress size that is sustained for many months. The dress size loss can be expedited by a logical and healthy reduced calorie diet BUT dieting limits strength gain so is not recommended here. It is much better to get fit and let your fit body reveal itself at the same time fitness is developed. People quit exercising so many times simply because they associate it so strongly with restrictive and unpleasant diets. Don't do unpleasant things to your diet without a just cause and a metabolic rationale (basic concepts about diet are laid out in a later chapter). It is inherently more important and more effective just to exercise as we lay out in this text and over time the body you desire will appear as a side effect of fitness.

There is another aspect of physiology that renders the concept that women will instantly bulk up to monstrously beefy proportions with just a few days of lifting completely false. That little debunking fact has to do with testosterone, the male sex hormone, the Yin to estrogens Yang. Women only produce at most one tenth of the amount of testosterone that men do. As testosterone is the major anabolic driving force for muscle gain (its why anabolic steroids a.k.a. synthetic testosterone is used so widely in sport), and women have so little of it, they are in very little danger of adding huge amounts of mass regardless of how hard they train. Although becoming a super-muscled female from simple weight training is an absolute myth, it is entrenched in the psyche of women so severely that it has become a rationalization of why not to exercise.

Another unfounded concern surrounding weight training is injury. If one considers the epidemiology objectively you will find that weight training is safer than grade school PE classes, and recreational lifting is eclipsed in injury rate by football (American soccer) and cheerleading, the two most dangerous sports on the face of the earth (5,6). Even walking and jogging produce tens of thousands more injuries than recreational and competitive lifting combined (7). In lifting we can add load in small increments and can quantify precisely the load. Both of these aid in proper progression in load and distributes those loads through a full range of motion safely and without injury.

The final concept relative to gaining mass from weight training is that specific set and repetitions schemes produce specific types of muscle adaptations. Not all weight training is intended nor can it produce a large increase in muscle mass. In sport, as in life in general, adding strength is beneficial in virtually all instances but adding mass is not necessarily needed.

Strength and mass, although produced with the same implements - weights, exist on opposites of a volume-intensity continuum. At one end is heavy weight training that by its physical nature can only be done in low volumes (low repetitions) and at the other end is training for mass done with lesser weights and higher volumes (high repetitions).

We firmly believe strength, not mass, is the most relevant fitness goal. As such most of our training time is spent on the high intensity-low volume end of the continuum. Yet here is another training fallacy for women. Simply look at the fitness books and magazines and examine the repetition and set schemes recommended. They are all biased towards low intensity and high volume training - mass gaining programs! The only reason that mass is not gained on these programs is because they are usually accompanied by low calorie and low protein diets which reduces the magnitude or negates any gains. Why not use the correct repetition and set scheme for the right purpose and not have to worry about starving or not getting strong?

Repetition - One complete raising and lowering cycle (or vice a versa) of an exercise through its complete range of motion. Also called a rep or a single.

Set - A cluster of repetitions with essentially no rest between each repetition. Historically sets are done in clusters of doubles, triples, fives, eights, and tens although any multiple of reps is a set.

Volume - A measure of how much work is done. In running volume is represented by mileage, in weight training it is represented by the total number of repetitions completed.

Intensity - A measure of how hard the work is relative to maximal ability. In running intensity is often represented as a percentage of maximal heart rate. In weight training it is represented as a percentage of the heaviest weight one can lift in an exercise.

1RM – One repetition maximum, personal best, PB, max, personal record, PR

High Volume
(Many Repetitions x Sets)

Low Volume
(Few Repetitions x Sets)

Mass Gain Bias

Strength Gain Bias

Low Intensity
(Low Percent of Max Single)

High Intensity
(High Percent of Max Single)

Figure 1. The volume-intensity continuum. Note that this concept is derived from centuries of practical evidence, not from laboratory experiments on beginners.

THE ANATOMY OF STRENGTH

Muscle is a wonderfully exquisite anatomical structure. Carefully integrated with the nervous and cardiovascular systems, muscle creates movement. Muscle is what we want to make fit and also what we use to make the rest of the body fit.

Muscle design

At the smallest functional level, muscle is an organized collection of proteins (chains of amino acids) that provide a scaffolding and some micro-machines that generate force against that scaffolding. There are two primary proteins active, actin the scaffold and myosin the force generating motor. When the millions of actin and myosin molecules inside of a muscle grab on to each other, myosin ratchets the two ends of the muscle - the tendons - closer together, a contraction is created. The work we do during any exercise begins with tiny little proteins binding and releasing each other over and over.

Not all muscle contractions are created equal. The repeated low force contractions produced in jogging and running are different from the high force contractions produced in maximal sprinting and lifting heavy weights. Not different in the actin and myosin interactions, but different in the type of adaptive stress created. Low force contractions do not create a need to add more actin and myosin molecules to the muscle in order to produce more force in the future, high force contractions do. Low force contractions are prolonged and are more of a metabolic stress rather than a high force architectural stress.

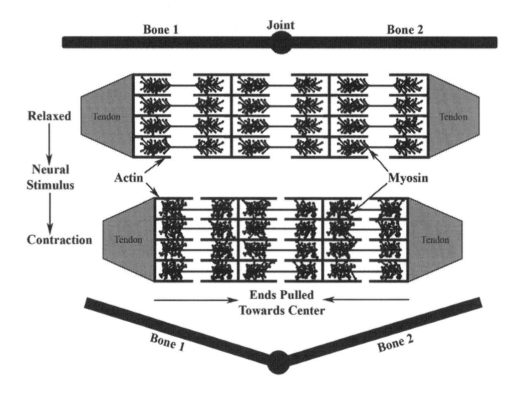

Figure 2. How a muscle works. When a neural stimulus tells the muscle to contract, the actin and myosin proteins present interact and cause a shortening of the muscle. Muscles are attached to two different bones and span at least one joint. When the actin and myosin generate force and pull the two tendinous ends towards midline, there is movement created around the joint.

Powering contraction

Metabolism plays a prominent role in muscle activity. And how we exercise influences how we power muscle contraction and where the power comes from. At rest, the majority of the energy we use comes from the break down of fat. If we do low force and continuous muscle activity, we use primarily carbohydrate and fat for power. If we do high force muscle activity, we use primarily carbohydrate for power. If we use maximal muscle force, we use energy coming from some stored phosphorous containing molecules called adenosine triphosphate and creatine phosphate (ATP and CP) while using virtually no carbohydrate or fat. So when we train with weights we are primarily using the last scenario, with each repetition consuming a little more stored ATP and CP until it is depleted. This takes about 10-15 seconds, meaning that a maximal set of 5 to 10 repetitions produces this specific metabolic stress. This is different than doing a maximal set of 25 reps that would create a carbohydrate dependent stress - we wouldn't use sets of 25 reps if we wanted to get strong though, this is just an example.

STATIC versus LOW VELOCITY versus HIGH VELOCITY STRENGTH

Not all strength training produces the same adaptive stimulus or targets those same biochemical constituents of the muscle cell. We've previously stratified strength into three sub-types; static, low velocity, and high velocity. Each of those possesses a few unique characteristics that imply differing training methods are needed to develop each type effectively.

Static Strength

During an isometric muscle action, the muscle is contracting as hard as it can. The persistent neural drive delivered additively recruits more and more motor units (a motor unit is a nerve that stimulates muscle contraction in all the muscle cells it touches) until virtually all motor units are being recruited. And neither fast twitch nor slow twitch muscle fibers are untouched, both general types are heavily recruited. If we also consider the overlapping of actin and myosin, we find that in a static position there are more possible interactions of actin and myosin possible than when the muscle is stretched or shortened. Combined, the high degree of motor unit recruitment of both fast and slow twitch motor units and the large overlap of actin and myosin make this type of strength the most forceful. Lots of muscle tension and pressure is applied against an object but there is no movement. This is the phenomenon that allows someone who cannot do a single pull-up to do a 90 degree flexed arm hang for many seconds.

In truth, a beginner cannot recruit all available motor units, only about 70-85% of them - but that is all the recruitment they are adapted to do. It is not until long into the advanced and elite levels of training progression when we see nearly 100% of the available motor units recruited. So neural recruitment is a trainable quality. It would be easy to suggest, based on this concept, that isometric training should be a mainstay in developing strength. And in actuality it can be a useful tool for stimulating adaptation in recruitment. However, it cannot be the primary means of training, isometric strength is specific to the joint angle in which the training exercise is executed. Such gains do not translate to greatly improved application of that strength to dynamic movement throughout the complete range of motion. This relegates isometric work to the category of an ancillary training tool, something we can use to address fitness shortcomings in intermediate and advanced trainees.

Low Velocity Strength

This type of strength is the kind we would normally conceive we are using during traditional weight training. We are using heavy weights and the weights are not moving very quickly. Basic physics and logic tell us that the heavier the weight is the slower it will move. As low velocity strength movements are slow, they share a bit of the same motor unit recruitment pattern as described for static strength. There is a large scale recruitment of fast twitch and slow twitch motor units but less than that of an isometric effort. This is due in large part to the moving target of actin and myosin interactions. At any given time there is less overlap and fewer connected actin and myosin molecules. This is why there is less absolute force generated in low velocity movement than in isometric actions.

It is important to develop this type of strength, it provides us the functional ability to apply force to environmental objects and overcome their inertia and move them. This is the realm of squats, deadlifts, presses, and such - exercises that tend to move at slow, sometimes grinding paces. They are essential weapons in the strength arsenal.

High Velocity Strength

Generating force in a fast movement is a display of high velocity strength. Accelerating out of the sprinter's blocks, swinging a sledge hammer, jumping over a roof gap carrying a load, and a simple Power Clean all represent movements expressing high velocity strength. In this type of strength there remains a high degree of motor unit recruitment, but due to the rapidity of the movement, it is primarily fast twitch motor units recruited. The slow twitch units possess conductive and contractile characteristics that proceed too slowly to contribute to a fast contraction and the ensuing movement. This is another essential type of strength to develop as many things we do professionally, athletically, and as part of life in general occur within this category of strength application. Inclusion of ballistic movements like Power Cleans, Power Snatches, Push Jerks, and more are valid exercises to address this need. There is an interesting study by Behm and Sale (8) that shows that if you do a slow strength exercise and actively attempt to move it as fast as you can, there will be a small, but measurable, improvement in high velocity strength. This technique is not as effective as simply doing ballistic weighted exercise but every little bit helps.

When we defined strength, we stated it was application of force across a spectrum of movement velocities. And if we consider, as we did above, only muscle force generation as a measure of strength we arrive at the relationship that the highest forces are produced with static strength and the lowest forces are produced with high velocity strength. There is a little more to it than this but the concept is sound.

High Force versus High Power

We haven't defined specifically what a force is other than it is something produced by muscles. For our purposes a force is a physical entity that possesses both a magnitude (how big) and a direction (which way) and can, if its magnitude is large enough, cause movement of an object. The bigger the force the muscle can produce, the stronger it is. This is an excellent concept relative to static strength - push against a digital scale to see how much force you produce. But we move when we exercise so strength should have an element of distance included in it. This is an easy order to fill. Physics has a nice definition for an entity called work. The product of a force acting across a known distance represents the quantity work. The formula we commonly use for this is:

$$\text{Work} = \text{Force} \times \text{Distance}$$

We can now suggest that the more work done relative to movement represents strength. The more weight you can move, the stronger you are. This fits nicely into the common impression of how strength exists in the real world. In this respect, slow velocity strength is reflective of strength. This works well except for one little detail, everything we do in respect to exercise, sport, and movement is associated with time of execution.

If we once again go back to our high school physics we can add the element of time into the formula for calculating work and arrive at a new entity called power:

$$\text{Power} = \frac{\text{Force} \times \text{Distance}}{\text{Time}}$$

You can look at this equation in another, more conceptual manner:

$$\text{Power} = \frac{\text{Strength}}{\text{Speed}}$$

Just as there is a relationship of strength to exercise and sport performance, there is a strong relationship between sport success and power output (9). This should be intuitive after looking at the last formula. If I increase strength (on top - increase the numerator) my power increases. If I improve movement speed (on bottom - i.e., go faster - decrease the denominator) my power increases. Both of these strategies - increase strength and increase speed - are viable means of improving power in the real world. However, increasing the strength expression of the power formula (getting stronger) is easiest to do and has the largest potential for improvement and influence on power. Increasing the speed expression of the power formula (getting faster) is more difficult to achieve and has limited trainability and thus a limited influence on power improvement.

Training the speed expression of the power formula is not so intuitive or easy. There are two strategies possible, both derived from the simple equation for power. Both involve improving speed by reduction of the value of the denominator in the power equation. If I can apply the force faster (smaller denominator) then power output goes up. This approach is extremely limited in how much improvement is possible. To understand this let's consider the two strategies:

(A) Nerve conduction velocity is approximately 50 meters per second … or about 5 milliseconds per 10 inches. Some people might propose that we can improve the rate of neural conduction significantly by doing "speed drills" and other things that have yet to be proven to improve speed performance. If we approach this objectively, without exercise professional conventional wisdom, we'll see that this is not really productive over the long term.

Think of how close most muscles are to the vertebral column. Once a sensory nerve fires in the hip musculature, impulses speed to the spinal cord, then exit to the motor nerve and muscle; it takes about 20, maybe 30 milliseconds to make the trip. With weight training and sprint training (high loads and velocity respectively) the motor end plates will adapt, and change structure as an adaptation, possibly to speed synapse. But the speed of conduction depends on the amount of myelination of the nerve axons, not really on motor end plates. And with only 20-30 milliseconds of total travel time, can we significantly increase nerve conduction velocity enough to actually record a movement velocity change with a stopwatch or see a power output change with a barbell? Not likely.

(B) Reaction time ranges from about 150 to 200 milliseconds (a simple stimulus yields a faster muscular response, a complex stimulus produces a slower muscular response).

We have to think consciously to make our bodies do what we want as a beginner. Think of the herky-jerky beginnings of you riding a bicycle as a kid. Wobbling every which way, your body was learning how to accomplish a complex movement task – your brain was trying to tell your body what to do but it couldn't get the job done fast enough with you thinking and then reacting. As technique was honed through riding practice (this goes for any exercise movement), reaction time became faster as the body began to sense the movement as a simple task rather than a complex one. Essentially, after much practice the body treats the learned movement or skill as a simple reflex (more or less).

You can improve quite a bit here, with the maximum amount of improvement being on the order of about a 50 milliseconds or so reduction in reaction time. BUT there is a bottom limit for reaction time of around 150 milliseconds. If our original reaction time was 250 milliseconds in a complex movement and our training can reduce it, once the bottom of 150 milliseconds is hit, there can be no more improvement on this side of neural adaptation.

This second approach above is the most applicable neural approach to all sport movement. Improve technical efficiency through repetition (read this as meaning skill practice), and speed in that movement will increase … to a limit specific to the individual. Increasing strength is what this chapter is about. The velocity component of this will be considered in later chapters.

Improving power may have a secondary benefit after improvement in performance. As previously discussed, there are numerous research reports that strength, of the slow velocity type, is associated with a reduced risk of death. There exists other data that also link increased power to improved survivability (10). Strong and powerful seems to be an effective means of living longer. Relative to this point, there is only one very short period in human history where strength training was not considered to be a contributor to physical readiness and longevity. In 1870, Dr. George Barker Winship, a very influential physician and quite public devotee of weight training, died at age 44. His early cardiac demise was attributed to his use of heavy weights and as a result, virtually all physical education programs, YMCAs, sport coaches, and physicians ceased recommending weight training for fitness and health. Even sporting goods catalogs and stores stopped carrying weights other than light dumbbells. It was not until 1940 when Dr. Karpovich of Springfield College, home of a historically prestigious physical education program, met with an actual experienced strength practitioner, Bob Hoffman (of York Barbell), that a turn around in professional philosophies towards strength training occurred. Unfortunately, the concept that strength training is an unhealthy, or at least an unnecessary undertaking, still persists in many professional enclaves in the health and fitness communities. We are not really concerned with the health and longevity aspect in this text (refer back to earlier definitions of fitness). The reason that the late nineteenth and twentieth century perspectives about weight training are relevant is that they created a void in the scientific and clinical literature relative to weight training methods and their fitness benefits. There is presently as much misinformation, probably more, about weight training as there is reliable information. Sometimes it would really help to have an event program to be able to tell who is who. Unfortunately, we are on our own.

MUSCLE IS MUSCLE

If you read the muscular fiction magazines you will find different training methods for virtually every muscle group - blast your bi's, shred your tri's, rip your abs - all with unsubstantiated, illogical, or untested presentations of set and repetition schemes promising to make you look like the current big thing in bodybuilding or perform like a champion.

We've already laid out how muscle adapts to specific volume and intensity loads in figure 1. Although this is a grey-scale continuum, not a black and white, either-or arrangement. Strength is best gained through lower to moderate volumes with high to maximal intensities. Mass is gained by training with higher volumes and moderate intensities. This basic relationship holds for all skeletal muscle, it does not magically change based on the location of that muscle in the body. Why would anyone expect their abdominal muscles to get stronger if they train them with endurance techniques? Millions of people have exactly that idea. "I'm going to get big, strong, and ripped abs by doing hundreds of crunches every day". There are several things wrong with this concept. Doing hundreds of repetitions is an endurance exercise that will increase exactly that, abdominal muscular endurance. It is a low intensity exercise - body weight and a very limited range of motion - so it cannot produce a strength gain stimulus. And similarly the low amount of muscle mass involved and low load is only a slight metabolic stress, even for a hundred repetitions, and will not significantly consume fat deposits exposing those sought after six packs. Treating sit ups, or push ups, as an endurance activity will not make anyone other than a brand new trainee stronger and it will only do that for a very short time. Every muscle and muscle group has to be trained in a manner consistent with the continuum if the desired goals are to be achieved. The abs and pecs are not exempt from this relationship.

THE TOOLS OF STRENGTH TRAINING

There are many names for strength training and many different tools used to develop strength, some are more effective than others.

Barbells

When people think of lifting weights they usually think of barbells either because of some TV or magazine exposure to the Olympic sport of weightlifting (one word), to another barbell sport, powerlifting (also one word), or in the form of weight training (two words) as part of high school sports preparation. No one in the general public uses the term barbell anymore, they just call them weights. Let's be precise and call them barbells for now. What is very interesting to note here is that the strongest people in the world used barbells to get strong and they still use them to stay that way. You use barbells if you are serious about getting fit and getting strong. BUT did you know that barbells were invented for the ladies? Well, maybe not invented for them soley, but the first use of the term is found in a book, Madame Brennar's Gymnastics for Ladies, in 1870. In it the author referred to an apparatus that was part "wand" and part "dumb-bell" and called it a "Bar-Bell".

A barbell is simply a bar with weights loaded on each end. There are any number of barbell types ranging from the discount store 110lb exercise set with a solid bar up to a calibrated international standard 308lb Olympic competition set costing more than $3,000. There are straight bars, bent bars, wavy bars, skinny bars, fat bars and many more. There are 1" hole plates, 2" hole plates, standard plates, international Olympic plates, iron plates, bumper plates, training plates, and more.

With the huge variation in quality and in type of equipment available to use, what is the right choice? The best choice is always the best quality product available and that is affordable. The most broadly utilitarian barbell set is an Olympic standard barbell set. The structure of an Olympic bar allows the bar portion (what you hold on to) to spin independently of the plates on the end. This makes doing exercises requiring wrist movements (like cleans) possible without releasing one's grasp on the bar. You can find a 310lb metal Olympic set for less than $150. If that is what is in your budget, you can make it work. But the bar will bend and the chrome plating will begin flaking off within the year, making it progressively harder to use until finally the bar's ability to rotate fails. Another limitation of cheap metal sets is that if per chance you do drop it, there will be floor damage unless a robust lifting platform is built. A better choice is an economy Olympic bumper training set. These sets generally run less than a thousand dollars for a 308lb set and have a higher quality bar and "bumper" plates. Bumper plates have rubber exterior elements that provide shock absorption if the barbell is dropped. This greatly reduces damage potential (to the bar and property) associated with dropping. In general this allows rubber matting or less expensive platforms to be used.

The bar is a crucial element of the barbell, after all, it is the part that comes into direct contact with your body. While there are a broad range of bar types, virtually everything that needs to be done relative to getting stronger can be accomplished on what is called an "Olympic" bar (the bar design used in Olympic weightlifting competition).

Standard Olympic bar dimensions (45lb or 20kg):

Total bar length	7.2ft (or 2.2m)
Bar diameter (the part you hold on to)	1.1in (28mm)
Outer sleeve diameter (where plates are loaded)	2in (or 50mm)

While this standard is extremely useful, not everyone is strong enough to where they can start with a standard 45lb (or 20kg) bar. This is not a limitation as there are two very useful variants of a standard Olympic bar, a 33lb (or 15kg) "women's" bar and a 22lb (or 10kg) "junior" bar. Having access to these bars makes learning and using the correct techniques for training possible even when extremely light loads are needed - a boon to child, female, and older adult training.

Women's Olympic bar dimensions (15kg):

Total bar length	6.6ft (or 2.01m)
Bar diameter (the part you hold on to)	1in (25mm)
Outer sleeve diameter (where plates are loaded)	2in (or 50mm)

Junior Olympic bar dimensions (10kg):

Total bar length	5.6ft (or 1.7m - varies by model)
Bar diameter (the part you hold on to)	1in (25mm)
Outer sleeve diameter (where plates are loaded)	2in (or 50mm)

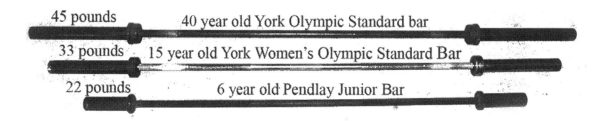

45 pounds — 40 year old York Olympic Standard bar

33 pounds — 15 year old York Women's Olympic Standard Bar

22 pounds — 6 year old Pendlay Junior Bar

Figure 3. Having the right weightlifting bar is important to progress. When well constructed they will provide a lifetime of service. If bought new today this men's bar (top) would cost $210, the women's bar $385, and the junior bar $310. These bars have been used hard for many years of indoor and outdoor lifting and have required no maintenance other than some minor seasonal brushing and cleaning. All have proven to be good products and good values.

For very strong individuals that will be using lots of weight there is another standard bar that is a useful tool, a power bar. Power bars were developed to not bend under very large loads (world record weights approach half a ton). These are very robust bars that can be used for most general training purposes as they can take lots of abuse and not bend. The disadvantage is the slightly larger diameter bar makes it a small bit more difficult for people with small hands to adequately grip the bar.

Power bar dimensions (45lb or 20kg):

Total bar length	7.2ft (or 2.2m)
Bar diameter (the part you hold on to)	1.1in (**29**mm - just a bit thicker)
Outer sleeve diameter (where plates are loaded)	2in (or 50mm)

Your personal selection of which of these bars to use or purchase should be based on your present abilities not on what you might be able to do in a few months or what someone else has. All of these bars are strong, with even the junior bar being able to hold up to 200kg (440lbs). This would not be optimal for junior bar maintenance but it should be evident that there is ample room to grow before you would need to buy your next, bigger bar.

The other component of the barbell is the plates. As mentioned earlier there are metal plates and there are rubberized "bumper" plates. Metal plates are always cheaper (we'll get to an exception in a moment) but having only metal plates places some restrictions on where and how you lift. Whether metal or bumper, you need to have standard size plates, 18in (or 450mm) in diameter, that place the bar in a useful starting position up off the floor and those plates need to be of weights across the spectrum. This allows you to assume a safe and efficient lifting position regardless of weight on the bar. There are Lexan or plastic "training" plates weighing as little as $2^3/_4$ lbs (1.25kg) that are precisely the correct dimensions. So for absolute beginners and basic learning and training purposes, a set of 1.25, 2.5, and 5kg training plates should be present along with pairs of 10, 15, 20, and 25kg bumper plates. With bumper plates be cautions of "rubber encased plates" they are not bumper plates that absorb shock, they just keep the plates from clanging. Also avoid non-round plates, drop one of those with the angle hitting the floor (or foot) and you have a decent amount of damage.

Then there are the "change" plates, small denomination metal plates - $2^1/_2$, 5, and 10lb plates (or 1.25, 2.5, and 5 kg). These are needed for progression in loading and are the cheapest plates to buy. If you buy an Olympic set, the small metal plates are generally included in the bundle. However, to be best prepared to train and progress correctly and efficiently another set of metal plates are useful, 1 kilogram rule plates. This set of plates comes in denominations of 0.5kg, 1kg, and 2kg. When added to the standard kilogram plates, this creates the ability to progress by 2.2lbs at a time rather than the 5lbs advances possible with standard sets. These plates are pricier than standard metal plates but they are well worth the money. With them there is virtually no population or rate of progression that cannot be accommodated.

Dumbbells

Dumbbells actually predate barbells. Some suggest that early Greeks used a version of dumbbells in training for a variety of purposes. However the dumbbells in that era were apparently used as calisthenic exercise aids and not as progressive strengthening tools. In more recent times, circa 1700, people would take the clappers out of bells, swing, and lift them (both the bells and the clappers can be used as a dumbbell) to train. A bell with no clapper is "dumb", not capable of ringing, hence the assumed origin of the name. Virtually every commercial gym in the US has a collection of dumbbells and often this is the most useful set of equipment in those gyms (this refers specifically to machine based gyms). Dumbbells can serve as a primary strength training implement if barbells are not available, but their most appropriate use is as an ancillary for developing independent motor control under load (developing mobility). If used as a primary strength tool, the programming of such will follow the same rules as barbell training advancement to be discussed later.

Dumbbells have evolved from their historic bell shape into two modern variants; dumbbells, the mini-barbells we commonly see in gyms, and kettlebells, a form that retains much of the original design elements of the original bells. Kettlebells have enjoyed a resurgence of interest in the past decade or so. It is interesting and important to note that historical and effective training tools persist and produce.

Dumbbells, as we know them - the characteristic mini-barbell shape, the escalating series of weighted pairs sitting in a rack - first appeared in an 1861 publication by Thomas Higginson. In that article in the Atlantic Monthly, he suggested that an ideal gym would have a set of dumbbells ranging from 4 pounds up to 100 pounds and that they could be used to exercise every muscle in the body in less than half an hour (No isolation exercises only multi-joint exercises!). The place of the dumbbell as a strength training implement was not superceded by the barbell until well into the 20th century. In fact, the weightlifting contest at the 1904

Olympics was conducted with dumbbells. The major advances in dumbbell design since the 1800's can be found only in materials and in the methodology of loading. Historically, having a series of fixed weight dumbbells has proven to be more durable and easier to use than having a single pair with changeable weights. The apparent ease of selecting weights and low breakage is why gyms continue to keep big selections of fixed weight dumbbells in stock as we approach a century and a half after their description by Higginson.

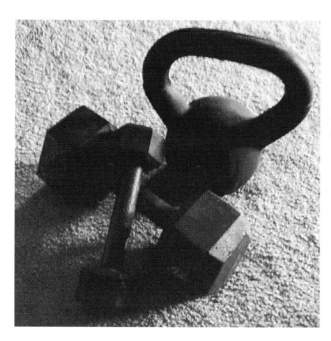

Figure 4. Dumbbells and kettlebells are useful strength tools.

Kettlebells have essentially the same history as dumbbells, however their use did not follow other European fitness methods across the Atlantic in the 1800s. Many of the famous strongmen of the 1800's used them in training and in shows across Europe. The recent assertions that they are solely of Russian origin are a bit off the mark as the Germans have as much of a claim for their popularization during that era as anyone. In fact, Scottish Highland games that were being revived in the 1800's also employed a relatively similar implement in their weighted throw events. British weight training instructional publications from the very early 1900's also included kettlebells as training implements (11). Regardless of who originated them, their use as a strength training tool was adopted very early on in the history of strength training. Their popularity only diminished once the development of the plate loaded barbell proved to be an even more effective tool for developing strength.

Kettlebells look essentially like big shot puts or cannonballs with metal handles molded onto them. They come in a variety of sizes, from as little as two pounds to over one hundred, are useful for asymmetrical movements (lifting the kettlebell with one hand) and for a variety of ballistic swings, lifts, and throws. The kettlebell's main advantage over the dumbbell is that it allows more mobility development across more movement speeds and in more joints and muscles. Some will say that the kettlebell has a disadvantage to dumbbells as it is more difficult to learn proper technique. This is not a disadvantage. Learning to use tools correctly is not disadvantageous, it's what you are supposed to do in order to use tools effectively. In this instance, the tools are intended to be used to create fitness.

Implements

Things as simple as rocks have been lifted to make people strong. This has been documented in man's earliest writings and depicted in art works for many millennia. People like to be strong and they will use whatever tools are available to achieve that goal. About 2500 years ago, the putative father of linear progression in exercise, Milo of Croton, is suggested to have lifted a newborn calf on his shoulders (assume a squat like motion) and then do the same thing with that same animal every day until it was a full grown bull. His intent was to become the strongest wrestler in all the world; where there is a will to get strong, people will find the means.

Implements have a place in fitness. In general they are less effective in developing strength than barbells but they can contribute to learning how to apply that strength in very functional real world environments. The key is that the implement used should mimic a desired fitness dependent activity and be scaled (made heavier or lighter). An example of a fairly new implement used in strength training is the tire. Popularized by World's Strongest Man contests where 500-800 pound tires are flipped along a known distance course for time, gyms across the country that have outdoor access are adding tire flipping to their repertoire. The ones that understand the concept of progression have a number of tires on site, from car and truck tires on up to tractor tires or larger. The activity can be scaled and the weight of the tire can be increased as fitness increases.

There are so many implements and variations of each type it goes beyond the scope of this book to describe them. However, at several points within we will suggest and explain the use of certain implements towards the development of fitness. In general, implements are used for many repetitions or for time making their inclusion into strength related endurance of primary value. One must develop strength to use them in their application as a conditioning tool.

Shoes

Much has been written on the topic of shoes for lifting. Some of it is even good. There are two critical elements regarding shoe choice for lifting; (A) the shoe must be constructed in such a manner that the forces created by muscle contraction are applied to the object lifted, not dampened by them and (B) the shoe must provide adequate stability in stance as to allow for consistently correct and repeatable technique. There are shoes made specifically for competitive lifting and they do their job quite well and can be used in fitness training (see resource list at the end of chapter). However, any shoe that meets those two criteria will also work for general lifting purposes (examples also provided in the resource list). To be blunt, any running or fitness shoe marketed to the general public, or advertises that it absorbs shock, or has a rounded sole, or touts its advanced technology is most likely not a good lifting shoe.

Machines

Many of our colleagues will eschew the inclusion of weight machines in this book. Machines effectively killed the viability of being a professional and well paid coach of strength. Previously "professors" of strength enjoyed royal appointments and presidential consultations. Today your local high school graduate who appears lean and fit and carries a clipboard is deemed an adequate fitness consultant as the skill of teaching weighted exercise is considered unnecessary on machines and the need for programming for progress is not a central mission of a commercial gym. They also make for very cheap labor. Stretching back to the 1910 writings of Max Unger in Intelligence in Physical Culture, machines for fitness have long been indicted for their lack of utility in not only driving fitness gain but for lack of relevance to real-world activities (12).

We present machines as a strength training tool because they are there. Every commercial and school gym has them. Instead of lamenting the fact that everyone should preferably use barbells, we want to enable people to use the tools at hand as best as possible to develop fitness. Wherever a machine may be useful, we will note how its use can be incorporated. And no, things like leg curls, leg extension, and pec decks are not the things we will be describing how to use. Multi-joint machines like the leg press and "shoulder press" (quotes because that's an improper exercise name - you do not press the shoulders) are potentially useful. Machines have their biggest value in the training of people who cannot yet do complete push-ups, pull-ups, sit-ups, or body weight squats. They offer a very limited physical stress and remove the motor control aspect of the movements. Very unfit people can do them safely and develop enough strength to allow them to control their body movements well enough to transition to free weights - dumbbells or barbells. But this also points out one major reason that we do not want to rely on machines, there is no element of motor control. If you train with machines you eliminate any mobility development during training. We do not want to do this. To recoup this lost opportunity for mobility development, additional mobility training would have to be added thus increasing training time. Everything in this book is bent on bang for your buck or maximum results in less time. Machines make everything slower; workouts and progress.

STRENGTH & MASS - THE COMMON GOALS OF WEIGHT TRAINING

The first step to training is learning how to train. The best and fastest way to learn how to lift weights is to find a qualified and experienced coach or trainer that has actually made other people strong. This is a tall task in even the most saturated personal trainer market. Word of mouth is probably the best means to find one. If the person you find doesn't have a certification from the National Strength and Conditioning Association, the American College of Sports Medicine, IFA, AFA, UFI, ACE, Fred's Online Certifications, or any of the 300 plus certifications for sale, don't worry. If they are good at what they do, they won't worry about pieces of paper stating that they meet minimum qualifications to practice in the field. Neither should you. A fitness certification is not like passing the Bar exam for attorneys or national boards for physicians. Any organization or any individual can legally certify any individual to be a fitness trainer. The common usage of certifications in the modern commercial gym is to lead the consumer to the notion that their trainers are experts. Some gyms actually certify their staff in house so they can say that 100% of their staff are certified - a purely promotional use. Certifications at best attest to meeting minimum standards, not to expertise. Certifications also assist in defending the gym against malpractice lawsuits - unless the plaintiff can demonstrate that the certification is simply a bought entity.

That's about it for the value of a certification. PR and legal defense. So until the certification system changes in the exercise arena, find professional coaches and trainers that have authentic experience and expertise, not an alphabet of letters behind their name. If they are confident in their knowledge and abilities they will probably have at most one set of letters behind their name, that of the degree or certification which they find most meaningful. They will also have a client list that have all improved in fitness and reached personal goals and will attest to their professional abilities ... this does not mean they will have famous athletes as clients and in fact you may need to be wary of some trainers whose only claim to competency is totally based on brief associations with professional athletes. Such a claim only has merit if the trainer played a significant role in the rise of the athlete to elite.

There are two times that it is essential that you are coached correctly and your time as a beginner is one of them. So if you can't find a local expert to teach you the "hows" of weight training, there are a number of experts that deliver high quality teaching of weighted exercises through workshops, seminars, or camps. High profile experts like Mark Rippetoe, Louie Simmons, Charles Staley, Mike Burgener, and Jim Wendler, to name a few, provide very sound instruction on how to safely and effectively lift to get strong (each with a unique approach or a specialty area). If you are going to pay to learn, why not learn from the best? The face of the field changes periodically with new experts emerging from time to time. Before you pay for a seminar, read about the coach, his/her philosophies, AND read things that the experts wrote. You need to be informed to determine if they really have a scientific AND practical base and if they fit your vision of what you need. Do not just sign up blindly. Mind you, at seminars and workshops these coaches will be teaching you HOW to lift to prepare you for training success, not providing a lifetime of coaching and mentoring (unless you subsequently hire them for such).

But not everyone has a coach in proximity or can afford the sometimes pricey seminars, workshops, or camps. This is still not too much of a problem because people have been teaching themselves to lift in isolation for centuries. A few good books and some accurate demonstration sequences or videos are all that is needed for the isolated trainee - that and lots of practice and patience.

After you are familiar with the execution of the lifts included in your intended training program, it's time to launch into the CORRECT program for you. Correct means that it is targeted on your specific goal. Here we are either assuming a primary goal of strength. We will also present relevant programs for gaining mass. Correct also means appropriate for your level of advancement - untrained, novice, intermediate, advanced, or elite. There are hundreds and hundreds of training programs and exercise routines on bookstore shelves and many more of them on the internet. Some are really bad, some are good. What we present here is a connected series of historically effective training programs that logically follow each other. Included are effective models or programs appropriate for beginners, along with information regarding altering their organization to accommodate different training goals. There are also programs provided for intermediates and for advance trainees with similar explanations of use and customization.

Realize that unless you have competed in weightlifting, powerlifting, or bodybuilding recently, we want you to begin with a beginners program. You will make gains with it because it is a novel stressor to you. If you have been training with isolation exercises or with machines for a year or two already, you are still a beginner because you are just beginning this system of training and it is different than what you have done before. You may out grow the beginners program in three to six months, but you will gain easy progress in that time. Don't give away progress because you don't want to be called a beginner.

We are getting to use the terms, "beginner" and "novice" in application now. It is important to remember that these terms refer to how a person adapts to stress. While those terms are often considered dependent on skill or strength level, it is specifically related to the ability to handle workloads relative to recovery. How do you know you should start as a beginner? If you have been sedentary or primarily been exercising with isolation movements, then increasing your strength through a beginners program will be the first step on your journey to better fitness.

BEGINNERS

The term for beginners frequently used in the weight training world is "novice". A beginners or novice program is based on the assumption that the trainee can correctly do the exercises included in the program. This means that they have been taught or have learned the correct full range of motion exercise techniques.

A beginner's level of ability is very far away from their genetic potential (or their maximum performance potential). Even though the weights they will use are heavier than they have used previously and will induce adaptation (remember the explanation of Selye's work), it is still light enough that the time required to recover and supercompensate is about 24 to 48 hours. A novice program capitalizes on this phenomenon and will add a little more weight to the bar in every workout. Progress is very rapid for beginners if this simple concept is applied - work a little harder every workout - a concept called linear progression.

Linear progression is a general term. When can make it specific for a strength program that consists of fundamental barbell exercises – squat, press, deadlift, and bench. These exercises are initially done with moderate volume and intensity then the weight used is increased steadily and consistently as rapidly as the trainee can tolerate. In linear progression different exercises get additional loading at different rates. A squat or deadlift might progress at about 10 extra pounds added in each squat or deadlift workout. These are multi-joint exercises with very large masses of muscle involved. Exercises working smaller muscle masses, like the press, will progress in smaller magnitudes. Adding 5 pounds in each subsequent workout might be appropriate. There is some variation between individuals with some people able to progress faster and some slower. The important thing to remember is to not get greedy. There is always a temptation to add more than the planned progression in weight. When progress is coming steadily with adding 10 pounds each time you do a squat workout, don't cave to temptation and jump 20 pounds, the magnitude and rate the additional load is added can easily overwhelm your ability to adapt and send you into overtraining (Selye's stage 3).

LINEAR PROGRESSION FOR STRENGTH

There are many well described and referenced training programs intended for beginners (13,14). There are literally dozens, if not hundreds, of on-line training programs putatively appropriate for beginners (*caveat emptor*). Many of the most effective programs revolve around a magic number of five repetitions for a variety of set numbers. Each wanting you to add a little more weight every time you do an exercise - on Monday if you are squatting 100 pounds, on Wednesday your expected to do 110 pounds (remember the exact increase depends on how well you recover and supercompensate between workouts). A simple explanation of why five repetitions seem to be preferred is that fives exist close enough to the strength end of the continuum to effectively produce a strength adaptation AND are a little ways out towards the mass end providing a small impetus for adding muscle mass. This is a nice initial set of desired adaptations. Fives also allow enough repetitions of an exercise to be done to move towards technique mastery without the inevitable technical failure induced by high repetition induced fatigue.

Most beginners programs that use sets of five use either three or five sets. Someone that has been previously sedentary (couch potato) will be best served by using three sets. Someone who has been active in other sports, other types of exercise, or has previously trained with weight machines, as they have some degree of work capacity, will most likely benefit from five sets. But when in doubt, start with three.

The most famous of the five repetition based beginner's programs is Rippetoe's Starting Strength program. In it there are five basic exercises; squat, press, deadlift, bench press, and power clean. The exercises are grouped into a repeating two workout sequence that distributes the exercises evenly over two weeks.

Week 1			Week 2		
Monday	**Wednesday**	**Friday**	**Monday**	**Wednesday**	**Friday**
Squat	Squat	Squat	Squat	Squat	Squat
Bench Press	Press	Bench Press	Press	Bench Press	Press
Deadlift	Power Clean	Deadlift	Power Clean	Deadlift	Power Clean

Each exercise is preceded by approximately three progressively heavier warm-up sets that are spread evenly in weight between the unloaded bar (45lbs or 20kg) and the target work sets. As the warm up sets get heavier, the number of repetitions done drop from 5 to 3 to 2. Then the work sets are done. Work sets are the highest weight to be lifted in the exercise during that workout. In Rippetoe's version, there are three work sets done with the same target weight ("sets across"). It is worthwhile to invest in your training, while we are presenting a conceptual overview of the program here, the original source book elaborates in much more detail the program and its navigation. You might want to buy the book (go do it right now). This goes for other source materials referenced in this text. Build a library to build your knowledge, its how you get good, its how you build your programming knowledge base.

An example of how this program might progress over a two week period is as follows:

Week 1

Monday		**Wednesday**		**Friday**	
Squat	165	Squat	175	Squat	185
Bench Press	135	Press	105	Bench Press	145
Deadlift	225	Power Clean	90	Deadlift	235

Week 2

Monday		**Wednesday**		**Friday**	
Squat	195	Squat	205	Squat	215
Press	110	Bench Press	155	Press	115
Power Clean	100	Deadlift	245	Power Clean	110

Note how rapidly the weights lifted increase. This is fairly typical of the rate of improvement when using this program in beginners. This program is so effective in progression that it sees gains in a matter of weeks, gains that other programs produce in months and years. The simple application of linear progression is quite powerful. One important issue here is that the program must be done as written to reap the best results. This means learning and doing all five exercises – it's not that hard. The authors have never seen any apparently healthy individual who could not learn and perform these exercises - ever. Many people have made excuses why they couldn't do them, but we got them to learn them safely, effectively, and quickly anyway.

Where to Start and Getting Over Plateaus

How do you know what weight to start the program with? Since this is a beginner, they are just learning how to do the exercises correctly. Learning the correct lifting technique precedes loading up with weights - always. So the beginning weight is a weight that can be done correctly and feels like a small challenge (it's a little bit hard). Whatever that weight is, that is the starting point. Because we start with a small magnitude stress (remember this is still more than the beginner has ever lifted before), progress in the first month or two seems to come effortlessly. That is where the temptation to take larger than planned weight jumps between workouts rears its ugly head. Repeated here for emphasis - do not cave in and jump. There is lots of difficult progression yet to come, do not give away future progress by bypassing your adaptive capacity. As one's time as a beginner comes to a close with this programming model, the rate of progression - how much weight you add each workout - will slow. At some point a few months into the program, there will be failures to get all five repetitions done in all three sets. This is indicative of getting close to the limit of one's ability to recover from an increased load within 24 to 48 hours. When a failure occurs, go home. Come back the next workout and re-do the workout that was done before the failed workout. Then come back next and do a workout with a lesser increase in weight (if the failure occurred by adding 10 pounds, this time add 5 pounds). If the workout is successful, then the next workouts will progress at a rate of five pounds increase instead of the addition of ten. At some point there will be a failure with a five pound increase in load. The fix is to step back, re-do the last successful workout and add less weight than five pounds. This is where having very small denomination metal plates comes in handy. They assist in maximizing the results possible from linear progression because they enable one to make maybe a dozen or so more progressions than possible with standard plates. When even small increases in weight can't be sustained from workout to workout, and this could be as soon as six months or as long as year or more after beginning training, its time to switch programs, you've become an intermediate trainee. Linear progression has been outgrown.

There is another approach to progression that may extend the duration and usefulness of the beginner stage. Assume a stalled progression of a five set by five repetition program. When the second plateau arrives after using the previous plateau breaking approach, a completely different repetition, set, and weight intervention is done. This stall is used as an opportunity to introduce a slightly different repetition and set scheme. Instead of going back to five sets of five reps with just a little less weight than before, a 20% reduction in weight used is implemented (if 200 pounds was the failure weight, we drop back to 160 pounds) and we change the repetitions to five sets of three repetitions. We then proceed back through progression with small jumps until reaching another plateau. What we are attempting to accomplish here is to capitalize on a break in training due to recovery as an opportunity to gently introduce a different volume of training to allow the trainee to push further out onto the strength end of the volume-intensity continuum. A plateau after this manipulation of the beginner's stage would also indicate its time to move to an intermediate program.

This program absolutely does not look like anything in the muscular fiction magazines. That's because it's not intended to sell supplements, apparel, or more magazines; it's intended to make you strong. It is not a three-way split isolation routine with 15 exercises per workout, just three basic, multi-joint, large muscle mass exercises per workout; exercises that produce big results in as little as an hour in the gym three times a week. It is those large muscle mass exercises that create the anabolic environment for strength adaptation (15). And really, won't you look way cooler squatting three wheels than doing curls with 45 pounds? The entire concept surrounding programming for a beginner is to select exercises that are large scale both in the number of joints and amount of muscle mass used. In that way the stimulus for adaptation is very potent, much stronger than if isolation movements are used. Wise selection of just a few exercises can lead to exemplary strength development in virtually all of the body's musculature. And a very desirable side benefit is that the time spent in the gym is much less than when using an isolation routine with a dozen exercises. It's not the time you spend in the gym that is valuable and productive; it's how you use that time to produce adaptations that is.

Double Time

Sets of five are not the only repetition scheme appropriate for beginners. Another option for increasing strength in beginners is to use lower repetitions for some exercises and a higher number of sets. There are a number of well respected coaches that prescribe doubles and triples for beginners. It's common for weightlifting coaches, who create some of the strongest people in the world, to never prescribe any more than three repetitions. They are only interested in lifting as much weight as possible, not getting big. The lower repetition numbers provide less of a stimulus to increase mass, focusing instead on strength gain. In the following example squats and front squats are alternated to provide a varied muscular stress on the hips and knees. Rows and pull-ups are alternated to provide exercises in axes complimentary to those in the press and bench press. This ensures complete development of the musculature around the shoulder joint - making it stronger, more stable, and less prone to injury. Weighted sit-ups and Romanian deadlifts are alternated to develop the abdominals, hip flexors, hip extensors, and the spinal erectors.

Week 1

Monday		Wednesday		Friday	
Squat	2	Front Squat	2	Squat	2
Bench Press	2	Press	2	Bench Press	2
Row	5	Pull-up	5	Row	5
Weighted Sit-up	5	Romanian Deadlift	5	Weighted Sit-up	5

Week 2

Monday		Wednesday		Friday	
Front Squat	2	Squat	2	Front Squat	2
Press	2	Bench Press	2	Press	2
Pull-up	5	Row	5	Pull-up	5
Romanian Deadlift	5	Weighted Sit-up	5	Romanian Deadlift	5

For the exercises using doubles for work sets, 8 sets should be done. The weights used will be heavy and at near limit with no less than two minutes rest taken between sets. This is essential in order to ensure between set recovery and repeated high quality work sets. For the exercises using five repetitions the standard three sets is used. As with the previous model, the weekly cycles are repeated until a plateau is reached. The plateau is broken with a single workout with a reduced workload then a slower rate of weight progression is used until the next plateau. At that point another run at progression can be made using very small additions in weight. After the third pass at progression, it is time to change to an intermediate model of programming.

Aside from those just interested in getting strong very quickly, these programs are likely the most effective off season strength programs for seasonal athletes. If an athlete is not in the gym year round, the case in many seasonal sports, these programs should be used during the months they are in the gym. It is likely that these may be the only strength programs a seasonal strength trainee may ever need.

Further, anyone who is getting ready to train endurance or is getting ready to undertake a program of general fitness training should start here. Getting strong before beginning the other modes of training will reduce the chance for injury and will facilitate faster gains in both endurance and mobility. Two months on a beginner's weight program will pay dividends in later training and performance.

The Machines that Fit

What if you only have access to a gym equipped with weight machines? Most gyms will have a leg press and a Smith machine. Use the leg press as it will not produce a motor pattern that distracts from efficient squat technique (when you get to squat in a good gym one day). Also add in work on the back extension or glute-ham deck to expand the muscles used to include most of those included in the squat. While this combination roughly approximates the musculature used in the squat, all of the stabilizers invoked with squatting are not used.

For the press and bench press, there are machines that mimic them. Use them. But every other press or bench press workout swaps in dumbbell presses and dumbbell bench presses to recoup some of the lost mobility stimulus from using machines.

The deadlift and power clean pose particular problems in machine based gyms. You can substitute in dumbbell deadlifts for standard deadlifts, but your progression will hit a wall at about 250 pounds since there will likely not be dumbbells heavier than 125 pounds. There is no machine equivalent of a power clean. A fast Smith machine high pull can work as a poor substitute. If there is a low cable row where an upright row starting with bent knees and hips can be done, that too can be somewhat of a substitute.

The mode of progression with machines is the same as with barbells. However, most machines have 10 pound increments in weight increase. If the gym does not have a $2\frac{1}{2}$ pound and a 5 pound weight that sits stably on top of the stack to aid in progression, get them yourself and keep them in your gym bag. With dumbbells the rate of progression can usually be accommodated with the collection of dumbbells normally in stock at most gyms.

The repeating two-week sequence that results would produce something like the following:

Week 1			Week 2		
Monday	**Wednesday**	**Friday**	**Monday**	**Wednesday**	**Friday**
Leg Press	Leg Press	Leg Press	Leg Press	Leg Press	Leg Press
Back Extension	Back Extension	Back Extension	Back Extension	Back Extension	Back Extension
Machine Bench	Machine Press	DB Bench	DB Press	Machine Bench	Machine Press
DB Deadlift	Cable Row	DB Deadlift	Cable Row	DB Deadlift	Cable Row

At some point you will be able to move the entire stacks on the weight machines. You are then faced with a tough choice; don't get any stronger or find a new gym.

LINEAR PROGRESSION FOR MASS

Although strength is a primary fitness goal, sometimes people just want to get bigger. If you refer back to the volume-intensity continuum, you'll note that mass is gained with higher volumes or more repetitions and sets. This is the domain of bodybuilding. Historically this type of training involves doing eight to twelve repetitions for up to five sets per exercise. There is some evidence suggesting that the peak stimulus for increasing mass is five sets of twelve repetitions done with as heavy of a weight as possible (16). Done as heavy as possible to invoke an increase in accumulated actin and myosin (increasing mass). Done with very short rests to increase the metabolic stress on the muscle in order to force an adaptation in carbohydrate storage inside the muscle cell (increasing its mass). Doing lots of repetitions with little rest makes this type of training very demanding training and time consuming. Also because of the duration of the sets, both fast twitch and slow twitch muscle fibers are active in generating force, and unlike our previous models the slow twitch fibers get bigger in bodybuilders, the only weight training group this occurs in. This type of training is very specific. It is very important to understand here that although most beginners with a goal of increasing mass also want to get "shredded", they cannot go on a weight loss diet and hope to achieve any kind of meaningful success. The goal of increased muscle mass cannot occur for as long as we want it to if there is a nutritional and caloric deficit.

For mass building you still do squats, you still do presses, you still do bench presses, and you still do deadlifts. These exercises drive muscle adaptations. They also set up the hormonal and structural disturbances that allow additional exercises, ones that provide more isolation on tangential muscle groups an opportunity to be effective. Basically, the isolation exercises only work well if they can ride the anabolic wave of the big exercises. You don't get big without doing the big lifts. No amount of leg extensions and leg curls can produce the same result as simply doing squats.

You won't see this is muscular fiction magazines, but a good beginner bodybuilding workout should start with a standard big barbell exercise. In this manner the muscles, nerves, and endocrine system (makes hormones) gets primed to facilitate gain in the following smaller mass exercises. It is also relevant to organize the exercises in a push/pull manner. If curls are done then a press variant or other triceps exercise would be appropriate to include as the next exercise. This increases the amount of mass worked and it ensures that the complete range of motion around a joint is being developed and this keeps or improves mobility.

A simple beginners program is barbell biased. We want the most progress possible. Bodyweight exercises, like chin-ups and dips, are also useful initially. But after you can do multiple sets of ten in them, its time to start doing weighted versions of them.

A beginning bodybuilding program will, like the strength program, consist of only three weekly workouts. It may actually be more of an imperative here. The higher volume of weighted work included in a bodybuilding workout requires more recovery in order to produce muscle growth. Having more than three workouts a week would reduce the available recovery time and gains would come more slowly.

In this beginners program there are five exercises included in each workout. Doing three sets of ten repetitions is recommended. We don't start the beginner off with five sets of twelve like the literature suggests as the rep-set scheme for maximum gain because a beginner is not adapted to attempt that magnitude of load - yet. If they did train more frequently, it would rapidly overwhelm their body's ability to adapt, they would rapidly hit a shallow plateau, then descend into over-training. Three sets of ten are far enough out towards the mass end of the volume-intensity continuum to produce the desired effects. A simple beginners program would look similar to the following:

Monday	3x	Wednesday	3x	Friday	3x
Squat	10	Bench Press	10	Front squat	10
Calf Raises	10	Row	10	Back Extension	10
Press	10	Dips	*	Curls	10
Lat Pull Downs	10	Deadlift	10^{Ω}	French Press	10
Shrugs	10	Weighted crunch	10	Chin-ups	*

* For dips and chin-ups, as many reps as possible for three sets until you can do three sets of ten, then begin adding weight on a harness.

Ω For deadlifts, the work sets are three progressively heavier sets that peaks in one heavy set of ten. The deadlift, due to its stressful nature can induce overtraining if included in too high of volumes.

Five exercises keep the total volume recoverable for the beginner and it keeps the amount of time in the gym reasonable. If a new set (either warm up or work set) is being started every minute and a half, these workouts take on the order of about an hour to complete. Everyone has heard the stories of strong or monstrously big people being in the gym for hours and hours a day. They didn't have to. More over, they were advanced and elite trainees when the big time investments occurred, not beginners. Don't let poor logic prevent you from doing what you should to reach your goals. You don't have to give up your day job or check out of all of life's fun events to get big.

Why aren't we doing an arm day, a back day, a leg day, etc? Because the goal is to add mass. Isolating the training to a small muscle mass does not disrupt systemic homeostasis enough to produce large adaptations; in this case the desired increase of muscle mass. Isolation exercises alone do not put us deep enough into Selye's Stage One to create rapid and measurable adaptations. As long as you follow the rule of including one or two of the big basic lifts in the workout, you can focus on body parts. Just remember that the smaller the focus area, the slower the results. Look at someone you know, a normal person in school, your job, or that has been training bodybuilding for years. Check out the biceps. Now hop down to your local competitive gymnastics club and find a guy that has been competing for a few years. Check out the biceps. You will note that the gymnast, who does not do 57 varieties of curls, has superior biceps development; way superior. Why? It is the volume of pull-ups and chin-ups, exercises that stress a large set of joints and muscles. He does it for function (performance), biceps development is just a side benefit. The large scale chin-up and pull-up exercises provide a larger anabolic stimulus than curls.

A critical point of distinction between training for strength and bodybuilding is that with body building you are attempting to push to NEAR the point of failure from fatigue. If you titrate the reps, sets, and weights correctly, you never miss a repetition. If you do miss a repetition it will be most likely because you have not allowed enough recovery time between workouts. You have not allowed your gas tank, so to speak, to fill back up between workouts. In bodybuilding failure from the weight being just too heavy within the first five repetitions should never happen. If it does, you are increasing the weight at too fast of a rate for your body to adapt.

Bodybuilding training is built for the addition of dumbbell exercises. In movements like pressing and bench pressing, the added mobility elements of independent motor control and coordination will actually assist in recruiting and working the stabilizing musculature peripheral to the primary movers - compared to the same movements with a barbell. This increased work can help stimulate mass gain. Doing the barbell variant uses heavier weights to produce a result, the dumbbell variant uses increased recruitment (although with lower weights) to produce a result. Nice, complementary methods.

Taking the example workouts above and subbing in dumbbell exercises would produce a repeating two week series of workouts:

Week 1

Monday	3x	Wednesday	3x	Friday	3x
Squat	10	Dumbbell Bench Press	10	Front squat	10
Calf Raises	10	Row	10	Back Extension	10
Press	10	Dips	10	Curls	10
Lat Pull Downs	10	Deadlift	10	French Press	10
Shrugs	10	Weighted crunch	10	Chin-ups	10

Week 2

Monday	3x	Wednesday	3x	Friday	3x
Squat	10	Bench Press	10	Front squat	10
Calf Raises	10	Row	10	Back Extension	10
Dumbbell Press	10	Dips	*	Dumbbell Curls	10
Lat Pull Downs	10	Deadlift	10^{Ω}	French Press	10
Shrugs	10	Weighted crunch	10	Chin-ups	*

* and $^{\Omega}$ see previous notations

But you look at this and say "just one day of curls?" Refer back to the gymnast passage. Just because there are no curls on Monday or Wednesday does not mean that they aren't getting lots of work. Consider the functional anatomy of the lat pull downs and rows. Are the elbows bending? Yes, and under a considerable load. Biceps even get a little work in pressing movements (you may want to refer to a good exercise anatomy book to confirm this). Considering the anatomical foundations of the exercises in this series of workouts; everything gets some work every single workout. That is why it is effective, there is a large magnitude and holistic stress rather than small magnitude and fragmented isolation training stress. Don't let preconceived hype prevent you from training as you should to get the gains you want.

Amping up Repetitions

Some individuals who have little strength and endurance may benefit from starting off at five repetitions of an exercise and progressing repetitions rather than weight. This practice has been used for centuries as a means to add mass and functional ability before a transition to advancing weight on the bar. In most programs used in recent and not so recent history, a repetition is added about every three days on weighted exercises. On bodyweight exercises, an additional repetition is added each day. When to change from increasing repetitions to increasing weight is a little bit of a gray area. We propose that once three sets of ten repetitions is achieved, then it is time to begin advancing in weight. Other authors have suggested as many at 25 repetitions before beginning to advance in weight. Such high repetitions are far in excess of that needed to induce strength or mass gain and in fact are an endurance stimulus and thus a misuse of time.

Hepburn's Repetition Advancement Program

In 1980 Doug Hepburn, a former heavyweight world champion weightlifter (1953) and professional wrestler, and John Myles collaborated on a book that claimed to be "the only weight training system that works with nature, not against it, because it progresses at a rate not beyond the body's ability to bring a full recovery before the next workout (17)." For the time, this was a forward thinking statement, essentially stating what we present in this text as what must occur with a beginner, recovery and supercompensation must coincide with the next workout. We include this program here as its progresses in load between each workout. There is a daily repetition progression that occurs for two weeks before an addition of $2\frac{1}{2}$ to 5 pounds is added to the work set weights.

Hepburn suggested that this very simple type of program, it only included seven exercises, would be useful for several years. He insisted upon very slow and methodical advancements and this likely protracted the beginners stage from lasting a maximum of 12-18 months as we perceive it, out to two or three years. We would suggest that larger increases in weight should initially be used, maybe 10 or more pounds, and increases made smaller as advancement becomes more difficult.

This is a nice example of manipulating repetitions and weights to produce a methodical and progressive increase in workload in every workout. The advancement one might use in the squat could be:

		Set								
	Weight	**1**	**2**	**3**	**4**	**5**	**6**	**7**	**8**	
Workout 1	200	3	2	2	2	2	2	2	2	
Workout 2	200	3	3	2	2	2	2	2	2	
Workout 3	200	3	3	3	2	2	2	2	2	
Workout 4	200	3	3	3	3	2	2	2	2	Week 1
Workout 5	200	3	3	3	3	3	2	2	2	
Workout 6	200	3	3	3	3	3	3	2	2	
Workout 7	200	3	3	3	3	3	3	3	2	
Workout 8	200	3	3	3	3	3	3	3	3	Week 2
Workout 9	205	3	2	2	2	2	2	2	2	
Workout 10	205	3	3	2	2	2	2	2	2	
Workout 11	205	3	3	3	2	2	2	2	2	
Workout 12	205	3	3	3	3	2	2	2	2	Week 3
Workout 13	205	3	3	3	3	3	2	2	2	
Workout 14	205	3	3	3	3	3	3	2	2	
Workout 15	205	3	3	3	3	3	3	3	2	
Workout 16	205	3	3	3	3	3	3	3	3	Week 4
Workout 17	210	3	2	2	2	2	2	2	2	
Workout 18	210	3	3	2	2	2	2	2	2	
Workout 19	210	3	3	3	2	2	2	2	2	
Workout 20	210	3	3	3	3	2	2	2	2	Week 5
Workout 21	210	3	3	3	3	3	2	2	2	
Workout 22	210	3	3	3	3	3	3	2	2	
Workout 23	210	3	3	3	3	3	3	3	2	
Workout 24	210	3	3	3	3	3	3	3	3	Week 6
Workout 25	215	3	2	2	2	2	2	2	2	

While this is a strength biased program, the methodology could easily be adapted to bodybuilding simply by starting with a higher base repetition count:

		Set			
	Weight	1	2	3	4
Workout 1	200	9	8	8	8
Workout 2	200	9	9	8	8
Workout 3	200	9	9	9	8
Workout 4	200	9	9	9	9
Workout 5	200	10	9	9	9
Workout 6	200	10	10	9	9
Workout 7	200	10	10	10	9
Workout 8	200	10	10	10	10

In workout 9, the weight would go up a very small amount and the cycle would start over with workout 1.

Biasing your Gains

The example mass gain programs provided will produce an even handed increase in muscle mass throughout the body. Some people would rather gain more mass up top and less down low. That is relatively easy to accomplish. In our example we would simply drop out the front squats and add in a second bench press session. We keep in squats as this is the most effective version of squatting. The front squat is removed as it is the lesser powerful adaptive stimulus. To distribute the workout load evenly over the week some adjustments to days and exercise order are made:

Monday	Wednesday	Friday
Squat	Press	Deadlift
Bench Press	Lat Pull Down	Dumbbell Bench Press
Row	Calf Raises	Curls
Dips	Back Extension	French Press
Shrugs	Weighted Crunch	Chin-ups

This can be done for upper versus lower body or for anterior or posterior. The above is just an example of what could be done. We DO NOT recommend anything other than a holistic approach and uniform development. Biasing development towards a single set of muscles or body part is a bit too cartoonish and reduces the functionality of the entire system of movement. An anatomical movement system can only function to the level of its weakest element.

Getting Over Plateaus

A plateau in mass building indicates the same thing it does in a strength building program; the body isn't recovering fast enough to supercompensate and handle the next higher workload. However, because mass building programs are volume based, it requires not just an offload (backing off) of the weight used, it also requires an offload in repetitions and sets. If, for example, the workout calls for three sets of ten repetitions with 200 pounds and there is a failure at the seventh repetition in the third set. We go home. We don't break it up into smaller sets to get all the reps planned, because smaller repetition sets produce a different adaptive stimulus than wanted. There is no reason to do them as there is no progress towards the desired goal. When we come back for our next scheduled workout, we use the last completely successful workout weights done (190 pounds if it was a 10 pound progression) and we drop back to two sets for the exercises - all of them, we want a systemic recovery. In this manner intensity is maintained and volume is reduced thus allowing the body to recover. In the next workout, we would go back to three sets of ten repetitions while advancing the weight to 195 pounds. If successful, future progressions would be at a rate of five pounds per workout. As with strength training, three plateaus and the successive reductions in the "rate of load increase" indicates the transition from beginner to intermediate.

There is another approach to progression that may extend the duration and usefulness of the beginner stage. Assume the progression described in a three sets by ten repetition program. When the second plateau arrives, a completely different repetition, set, and weight intervention is done. This break, caused by the need for recovery, is used as an opportunity to introduce a slightly different repetition and set scheme. Instead of going back to three sets of ten with just a little more weight than before, a 20% reduction in weight used is implemented (if 200 pounds was the failure weight, we drop back to 160 pounds) and we increase the repetitions to 12 and the sets to four. We then proceed back through progression with small jumps until reaching another plateau. What we are attempting to accomplish here is to capitalize on a break in training due to recovery as an opportunity to gently introduce a higher volume of training to push further out onto the mass end of the volume-intensity continuum. As this is the third recovery manipulation of the beginner's stage, a plateau here also indicates its time to use an intermediate program.

Do not set a time limit for your time as a beginner. Some people out grow linear progression in six months or less, some take more than a year. In actuality, a longer time spent as a beginner means lots of progress at a relatively fast pace. So don't hurry it. Try to break plateaus at least twice. Get tiny weights and use them to try to extract as much progressive improvement as you can. Progress only gets harder to come by as an intermediate.

Don't Go to the Cafeteria

It is forever frustrating to see beginning trainees do what we call cafeteria training; changing from program to program after just a couple weeks based on whim or because they don't feel like its working or they see a new program that looks cool in a muscular fiction magazine. Or they select what looks easy for program A and couple that with part of program B that is heavy on their favorite lifts and then use the sets and rep scheme from program C for part of their program. You will not make gains if you do not stick to the program. Patience with your training program is a virtue. Adaptation takes time and if you are constantly altering the nature of the stress applied to the body, adaptations will be slow or absent. Even bad programs will produce some positive results if you put in the work and do them as written. Lyn Jones, a former national coach in the British, Australian, and American coaching systems (coach of Olympic Champion Tara Nott) once told one of the authors that it is more important to simply have a plan, believe in it, and do it than to have the perfect plan. Failing to plan is planning to fail.

The basic concept of beginners training

1. Honestly identify your goal.
2. Select the repetition scheme based on your goal and the volume-intensity continuum.
3. Begin with a routine based around the big lifts.
4. Use slow and steady progression of weights in every workout (don't get greedy and add weight or repetitions too fast).
5. Stick with the program.
6. When a plateau is encountered, off load then use smaller increases in weight.
7. When a plateau cannot be overcome with offloading and smaller progression, it is time to transition to an intermediate program.

INTERMEDIATES

Having spent considerable and regular time in the gym using a linear progression program as a beginner, an intermediate's ability to recover from a new workload takes longer than the time between workouts. So instead of increasing loads a little in every workout, we now begin to increase workloads once a week. We will pick a day and that will be the "heavy day" for the duration. We also begin varying the loads used for each workout during the week. Together this is the simplest form of periodization, manipulating the stress placed on the body through periods of increased work interspersed between periods of reduced work. The intention is to increase the weight on the bar on the day of the week when supercompensation occurs. Ideally this is the heavy day of training.

Even before anyone had hypothesized about adaptation, peaking, and supercompensation people were using versions of simple periodization. Not because they understood it but because it worked. The versions used at the beginning of the 20th century are as useful today as they were then, more so because we now understand how they work. The fact that it is so useful means that virtually every intermediate program is a permutation of this single theme.

Three Days - Three Different Loads

One of the oldest and most widely used of these versions was the Medium-Light-Heavy model in Bob Hoffman's Simplified System of Barbell Training (18) and Daily Dozen booklet (19). In this model Monday is a medium load day, Wednesday is a light day, and Friday is a heavy day. This model worked very well and was built to accommodate weekend competitions and the York Barbell picnics, periodic Saturday events sponsored by Hoffman where those training with him or near him would assemble for maxing out and food (20). By moving the Friday workout to Saturday provided an additional day of recovery that likely aided in further supercompensation and high performance on Saturday picnics. One point comes to mind when thinking about a Saturday workout/competition/extravaganza/picnic – training is supposed to be fun and have a point.

The order of loading used in the version of simple periodization described here is Heavy-Medium-Light (Monday-Wednesday-Friday), a bit different than Hoffman's. There are a number of definitions of heavy, medium, and light relative to a personal best, personal record, max, or 1-repetition maximum. Most of those found on the internet are reflective of Prilepin's tables regarding the appropriate numbers of repetitions of specific percentages to include in workouts (21). Here we will call anything below 70% light, anything between 70 and 85% medium, and anything from 86% to 100% heavy. For this program to work, heavy really should be synonymous with maximal or going all out. Some people suggest that using "how the weight feels" to you during the workout to determine heavy, medium, and light. We strongly argue against this as there is no room for subjective feelings in a quantitative training program.

With this model of training, the first training day of the week is a heavy day. It is assumed that you are coming off of a two day recovery period and are ready to successfully handle an increased load. So on day one of every week, the weight goes up a little - a little - but this is still a maximal work day and is disruptive of homeostasis. In our example this occurs on Mondays. On Wednesday we back off a bit to a medium load. The medium load is still enough stress to provide an additive stress on top of Monday's heavy load. On Friday it is a light day, actively transitioning into our recovery weekend. On the following Monday we add just a little bit of weight and repeat. This continues for as long as gains continue to be produced.

This system works very well if the same exercises are included in all three weekly workouts as all lifts get equal attention. If there are different workouts for different days, a rotation must be made in order to provide gains in all lifts. If an exercise is only done on Friday the light day, you cannot expect to make any progress in that lift. It must at some point be done heavy in order to progress. An eight week cycle seems to be long enough to reap gains before switching the exercises on the heavy day. The most important lifts should spend the most days on the heavy days but a strict application of such a rotation would look something like:

Week 1

Monday - Heavy	Wednesday - Medium	Friday - Light
Squat	Dumbbell Bench Press	Front squat
Calf Raises	Seated Row	Back Extension
Press	Dips	Curls
Lat Pulls	Deadlift	French Press
Shrugs	Weighted crunch	Chin-ups

Week 8

Monday - Heavy	Wednesday - Medium	Friday - Light
Dumbbell Bench Press	Front squat	Squat
Seated Row	Back Extension	Calf Raises
Dips	Curls	Press
Deadlift	French Press	Lat Pulls
Weighted crunch	Chin-ups	Shrugs

Week 16

Monday - Heavy	Wednesday - Medium	Friday - Light
Front squat	Squat	Dumbbell Bench Press
Back Extension	Calf Raises	Seated Row
Curls	Press	Dips
French Press	Lat Pulls	Deadlift
Chin-ups	Shrugs	Weighted crunch

There are other versions of this basic training premise. There are four day, five day, and six day manipulations of heavy, medium, and light. However, most recreational and professional trainees will not need more training days than four, nor will they have the time to spend in the gym. If a trainee's goals center specifically on getting stronger or gaining mass and nothing else, then more than four workouts per week are useful at this stage. A conservative schematic of how one would add workouts and loads follows:

Workouts/Week	Monday	Tuesday	Wednesday	Thursday	Friday	Saturday	Sunday
Three	Heavy		Medium		Light		
Four							
Entry	Heavy	Light		Medium	Light		
Progression	Heavy	Medium		Medium	Light		
Progression	Heavy	Medium		Heavy	Light		
Five							
Entry	Heavy	Medium	Light	Heavy	Light		
or							
Entry	Heavy	Medium		Light	Heavy	Light	
Progression	Heavy	Medium		Medium	Heavy	Light	
Progression	Heavy	Heavy		Medium	Heavy	Light	

Each progressive level of organization introduces an additive stress ... gradually. It is important to stay in each level of progression for at least three training cycles (or at least three months) in order to reap adaptation and preparation for the progression to the next, more difficult level. Direct addition of a heavy workout is never done without transitioning through light and medium progressions first. We want to avoid overtraining and we want to get the most performance boost possible out of every training organization.

As the beginner is often tempted to change programs due to impatience, the intermediate is often tempted to workout too frequently for the same reason - impatience because of the problematic axiom; if a little is good, more is better. By this stage in their training career, a beginner has achieved a good deal of strength success from spending time in the gym. So there is a temptation to add more time in the gym, much more than necessary, with it being a common occurrence to see people attempting to train six or seven days per week. It is a physiologic necessity to have ample time for recovery. There is never a valid reason or a physiological benefit for a normal person to train seven days per week. Essentially, a decision to train seven days per week means that you are planning on not recovering and supercompensating. This is an instance where you have not failed to plan, you have planned to fail.

For the general population - those who are training for strength as a fitness goal - there is a rough correlation between the number of workouts that should be done and the years of consistent and progressive training you have done. If you have less than three years of training it is recommended to do three workouts per week. Four years of experience builds enough base to tolerate four workouts per week. Five years makes you ready for five workouts per week. This is a broad generality for those who have fitness goals, not for competitive weightlifters, powerlifters, or bodybuilders who must progress faster by necessity or fail to be competitive.

Repetitions and sets for this program are once again tied to the specific goal of training. The same relationship to the volume-intensity continuum holds. A strength focus has very few reps per set and a mass focus has many reps per set. There is often a worry about how many repetitions of a certain weight are completed in a training cycle. This is usually driven by someone reading Soviet training literature from the 1960s through the 1980s and seizing upon a little factoid to apply to their own training. The Soviets simply assumed that total repetitions in a normal program should conform to a Gaussian distribution (bell curve) with fewer very light repetitions (no contribution to fitness), more moderate intensity repetitions (technical practice and mass building), and few repetitions with heavy weights (limited due to large stress factor). While they did seem somewhat anal retentive in their programming, if you just simply follow the volume-intensity continuum and the heavy-medium-light system, then the distribution of repetitions will work out without any special consideration. That's one less thing to distract you from simply training to get strong (or big). And although it cannot be disputed that the Soviet sports scientists and coaches were excellent programmers, the real concept behind the success of the cold-war Soviet system was eloquently summed up by Pavel Pervushin, "The point is to train and train very earnestly".

The basic concept of intermediate training

1. Honestly identify your goal.
2. Select the repetition scheme in reference to your goal and the volume-intensity continuum.
3. Begin with a routine based around the big lifts.
4. Use slow and steady progressions of weights once a week (don't get greedy and add weight or repetitions too fast).
5. Stick with the program and train hard.
6. When a plateau is encountered, off load then use smaller increases in weight.
7. When a plateau cannot be overcome within one training frequency, off load for two weeks then attempt a different frequency with small weight increases over a longer time.
8. When progress stalls despite transitions to more training days, small weight increases, and two week offloads between transitions, it is time to move to an advanced program.

BEYOND INTERMEDIATES

Once intermediate programs come to an end of usefulness, then come advanced programming where we increase loads - or go maximal - about once a month. The more advanced you become, the longer it takes to recover from the big and heavy workloads you can now produce. Advanced training methods are rooted in accumulated stress over weeks (or months as you become more advanced) in order to provide an adequate disruption of homeostasis. In all viable models of this type of training a short period of off loading (or unloading or taper) follows. There are a tremendous number of these programs out there all with different names, rep and set schemes, included exercises, and names, but they all share a common history and training intent.

In general, advanced programs are percentage based, meaning that how much weight used for each exercise in a workout is calculated from a known maximum lift. The percentages used start off relatively low and progress over the weeks until at some distant point a new maximum is achieved and the process starts over again with percentages of the new maximum. These programs also include a relatively short period of reduced work that is intended to ensure supercompensation before the addition of the next load. Another characteristic is that there is generally an inverse association of volume to intensity. As the intensity of the training increases, the volume decreases.

Heavy-Medium-Light on a Bigger Scale

One of the simplest manipulations to make for a newly advanced trainee is to create a three week cycle heavy, medium, and light training. The logic and design of the program parameters are exactly the same with the intermediate program, but entire weeks are spent at the specific loads rather than just a day. This particular manipulation is useful for early stage advanced trainees as it produces a two week homeostatic disruption followed by an entire week of recovery before advancing in weights used.

			Strength		Mass	
Week	Load	%	Sets	Reps	Sets	Reps
1	Heavy	Maximum	8	2	5	10
2	Medium	85%	8	2	5	10
3	Light	70%	6	2	3	10
4	Heavy	Maximum	8	2	5	10
5	Medium	85%	8	2	5	10
6	Light	70%	6	2	3	10

Progression should be small denominations, using small end plates. A one kilogram (2.2 lb) advancement is absolutely OK. Tracking of advanced and elite weightlifters and powerlifters tells us that a ten kilogram gain in a year is quite good. So at this stage of the training game it is important to maintain small gains in the shortest duration of time possible, thus this three week cycle is useful for a new advanced trainee. As this program diminishes in return, a slightly longer cycle program becomes viable. There are any number of four week cyclic programs, some have proven to be more effective than others.

5-3-1

A program that manipulates loading on relatively short four week cyclic basis is the 5-3-1 program developed by former University of Arizona fullback and powerlifter with a 2375lb total (that's big), Jim Wendler (22). Although primarily designed for powerlifters from beginners on, it is included here as an intermediate program as it is organized as such. This program has some interesting nuances, the first being that the intensity or weights to be used in the work sets are calculated as a percentage of 90% of an individual's maximum at entry. This diverges from most programs as they calculate loads based on absolute maximums (100%). This manipulation was developed from Wendler's own experiences training and coaching and is a method of ensuring the load is not overwhelming to recovery and adaptive capacity.

The main set and intensity scheme within each workout is a simple 5% ladder - with each work set, the intensity percent goes up 5%. Each workout of the week has a consistent repetition number per set and the same target intensity percent; week 1 85%, week 2 90%, and week 3 95%. The second nuance comes in week three where there is a down ramp in repetitions in the work sets, from five to three to one (thus the name of the program). Now the third nuance, the last set of weeks one through three is actually as many reps as you can do. For example in week three getting one is good, but more is better - a more potent stimulus to disrupt homeostasis as you transition into the fourth week of the program, the off load week of very light work at 60% intensity.

Progression through the system in terms of weight used is done by adding 5 pounds to the 90% of maximum calculation for upper body exercises and 10 pounds for lower body exercises. The program does not test one repetition maximums every four weeks and that is just fine. You are building strength over time for a purpose, to be stronger. Having a monthly max weight data point is likely disruptive to the design of the program. It's more important to think about where you want to be six months or a year from now and test then.

As so many other successful programs, the 5-3-1 is built around the big lifts, the basics work. One major exercise (squat, press, deadlift, bench press) is done in one of four workouts each week. The volume of the strength version of the program is low with only two exercises each day, one of the major exercises and one assistance exercise complementary to the big lift. The accessory exercise contributes to the stress produced. The bodybuilding version uses the same programming of the big lifts but adds four assistance exercises instead of one and uses a much higher repetition volume (>10) for each of them. The basic scheme for the major lifts is:

Week	Repetitions	Sets	Intensity
1	5	3	85
2	3	3	90
3	5-3-1(AMRAP)	3	95
4	5	3	60

AMRAP = As many repetitions as possible

Weightlifting Models for Bridging Advanced to Elite

We generally suggest that when one moves from being an intermediate to being an advanced and then an elite trainee, the duration between distruption of homeostasis and supercompensation has moved from being doable in one weeks time to one months time then to more than a months time. This makes for easy programming as a weekly program cycle and a monthly program cycle are in handy units of time. But individual recoverability does not always like handy units of time. One of the most widely known versions of advanced/elite programming is that included in the club coaching manual of USA Weightlifting (23). Depending on interpretation it could be suggested that the program could be accommodate a six, eight, ten, or twelve week adaptive capacity. In USA Weightlifting's strict application of the program, individual four-week submaximal cycles are strung together to create a stair-step to 100%. The starting intensity is based on how many weeks are allowed to reach the maximal week:

Week	%	Set/Rep	%	Set/Rep	%	Set/Rep	%	Set Rep
1	85	5/5	80	5/5	75	5/5	70	5/5
2	95	5/3	90	5/5	85	5/5	80	5/5
3	90	4/2	85	4/3	80	5/5	75	4/5
4	100	5/1	95	5/3	90	5/3	85	5/3
5	Offload	5/1	90	5/3	85	5/3	80	5/3
6	Test	4/1	100	4/1	95	4/3	90	4/3
7			Offload	4/1	90	5/3	85	5/3
8			Test	4/1	100	5/1	95	5/1
9					Offload	4/1	90	4/1
10					Test	4/1	100	5/1
11							Offload	5/1
12							Test	4/1

Test = continued taper to maximum attempts or competition

We don't recommend using the six week version repeatedly because four of the six weeks are at 90% or higher. This is likely too much intense training with not enough recovery to allow repeated use of this model. If used to fill in odd durations of training prior to events it could be occasionally useful. The eight, ten, and twelve week models are much more appropriate.

Another program model of interest is the three month duration program from USA Weightlifting's senior coaching manual (24). Although this program is directed at competitive weightlifters it, like the other weightlifter's programs, can be easily manipulated to accommodate those interested in non-competitive development of strength simply by using a different exercise menu. The set structure of this program is a basic ladder. In a ladder, the weight is increased by about 5% with each set until the target weight is reached. A ladder is calculated from the target weight for the day. If the target weight is 200 pounds, then the ladder for five sets would be something like 180-185-190-195-200. In this program the work sets are followed by a back off set, a reduction of 10%, where technique is reinforced. In many versions of this program, the back off set is absent because the downward arm of a pyramid (an upward ladder - 10/20/30 - followed by a downward ladder - 30/20/10) produces a negligible effect on strength. If the intent of the program is strength, then the absent back off set is appropriate. If the intent of the program is mass gain, it should be included as it adds a training volume stimulus. In the programs original intent, improving weightlifting performance, a back off set can be included as technical skill practice is important.

Week	Repetitions	Sets	Intensity %
1	5	5	70
2	5	6	75
3	5	4	65
4	5	6	80
5	3	5	75
6	3	6	85
7	3	4	70
8	3	6	90
9	2	6	85
10	2	9	95
11	1	5	75
12	1	8	100

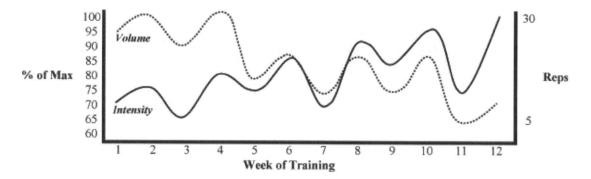

Figure 5. Plotting the volume and intensity variations for the USA Weightlifting senior course periodization model.

As you can see there are much larger variations in loading and offloading percentages. The offload between week ten and eleven is 20% and represents the need for more recovery in this model for more advanced lifters. These longer duration competitive weightlifting based models can serve as the transitory programs between an advanced trainee and true elite. But with late advanced and early elite trainees, there is an expected uncertainty of programs due to individual differences. This means simply that a given program may be perfectly structured BUT it just may not work for you. Programs at the elite level rapidly become one-off programs built specifically for the individual trainee in order to conquer shortcomings, capitalize on known recovery patterns, and ultimately achieve individual specific goals. At this point in a trainee's career it becomes worth the money, maybe even essential, to recruit an expert coach to create your programs and supervise your training. Sir William Osler's counsel for physicians in the 19th century, "a physician who treats himself has a fool for a patient" can easily be modified for those elites training themselves. Objectivity is lost when you look in the mirror.

What Exercises Should I Use?

No one can answer that question specifically for you. You have to choose whether or not you want to follow the advice of literally hundreds of experts with combined thousands of years experience and acquired knowledge. Since the advent of the barbell, the squat, the deadlift, and the press have been the backbone of every major successful training program - for athletes, for the everyman, for the everywoman, and for the healthy. Do not design a program without them. Since the introduction of the bench press in competition and the availability of inexpensive benches, the bench press has proven to be a valuable contributor to strength gain. It is not a substitute for the press; they both warrant being considered major exercises. If you do nothing but these four exercises progressively and consistently over time, you will become strong in all the right places. In fact, that would be a nearly perfect place to start.

If you choose to do additional exercises there are a number that also prove useful, just to a lesser extent than the four major strength exercises. It is important to remember that you do not need a dozen exercises in your daily program, just at least one big basic exercise and a select few contributory exercises. We would not recommend more than six exercises in any workout in any training program and even then that is specific for mass gain. Two to four exercises is much more typical and useful for developing strength.

Ballistic or Power Exercises	**Calisthenics Based Exercise**
Jerk	Pull-ups
Push Jerk	Chin-ups
Push Press	Dips
Power Clean	Push-ups
Power Snatch	Weighted sit-ups

Isolation Type Exercises	Machine Based Exercises
Rows (old school name - bent row)	Lat Pull Downs
Good Mornings	Leg Press
Shrugs	Back Extension
Calf raises	
Curls	
French Press	
Romanian Deadlift	

Inclusion of the above exercises into a workout program should occur when and only if there is a legitimate need for them to meet training goals. For example, athletic or military populations would likely want to include exercises from both the ballistic and the calisthenics groups in their training at the earliest possible convenience (after learning the movements and basic conditioning). Exercises therein mimic both the metabolic demands and movement types experienced in those endeavors.

Minimizing Strength Gain?

Everything presented in this chapter assumes a SPECIFIC and exclusive training focus on getting stronger. While this is quite a valid approach, many people will include endurance type training in their workout programming. Either doing endurance work in the same workout with lifting or doing it on alternate days. There are some relatively large limitations placed on the body in terms of rate of fitness gain when we put multiple and different training modes into a single workout or over multiple workouts (see chapter 2). If we wish to maximize strength rapidly, 100% of the focus should be on strength as inclusion of other modes of training slows the rate of strength gain over time (figure 6).

It should be intuitive that the training program undertaken must match the fitness goal or goals of the trainee. Specialization in strength is easy to program if you match the training program to the level of fitness progression of the trainee. Weight training is specific training for weightlifters, powerlifters, and bodybuilders. All of their attention and training time is focused on a single training mode and adaptive stimulus to achieve a strength goal. Spending long hours in the gym is a given and becomes more and more necessary over the training career. This is tremendously different than general fitness populations and athletes. For those populations, weight training is general physical training, a contributor to the big picture. It is not THE big picture. Therefore, in non-strength sport trainees, the degree of programming invasiveness, attention, and time devoted to strength is lower, especially if multiple fitness components are in need of development to support sporting/occupational success or if significant skill practice is required as part of achieving the goal(s). The bottom line is that precisely copying a competitive lifter's program is not a relevant practice for general fitness trainees or many sportsmen and women. The concepts and principles of the training of competitive lifters are relevant, they just need reframed to allow achievement of multiple training goals without pushing the trainee into overtraining. This generally means that we should not be in the weight room for more than 3-4 hours per week if we are not strength athletes. We should distribute the training of the multiple fitness elements according to importance to our fitness or sport preparatory demand. Programming multiple or combined fitness goals is more difficult to manage and as such we later devote an entire chapter (chapter 6) on how to best accomplish achieving broadly scoping fitness through multi-element training.

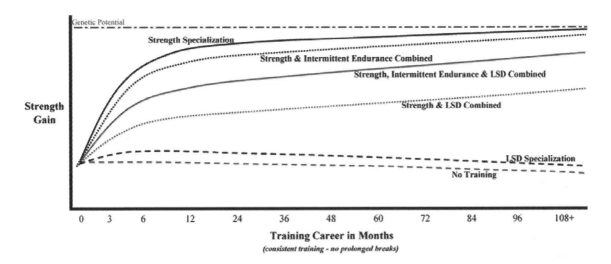

Figure 6. Including only strength training in programming yields the fastest and largest magnitude changes in strength. Note that intermittent endurance work (like intervals) interfere with gains to a much lower degree than combined strength training and long slow distance endurance work.

Can I get too strong?

No.

But in many instances individuals will have a specific strength target in mind that they reach and have no further interest in advancing. This is OK as long as your goals put you in the top third of population strength levels. Remember we want to reap the survivability benefit of strength.

If an appropriate strength goal is reached, then it is fairly straightforward to maintain strength levels. Hitting one or two sessions per week of low volume training with 85 percent or more of 1RM has been shown to maintain strength levels over time (25). The simplest approach here would be once the target 1RM is achieved, the training days and loads would be rolled back as just described. At some point after this, many weeks or many months, the slow decay of fitness from using submaximal loads exclusively will result in a small but noticeable loss in strength. The solution is very elementary, simply spend a couple months working through a basic linear progression strength program to regain any lost strength, the roll the days per week and training load back again. This process will need to be repeated periodically over the years and this should maintain strength at goal levels without a huge investment in time.

REFERENCES

1. Ruiz, J.R., et al. Association between muscular strength and mortality in men: prospective cohort study. British Medical Journal, 337(7661):92-95, 2008.

2. Hickson, R.C., M.A. Rosenkoetter, and M.M. Brown. Strength training effects on aerobic power and short-term endurance. Medicine and Science in Sports and Exercise, 12(5):336-339, 1980.

3. Marcinik, E.J., et al. Effects of strength training on lactate threshold and endurance performance. Medicine and Science in Sports and Exercise, 23(6):739-743, 1991.

4. Hoff, J., J. Helgerud, and U. Wisloff. Maximal strength training improves work economy in trained female cross-country skiers. Medicine and Science in Sports and Exercise, 31(6):870-877, 1999.

5. Hamill, B. Relative Safety of Weightlifting and Weight Training. Journal of Strength and Conditioning Research. 8(1):53- 57, 1994.

6. Shields, B.J. and G.A. Smith. Cheerleading-related injuries to children 5 to 18 years of age: United States, 1990-2002. Pediatrics, 117(1)122-129, 2006.

7. Hreljac, A. Impact and overuse injuries in runners. Medicine and Science in Sports and Exercise, 36(5):845-849, 2004.

8. Behm, D,G. and D.G. Sale. Intended rather than actual movement velocity determines velocity-specific training response. Journal of Applied Physiology, 74(1):359-368, 1993.

9. Stone, M.H., et al. Maximum strength-power-performance relationships in collegiate throwers. Journal of Strength and Conditioning Research, 17(4):739-745, 2003.

10. Metter, E.J., L.A. Talbot, M. Schrager, and R.A. Conwit. Arm-cranking muscle power and arm isometric muscle strength are independent predictors of all-cause mortality in men. Journal of Applied Physiology, 96(2):814-821, 2003.

11. Pullum, W.A. Weightlifting Made Easy, Athletic Publications LTD, London, UK, 1922.

12. Unger, M. Intelligence in Physical Culture, Health & Strength Institute, NY, NY, 1910.

13. Starr, B. Strongest shall survive: Strength training for football. Five Starr Productions, Baltimore, MD, revised 2007.

14. Rippetoe, C.M. and J.L. Kilgore. Starting Strength: A simple and practical for coaching beginners. Aasgaard Company, Wichita Falls, TX, 2005.

15. Rønnestad, B.R., H. Nygaard, and T. Raastad. Physiological elevation of endogenous hormones results in superior strength training adaptation. European Journal of Applied Physiology, Online First[TM], February 16, 2011.

16. Stone, M.H., H. O'Bryant, and J. Garhammer. A hypothetical model for strength training. Journal of Sports Medicine and Physical Fitness, 21(4):342-351, 1981.

17. Hepburn, D. and J. Myles. Hepburn's Law. Kodiak Super Strength Enterprises, Vancouver, BC, Canada, 1980.

18. Hoffman, B. Bob Hoffman's Simplified system of barbell training. Strength &Health Publishing, York, PA, 1940.

19. Hoffman, B. Bob Hoffman's Daily Dozen. Strength & Health Publishing, York, PA, 1958.

20. Thomas, A. Remembered pleasures of another world and time: The great Strength & Health picnics. Iron Game History 1(4):15-17, 1991.

21. Laputin, N.P. and V.G. Oleshko. Managing the Training of Weightlifters (translated by Andrew Charniga). Sportivny Press, Livonia, MI, 1982 (reference to Prilepin's tables).

22. Jim Wendler. 5/3/1: The Simplest and Most Effective Training System to Increase Raw Strength. Jim Wendler, Columbus, OH, 2009.

23. Jones, Lyn. Club Coach Manual. US Weightlifting Federation, Colorado Springs, CO, 1988.

24. Jones, Lyn. Senior Coach Manual. US Weightlifting Federation, Colorado Springs, CO, 1991.

25. Baker, D. The effects of an in-season of concurrent training on the maintenance of strength and power in professional and college-aged rugby league football players. Journal of Strength and Conditioning Research 15(2): 172-177, 2001.

CURRENT INFORMATION AND EQUIPMENT RESOURCES

Strength Training Books
Starting Strength: Basic Barbell Training - Rippetoe and Kilgore
Practical Programming for Strength Training - Rippetoe and Kilgore
Science and Practice of Strength Training - Zatsiorsky
5/3/1: The Simplest and Most Effective Training System to Increase Raw Strength - Wendler

Powerlifting Books
A Practical Approach to Powerlifting - Sheppard and Jamison
International Powerlifting Federation Rulebook

Weightlifting Books
Olympic Weightlifting: A Complete Guide for Athletes & Coaches - Everett
International Weightlifting Federation Rulebook

Weightlifting Bars & Sets
Elieko - Men's and Women's Olympic standard bars
Pendlay - Men's, Women's, and Junior Olympic standard bars
Rogue - Burgener-Rippetoe Bar (hybrid of Olympic and Power bars)
York - Men's and Women's Olympic standard bars

Powerlifting Bars & Sets
Elieko
Ivanko

Olympic Bars, Plates, & Sets (Metal, Bumper, and Training)
Elieko
Pendlay
Rogue
York

Dumbbells and Kettlebells
MuscleDriver
Rogue
York

Implements
VS Athletics
Getstrength
Rogue

Power Racks, Squat Racks and Benches
MuscleDriver
Promaxima
Rogue
York

Weightlifting Shoes
VS Athletics
Adidas
Nike
Pendlay
Rogue DoWin

Shoes that can be used for Weight Training
VS Athletics Hybrid Trainer
Adidas AdiZero Shotput
Converse All-Star (old school)
Nike Zoom SD3
Spikeless Racing Shoes (any brand with virtually no heel)

More often than not, a hero's most epic battle is the one you never see.

Kevin Smith

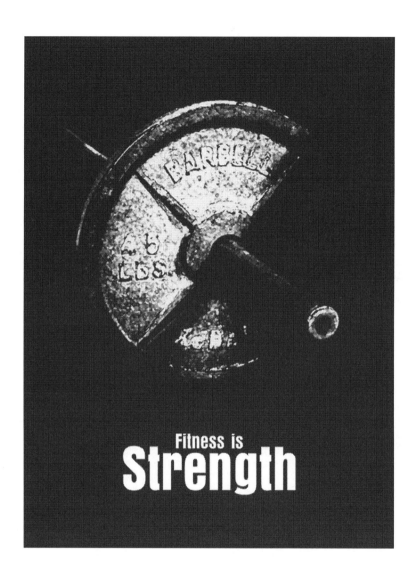

ENDURANCE

Endurance is one of the most difficult disciplines, but it
is to the one who endures that the final victory comes.

Buddha

We define endurance as the ability to sustain a task over time. Have you ever thought about what it is exactly that drives improvement in endurance? If you are like most people you really haven't felt compelled to ponder this. If you are like most fitness writers and academics, when asked that question you would probably pull the answer out of some old aerobic dogma buried in your brain somewhere, obtained from reading texts and research journals or from sitting in a lecture hall somewhere. Most people accept, fairly unquestioningly, the conventional wisdom of aerobic training physiology - just go walk or jog and all will be well. Those things are easy enough to do and the experts say endurance improves when you do them, so why be quizzical?

As it turns out, being quizzical would have been frustrating. As mentioned in an earlier chapter there is no consensus scientific data that tells us what to do in order to improve endurance (1). In a search for a scientific explanation of how endurance improves or even which training methodologies contribute, it will be quickly demonstrated that the state of endurance training theory is not as advanced as one would assume. The answers to simple questions are hard to find and most of the literature doesn't stand up to scrutiny in respect to quality and utility. There are lots of diverse factoids but very little cohesive research data. It seems as though instead of asking what drives adaptation in endurance, most researchers in exercise academic circles have been interested in what limits it, two different entities. Understanding human limitations is a noble effort but fairly futile if you do not understand the process of inducing the physiological adaptations that move the body towards those limitations.

To understand endurance adaptation, we must remember the crux of the correct application of Selye's theory, to understand that a disruption of homeostasis must occur in the physiological system of interest in order for adaptation and fitness improvement to occur in that same system. Endurance is not just walking and jogging. One of the most apparent examples of the misuse, or more precisely, ignorance of the appropriate use of Selye's theory can be found on the holy ground of aerobic fitness. The fitness boon was born in the late 60's under the guidance of Jim Fixx, Thomas Cureton, and Kenneth Cooper. The idea was, and still is, simple. Run a lot and you will be fit and healthy. Over the decades, the mythology of running has firmly entrenched into conventional wisdom the idea that developing aerobic fitness (endurance) requires you to run - run long and run slow. The American College of Sports Medicine (ACSM) recommends 30-60 minutes of continuous low-to-moderate intensity aerobic activity in order to develop aerobic fitness. A problem immediately presents itself with this training concept. With low to moderate intensity running, the ultimate marker of aerobic fitness VO_2max - the maximum amount of oxygen the body can consume at maximal effort - is not challenged. In the classical aerobic exercise prescription for improving aerobic fitness for the masses, the demand for oxygen at the working muscle is met by supply. The name itself says it all - aerobic - in the presence of oxygen. This means that by definition, this type of training cannot provide a disruption of oxygen homeostasis. With no homeostatic disruption there can be no oxygen-related adaptation and fitness gain. That is IF we believe Selye's theory. And of course we do. So it is obvious that the accepted prescription of long-slow-distance exercise for improving aerobic fitness lacks both substantial theoretical support and logic.

Let's take this to the field, out to people who train people to have more endurance. Coaches do not use ACSM recommendations to improve VO_2max and performance in their athletes - in fact they don't even worry about VO_2max they only worry about performance. They do not and would not have a trainee run at 70% of VO_2max for an hour in every training session. They know that performance is unaffected by this. And what does not work in the field is abandoned in the field. Practical experience from more than a century past has demonstrated that this is an ineffective means of increasing VO_2max and performance. The only time you will see 70% runs being used is on a training day designated for recovery. A 70% workload cannot disrupt oxygen homeostasis. It is used for recovery training as it is thought to be easy enough on the body to allow for physiologic recovery from more rigorous training methods without losing neuromuscular condition.

But endurance is a good thing

Endurance is a very good thing. Lots of simple things that we do day-to-day and for sport require some degree of endurance - walking across campus, carrying groceries up to a fourth story walk up, lasting an entire soccer match without having to walk, or even running a marathon. When thought of in this manner, endurance contributes to mobility by allowing one to maintain steady and sure repeated or sustained efforts in the activities in which we engage. Whenever we have to stop doing something before its done because we simply could not do it any longer means that we don't have enough endurance. Since not everyone wants to do the same thing for the same duration of time means that how much endurance someone needs is based on an individual's desires and on the activity in which the individual engages.

Endurance is primarily a bioenergetic entity, related to the ability to deliver both oxygen and energetic nutrients to the working muscles at adequate rates and for long enough of a duration to accomplish the task at hand. However, it is not just important to things we do and want to do, it is important in keeping us alive. Any number of research studies have produced a correlation between cardiorespiratory fitness (endurance) and death from cardiorespiratory disease, cancer, and in several papers, all-cause mortality (2,3,4). As with the strength research relevant to mortality, these are correlational papers and do not establish causality, just that condition A is often present at the same time as condition B. Regardless, it has been well established that those with the lowest degree of endurance are likely at the highest risk of mortality. We can loosely suggest that those in the lowest 25% of the population are at the greatest risk. There is a fairly significant reduction in deaths in the next higher 25% in fitness, essentially those that are exercising but not very much but that are little more fit. In the top 50% of fitness the death rate does not drop much at all compared to the transition from untrained to minimally trained. This particular observation, coupled with the fact that getting 300 million people to go out and run long distances is a losing proposition, is why so much of the research in the exercise arena is focused on how little exercise is needed to stave off disease and death, not on how to get fit. The research and government perception is that public health would be better served by identifying a minimum amount of physical activity rather than identifying the most effective exercise means to create the minimum change desired.

So what do we need to do to develop endurance?

To more fully examine the methods used in the field to make people more enduring, let's divide training for aerobic fitness into two basic types of training, long-slow-distance and interval training. There are many variations of both of these types but in large part the variants are fairly similar (table 1) and can be described as follows. Long-slow-distance work is intended by convention to improve cardiovascular efficiency and VO_2max and interval training is intended to improve lactate tolerance/clearance and VO_2max. Both of these types of training have been demonstrated to improve endurance performance and VO_2max and this is where it gets tricky. Two different training methods, two different sets of metabolic demands, and they both yield the same result. How can this be? Part of the answer can be found by considering the population on which the majority of research has been done, usually low to average fit individuals just starting a training program. In other words, a beginner. A beginner is very far away from their genetic potential for performance and as such a very low level and non-specific stress can induce positive adaptations. We can basically have a beginner walk, jog, sprint, jump, twist, flex, wiggle, dance, swing, hang, roll, bounce, do virtually any activity, and improve endurance. This is so because any advancement of metabolic and oxygen demand beyond their sedentary lifestyle is a novel and disruptive stress and will induce an improvement in endurance and VO_2max. This concept of beginners responding to a non-specific stress is not unique to aerobic exercise. In the realm of strength development, you can have a beginner ride a bike and they will improve their squat performance. But put an intermediate, advanced, or elite trainee on a bike and they will not improve their squat. They need to do Squats, they require specificity. Considering data from beginner populations to be relevant to trainees at every level of training advancement is a gross and progress defeating mistake.

If much of the data we have is flawed or uninformative, how are we supposed to know how to train people? We use our brains. Let's consider what specifically each of these two field methods of training do to the body. We've already established that long-slow-distance training cannot, by definition, disrupt oxygen delivery and utilization to a point of homeostatic disruption. But we also know that endurance can be enhanced by this type of training. Why the incongruity? It's not really incongruent it's just confusing because of lax and complex terminology academics and clinicians have devised over the years. Endurance isn't just VO_2, there are more facets to it than that. But let's keep it simple here and examine the two major facets of endurance, (A) energy and (B) oxygen.

Training Method (Common Name)	Description	Accepted Intent or Disturbed Variable	Degree of VO₂ homeostatic disruption	Actual Disturbed Variable	End Result in Trained Individuals
Recovery	20 to 60 minutes at approximately 70% of VO₂max	Warm-up, Cool-down, recovery day NOTE: 20-60 minutes of aerobic activity is not a warm-up or a cool-down it is a workout (but not a very effective one)	None	None	Recovery of previous levels of performance, no improvement induced
Long-Slow-Distance	60 to 120 minutes at approximately 70% VO₂max	Cardiovascular efficiency improvement	None	Oxidative Metabolism (Carbohydrate & Fat)	Improvement in stores of oxidative energy substrates and associated enzymes, can run longer but not faster
Tempo (Interval type)	20 minutes at approximately 85% VO₂max	Improve lactate kinetics	None	Aerobic Glycolytic Metabolism (Carbohydrate)	Improvement in stores of aerobic glycolytic energy substrates and associated enzymes, delay of switch to anaerobic metabolism, can run a little longer a little faster
Interval	Up to 5 minutes at 95-100% VO₂max	Improve VO₂max, Improve lactate kinetics	Small	Primary - Aerobic glycolytic metabolic system, Secondary - Anaerobic Glycolytic Metabolism	Improvement in stores of aerobic glycolytic energy substrates and associated enzymes, delay of switch to anaerobic metabolism, improvement in anaerobic enzyme stores and function, can run a little longer a little faster (does not significantly improve VO₂)
Reps (Interval Type)	30 to 90 seconds at slightly greater than VO₂max	Improve speed and economy	Large	Anaerobic Glycolytic Metabolism and VO₂	Improvement in anaerobic glycolytic storage and function, increased efficiency in O₂ consumption at the working muscle - Increased VO₂max

Table 1. Comparison of contemporary endurance training methods.

Long-slow-distance training is energy substrate depleting in nature. It has been shown many times over that glycogen stores can be totally depleted with this type of training, and depletion of an energy substrate should be considered a fairly significant homeostatic disruption of metabolism. It would not be prudent to consider only complete depletion as a disruptive stress, partial depletions should be considered disruptive as well IF AND ONLY IF the depletion is larger than previously experienced by the trainee. This type of training can also exceed the body's ability to metabolize fat for energy. Driving a metabolic system beyond its normal range of operation or to failure is definitely a disruption of homeostasis. Combined, the stress of glycogen depletion below normally experienced levels while simultaneously exceeding fat metabolic capacity drives an improvement in storing and utilizing these two energetic substrates and results in being able to run longer - thus endurance has improved but VO_2max has not improved. This is a specific adaptation to a specific stress in a previously trained subject. This seems obvious, but most people fail to see this connection between aerobic exercise, metabolism, and performance and automatically, and incorrectly, attribute the improvement in endurance from an energy depleting training protocol to an improvement in VO_2max. It is important to note here that if the ability to maintain unrelenting and constant movement for two or more hours is a goal, it is quite appropriate to include some long slow distance in a training protocol. It would be a mistake for endurance athletes to eliminate it simply because it does not advance VO_2max. Similarly, if you are planning on doing sustained multiple hour physical activity of any kind there is a need for intelligently included LSD in your program.

The second common type of training done for aerobic fitness is interval training – shorter and more intense segments of effort with little rest between repeats. It has been observed that lactic acid accumulates during this type of training and thus it is commonly accepted that intervals push the body to adapt to the presence of lactate by enabling it to tolerate higher concentrations. Alternatively, it is suggested that interval training may enable a quicker removal of lactate from the tissues and blood. This seems nice and logical, but it is off base. Although we are inundated with (mis)information that lactic acid is bad, lactic acid is an essential hydrogen ion acceptor in glycolytic metabolism. Sure the exercise conditions that are associated with its accumulation are a bit uncomfortable but correlation is not causation. So do we really care that lactate has accumulated? We really shouldn't, lactate isn't even part of aerobic metabolism and VO_2max, it is simply an inevitable consequence of the really important things happening here. With interval training, producing lactate is not important per se, exceeding oxygen consumption capacity is. Intervals are done in the glycolytic realm, whereas long-slow-distance is primarily oxidative. Running fast enough to require the primary metabolic systems for exercise support to be glycolytic, specifically anaerobic glycolysis, means that the working muscle cannot take up and use oxygen fast enough to meet exercise driven demand. If anything, significant lactic acid accumulation occurs coincident with disruption of oxygen homeostasis. The level of exertion where lots of lactate is produced is the level of exertion needed to drive improvements in VO_2max. It's the level of exertion where we have exceeded oxygen consumption capacity. The body will adapt to this stress by augmenting its ability to take up oxygen and to use it in the muscle - if this type of training is repeated chronically and progressively. It has been traditionally suggested that interval training should account for about 5% of a runner's total mileage and this is a gross under-use of this training method. Lots of aerobic athletes use intervals. Many use them for the wrong reason. Regardless of the decision process used to justify their inclusion, they should likely do more, lots more. Most runners use interval intensities of between 85% to 105% of VO_2max (usually calculated as a speed just slightly faster than race pace). Intervals need to be short and intense. Trained runners can run many miles at 85-90% of VO_2max, so the low end of the common interval prescription is not useful. At the upper end, 105% is just barely enough intensity to drive any type of positive oxygen handling adaptation. Productive intervals will have intensities in the range of 150% or more of VO_2max. To maximize endurance gains, trainees should run faster, a lot faster. Support for this concept comes from many practical observations of successful athletes. And recent pilot data from the laboratory of Dr. Julien Baker of the University of the West of Scotland demonstrates that four (4) thirty second sprints at peak velocity separated by thirty seconds of rest, when done three days a week improves endurance significantly. Several other papers by various authors back up this finding. Clearly, this type of training is the meat and potatoes of endurance.

THE ANATOMY OF ENDURANCE

As endurance is time dependent, it is easily measured with a watch and measuring tape or any number of other common or laboratory measurement devices. Endurance can be subdivided into continuous endurance, where the activity is sustained, as in jogging - and intermittent endurance, where work-recovery cycles are repeated for long durations, as in digging post holes for a fence row. Intermittent endurance training is more important than continuous endurance training, but we have to do a little dissection to get to the why of this non-intuitive statement.

Powering Continuous Endurance Exercise

If we are going long, going slow, and going for the distance there has to be a sustained delivery of energy to the muscle. In this type of endurance, the storage, delivery, and break down of glycogen (chains of glucose), glucose, and fat is of primary concern. These metabolic processes are the limit to performance, when we run out we have to slow way down in order to use the next available source of energy, protein. Using protein as an energy source is very slow and not very productive. If you've ever seen a marathoner or ultra-distance runner crawl across the finish line, its primarily because they have run out of readily available carbohydrate and fat and have switched to protein as an energy source. This is different than "hitting the wall" or "bonking" during a distance race. That occurs simply because the runner has adopted a race pace that requires energy at a rate that his aerobic capacity cannot deliver. At some point he will have to slow to a much much lower velocity pace where aerobic function and hopefully recovery can occur and allow for completion of the race. There is a gray area between outstripping the metabolic ability of the body and the total depletion of normally available energy sources with many variations of how they can occur. However they both have the same end result, slowing down or stopping.

One of the previous scenarios is not usually experienced by the average endurance exerciser who's normal training run, ride, or swim is generally much shorter than the two to four hours of 70% plus of maximum running velocity required to strip out the body's stores of glycogen. But the other, going too fast for aerobic metabolism to keep pace does occur. When one does long slow distance, it needs to be just that, long and slow. You want to keep a metabolic pace that consumes carbohydrate.

There are two basic locations of carbohydrate (glucose) in the body. The first is muscle glucose that is on site inside the muscle and is very quickly available for use. The other source is liver glycogen, a large repository of carbohydrate. When muscle glucose starts being depleted, the body starts breaking down glycogen into glucose and mobilizing into the blood. As blood glucose it gets moved to the muscle where it gets used. When we do a novel effort in long slow distance training and cut deeper into our carbohydrate stores, this system is moved into disequilibrium and Selye's adaptation theory becomes applicable. The body begins to store more carbohydrate and to augment its ability to break down carbohydrate and deliver it to the muscle.

The other component of powering aerobic exercise is deriving energy from fat. Fat is a very energy rich metabolic resource with more than twice the amount of useable energy in one gram of fat compared to one gram of carbohydrate. Although it is a very energy dense substance, it takes a lot of time to break it down from its triglyceride form in your fat cells into fatty acids, move those fatty acids to the blood, move them into the cell, then further break them down, move them into the mitochondria, then derive their available energy. To use fat significantly one needs to go very slow - from sitting still up to a moderately paced jog (5). A benefit of long slow distance training is that it does enhance ones ability to break down and deliver fatty acids in support of endurance activity. Enhancement of the body's ability to mobilize and use fat to power exercise is a primary adaptation generated relative to continuous endurance. Luckily we never really eat into our fat stores (Get it? A pun!) and disrupt homeostatic fat storage conditions during exercise. If we did, the adaptation would be to add more fat. Humans have a well developed ability to store fat, an ability developed over potentially millions of years in order to survive periods of low food supply (such as winters), we can literally store enough calories in the form of fat to survive for a couple months of no food. A mere few minutes or even a few hours of exercise do not provide a significant stress of our abilities to store fat. That's a good thing since modern man frequently manages to enhance fat storage through another process, over eating.

Both of these sets of adaptations, one set specific to carbohydrate and one set specific to fat, have common results. They enhance our ability to exercise for longer times or cover longer distances, or essentially how much endurance work we can do. This is where the greatest magnitude of fitness improvement lies with this type of training, our gas tanks have a few extra gallons of gas in them as an analogy. A much smaller but still performance enhancing adaptation is the augmentation of the metabolic machinery that breaks down aerobic energy sources and powers continuous muscle activity. The closest automotive analogy here would be that we just got an engine tune up and we can now squeeze out another mile per gallon from the gas we have on board.

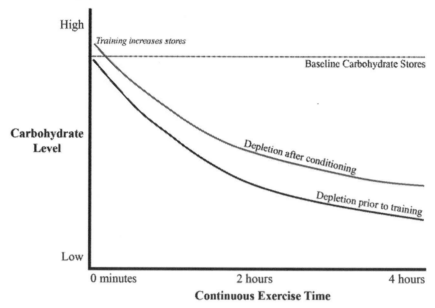

Figure 1. Total body carbohydrate is depleted significantly with prolonged exercise before and after a program of continuous endurance type training. Appropriate training protocols provides us a higher baseline amount of storage thus extending the length of time to exhaustion. The graphic depicts the cumulative amount of storage in muscle and the liver. Muscle glycogen can be completely depleted within four hours, liver glycogen can be reduced by 50 to 75% in the same time frame (6).

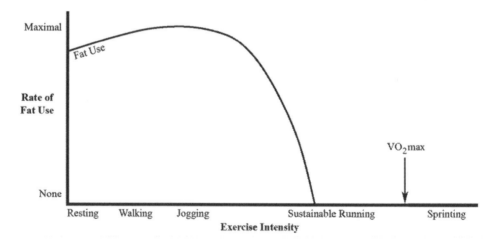

Figure 2. Lipid utilization occurs during rest (about 80% of total energy used at rest) and low to moderate intensity endurance activities.

Powering Intermittent Endurance Exercise

Humans evolved in hypoxic (low oxygen) environments (7) and as such the human race developed an ability to extract oxygen from the atmosphere and deliver it to the working muscle where it is used as a key component in the break down of carbohydrate and fat to produce energy - even when there is low oxygen availability (altitude). The ability to extract and deliver oxygen to the muscle AND the ability of the muscle cells to internalize and use the oxygen affects the rate of endurance work we can do. An untrained individual can only do so much work so fast before he becomes "out of breath", "winded", or in other words he is going too fast for his cardiorespiratory system AND his muscle cells to deliver AND extract oxygen for use in metabolism.

The intermediary in oxygen movement from the air and delivery to the muscle where it is taken in by the cell is the blood. Most of us are fairly familiar with the fact that the blood carries oxygen to where it is needed in the body. All of those red blood cells (erythrocytes) that are part of our blood contain a chemical, hemoglobin, that draws oxygen out of the air and binds it as it circulates in the body. As such, blood has a characteristic amount of oxygen, or oxygen saturation, under normal conditions. Oxygen saturation is generally reported as a percentage with normal resting values ranging from 97 to 99%. Lower resting values to 95% are generally of no clinical consequence, however, as values approach 90% the likelihood of pathology and need for intervention increases. Pathologically, low oxygen saturation is generally a problem of something interfering with oxygen getting into the blood not of us taking too much out of the blood. But we can depress oxygen saturation through exercise.

Exercise induced hypoxemia is generally defined as a reduction, as a result of exercise, of blood oxygen saturation to either 94% or a reduction of 4% below resting saturation.

We can make the muscles consume lots of oxygen by exercising at a very high work rate for relatively short durations. The exercise has to be done at a rate higher than the rate where we are at VO_2max, the maximum ability of the heart and lungs to deliver oxygen to the working muscle. We have to exceed delivery capacity in order to desaturate the blood of oxygen and disrupt oxygen homeostasis. In practice this means running faster than your best mile time, maybe better than your best 800 time, for as long as you can for repeats in order to accumulate a reduction in blood oxygen saturation. It means that you have to push into the edge of discomfort and distress to produce a fitness gain in this area. To develop intermittent endurance and to develop VO_2max, interval training has to be done, it is a very specific training tool that produces a very specific adaptation. An adaptation that increases how much work you can do in a given amount of time and when coupled with enhanced continuous endurance makes you able to go much faster for much longer.

	Oxygen Saturation %	Heart Rate Beat/Min	Respiratory Rate Breath/Min
Rest	98	72	12
After Warm up	98	87	12
After 4 Sprints	93	162	50
After 8 Spints	91	164	50
After 12 Sprints	87	168	48
5 Minute Recovery	96	113	20

Table 2. Oxygen saturation can be depressed significantly by repeated maximal intensity efforts such as repeating 50 yards sprints on the minute for 12 minutes. Note that the reduction in saturation percent was the result of cumulative efforts. The maximum predicted heart rate for the subject here was 169 beats per minute (220 - age).

Oxygen desaturation however is a variably responsive entity. There will low responders and high responders based on muscle fiber type profile and the degree of existing metabolic conditioning. The largest desaturations will likely occur in those individuals who are strong, are fast twitch muscle fiber dominant, have well developed phosphagenic pathways, and poorly developed glycolytic and oxidative pathways. This set of physiological characteristics allows an individual to work at a very fast rate and consume oxygen much faster than it can be delivered. At the other end of the spectrum is the individual that is more slow twitch muscle fiber dominant, has well developed oxidative metabolic pathways, is weaker, and has poorly developed phosphagenic and anaerobic glycolytic pathways. Such an individual will not be able to exercise at a fast enough (because of poor phosphagenic and anaerobic glycolytic development) and large enough (because they are not strong) work rate to create a large desaturation. The continuum in between these polar opposites is rather messy given the individual and unknown nature of individual fiber type profile and degree of metabolic development. However, it should be apparent that strength is a key element in developing endurance. It should be equally apparent that low to moderate intensity exercise - that develops the ability to store and utilize carbohydrate and fat in support of long duration activity - is not the driving force of aerobic fitness gain if measured as VO_2max.

THE TOOLS OF ENDURANCE TRAINING

As with strength, the first step in training is to learn how to effectively do the exercises you are planning on including. By far and always, the most popular form of exercise is jogging (running at a pace of 10 minutes per mile or slower, but faster than a walk). However, as any high level sport coach will tell you, there is a tremendous shortcoming in the teaching of running technique at every level of physical education. Just think about your own personal history in running, when did you learn to run and did anyone ever actually watch you and teach you how to run efficiently? If someone did, how do you know they taught you correctly? The assumption that one innately knows how to run simply by virtue of being human is not justified or appropriate. Let's consider a parallel, although anyone can squat down and pick something up off the ground, we know that virtually everyone needs to be taught how to squat with weights correctly to be safe and productive. This relationship holds for every exercise we do and for the use of every piece of exercise equipment. We need to learn how to do endurance exercises correctly as the best results come to those with good technique. And we need to be able to use the tools of the trade to their best application.

On your feet

Running is considered an intuitive exercise modality by virtually everyone. The common exercise prescription given to most people just beginning to exercise is simply to go out and walk or jog in a pair of comfortable shoes. Very few people are ever appropriately instructed on how to run or in what type of shoes are suited for the activity.

Let's first consider running technique. One would think that everyone runs pretty much the same way and that good technique is an accepted and defined set of anatomical and mechanical statements describing efficient movement. They don't and it isn't.

Running technique is usually taught in simple terms if it is taught at all. Look on the web and you will see some "experts" stating that running technique is inherited and the only way to improve running performance is to get more fit. They don't even bother with technique. Most people don't think this way. In fact, since the 1960s experts have been teaching fitness runners to run in a heel first technique. The heel contacts the ground first, the ankle moves from flexion to extension (dorsiflexion to plantar flexion), the knee flexes to absorb shock then extends. There have been studies done on how well people can learn this technique, and have demonstrated that this technical model can be learned in as little as 15 twenty-minute coaching sessions (8). Spending this time learning the heel strike method might not have been the best use of time. In recreational runners who almost exclusively use this technique, the frequency of injury has been conservatively reported to be three injuries per every 100 hours of running or that more than half of all runners experience injury within any given training year (9,10). This makes it one of the more dangerous training modalities recommended by fitness and medical professionals - one where technique and equipment should be carefully assessed and prescribed in a scientific and logical manner.

There has been much recent attention on running technique and appropriate footwear in recent years. The high incidence of injuries in heel strike runners in spite of advanced heel cushioning technology in modern running shoes has prompted a re-analysis of both technique and footwear. Several papers have been written, both theoretical and data driven, suggesting that the heel strike technique should be replaced with a fore-foot strike technique (11,12). The recent analyses are not revolutionary in the least. In 1955 John Bunn described the basic mechanical and practical benefits of a fore-foot running technique versus a heel strike technique, with the heel strike described as more shock producing and containing a velocity retardation (deceleration) component (13). It has been frequently stated that the slower you run the more you shift the point of foot impact towards the heel, it is more likely that you run slower because you impact on your heels. Running on the forefoot is a learnable skill, arguably taught in a weekend seminar or through repeated practice over three months (14). What the rest of the body is doing during running is also fairly loosely described. It is commonly recommended to "run tall" maintaining a vertical posture with the back perpendicular to the ground (15). This is in direct contradiction to the historical mechanically derived concept that the body must have a forward lean, up to twenty degrees, in order for propulsion to occur effectively (16). If the center of mass is not in advance of the point of foot contact, we slow down or stop. Instructions for the carriage of the arms is also variable, ranging from being carried at 90 degrees at the elbows and swinging the hands from just behind the buttocks (same side as the hand) then across the body to anterior of the opposing hip or alternatively a similar elbow angle with restricted range of motion of the arm directly forward and backwards with no lateral arc. The mass of running advice available to the general public is conflicting and much of it is derived not from objective data or observation rather from personal perspectives from perceived authorities that have become ingrained as fact over the years (17). Although it would be tempting to blame self-appointed authorities for any error ridden concepts about running and running technique, we can't, they are operating in an informational vacuum. A search of the scientific databases will not provide one any means to create a picture of appropriate running technique, only an assemblage of diverse data that cannot produce a systematic means of teaching running. In the realm of physical education one of the most cited resources for teaching running is a nearly thirty year old 32 page pamphlet put out by the British Amateur Athletic Board (18). In the track and field literature, even very extensive treatises on the training of competitive track athletes minimally explain running technique, usually as a brief few sentences regarding each; torso angle, arm swing, and footstrike (19,20). More time is spent describing peripheral science issues than on actual coaching methods. If we move into the commercial fitness world you will find another famine of information with only two relative newcomers contributing to the teaching of running, the POSE running system (1997) and the Chi Running system (2004), the only commercially available systems of running technique instruction available.

How do we know what technique to use if there is no consensus? We go back to science and basic logic. Bunn's 1955 physics based explanations of running technique are in line with those found in competitive coaching manuals, telling us that what worked in the 50s is still working today, it just hasn't been articulated very well to the running public. So here we'll divide running technique into four anatomical areas - torso, arms, legs, and feet - and describe the basic movement patterns that constitute appropriate running technique. Realize that not everyone will look the same even though they are following the same pattern of movement, anatomical differences mean that body segment position will vary between individuals. Someone with a 28 inch inseam will look different than someone with a 36 inseam when doing the exact same movement. Don't look for precise angles and absolute descriptors, look for patterns and relationships.

The torso has to be oriented so that the center of mass of the body is slightly ahead of a point on the ground where the feet would be if you were standing still. Walking and running can be described as a controlled loss of balance forward, so there is a narrow margin of control. Luckily this is one of the things we have learned during a lifetime of walking and running around - controlling our balance. We do this part fairly intuitively once we get started running BUT if you take a novice runner out and tell them to accelerate as fast as they can, about ten percent of the time or so, they will lean too far forward and end up sprawling across the ground. Learning the appropriate amount of lean for a given acceleration takes some practice, experimentation, and feedback. When observing someone running correctly at a steady pace, the angle of a line from the hip joint to the top of the sternum will be at about a twenty degree angle (not the same in every one). If we look at anatomical relationships, the neck will be just in front of the hip. This orientation keeps the center of the body's mass in a forward position to facilitate maintenance of forward momentum without being so far forward to lose balance or introduce unnecessary compensatory movements. There will be a little rotation of the shoulders and chest forward and back around the axis of the vertebral column, but it should not be any more than the thickness of the shoulders themselves. As the position of the head affects the position of the torso, the neck should be kept in normal postural extension. In fact, the entire vertebral column should be held in normal extension – this is the source of the oft heard mandate that you must run upright, it is a CUE to get people to maintain normal posture and not look down, hunch over, or assume any other non-extended vertebral orientation. This accomplishes two purposes; (A) it prevents the head from slowing pace (head back) or speeding pace (head forward) and (B) it enables a complete and safe field of vision.

> *Cue* – A word, phase, or simple instruction that is used to get a trainee to assume the correct position or execute an exercise skill in the correct manner. They are generally only effective when they are short and simple. Exaggeration is frequently useful. For example, telling a runner to run with their body straight up and down is an exaggeration, as efficient forward movement during running requires a minimal forward lean. However, the runner's mental image of an erect torso gets the runner to assume normal vertebral extension from the lumbar region up to the skull.

The arms, at the elbow, are in flexion. By bending the elbows to about 90 degrees, the length of the lever arm (actually the moment arm) that is being moved at the shoulder is decreased. This makes it less energetically costly to move the mass of the arms as a counterbalance to the movements of the legs. In their role as a counterbalance, the range of motion of the arm should place the hand, at the arm's peak backward excursion, just superior and lateral to the hip joint. The hands of people with shorter arms will swing back to a position at about the peak of the iliac crest. At the peak of the arm's movement forward, with elbows still bend to 90 degrees, the fingers will rise to about the level of the shoulder (about the height of the deltoid). The motion of the arms affect the rotational movement of the shoulders and torso so it is important to maintain as linear of motion as possible with the arms - straight forward and straight back. While it is important to hold the arm's in the correct position, this does not mean that a great deal of muscular exertion is called for, rather the minimum amount of effort to maintain the position and movement pattern is needed. It is frequently recommended to "relax" the upper body, arms, and hands when running. This is not precisely achievable since we are actively contracting these muscles for balance but the concept is valid, use only enough force to maintain correct form.

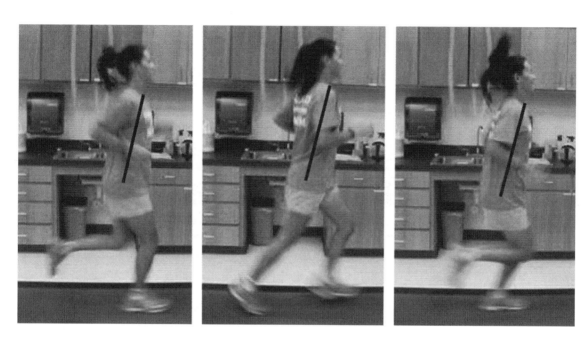

Figure 3. Throughout the running stride the torso maintains a consistent forward lean.

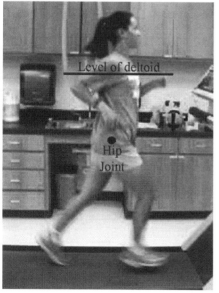

Figure 4. At their peak excursion forward and backward, the hands reach the line of the hip joint (near hand) and the level of the shoulder (far hand).

The legs (hips, knees, and ankles) are key elements in effective running. They have to flex and extend at the right time for it to work right and produce safe and effective technique. When we step off, we push one leg backwards (we are actually pushing the body forward) through a combination of hip extension, knee extension, and ankle extension (plantar flexion) - that leg is the trailing leg. The other leg, the lead leg, is flexing at the hip, knee, and ankle (dorsiflexion) and swinging forward. It is important to adequately bend the knee as this shortens the moment arm and reduces the force required to move the entire leg forward to where the foot is under the center of mass at touch down. If the point of touch down is in front of the center of mass, overstriding, the forward disequilibrium required to maintain forward momentum is destroyed and a braking effect is produced. Overstriding appears as the lead leg being very extended in front of the body (close to being a straight knee - entire leg angling up and back towards the torso). When overstriding occurs, the trailing leg must produce more propulsive force to move the mass of the body in front of the lead foot. With overstriding, the center of mass will drop quite a bit after touch down in order to maintain a degree of momentum. These are both ineffective movements and increase the energy cost of running (you tire faster). This is also why most beginning runners do not run smoothly, rather they look interrupted and jostled in their stride - the result of the trainee trying to reach out too far with their lead leg. It is tempting to try to show the average Joe the long elegant strides of an Olympian and say "do that", but that image of long legs striding out over meters can be misleading unless you point out where the center of mass is relative to touch down. Fixing this at the outset of training will pay dividends in lower injury rates later. If everyone tends to overstride, where should we try to touch the foot down to prevent it? The foot should touch down at a point on the ground where the heel is fairly close to being directly under the chin and the shin is close to vertical. OK but what part of the foot should touch down first? This leads us directly into the next important element to be considered, the foot.

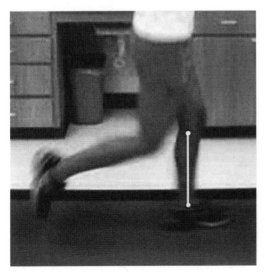

Figure 5. When the foot touches down, the shin will be approximately vertical (knee joint over ankle joint).

The feet are our interface with the earth. We push off of and touch down on the ground with our feet. The anatomical structure of the foot has developed over the eons to provide us with a robust shock absorptive system that can also assist in transferring muscular force generated in the legs to the ground. When we consider how we land with every footstrike, there are three basic categories; forefoot, midfoot, and heel strike. The forefoot and midfoot strikes are variations on the same theme with both having initial contact between the ball of the foot and the ground. With forefoot strike technique, the distribution of the body's weight on the foot stays forward but with midfoot strike technique the body's weight settles backwards towards the ankle and in fact the ankle flexes and the heel comes close to touching the ground. In both cases, the ball of the foot remains the only weight supporting element. The term "midfoot" is a misnomer as the middle of the foot does not strike the ground first (or at all - unless there is inversion of the foot, and then the lateral aspect of the fifth metatarsal would come into contact with the ground as well). The third type of footstrike is heel strike. In this technique the calcaneous, or heel bone, strikes the ground, then the ball of the foot levers down to strike the ground, after which the heel rises, and then there is a push off. This long series of events keeps the runner on the ground a long time and this is also inefficient. To make a heel strike happen, the beginner essentially has to overstride and extend the knee beyond the center of body mass. This will appear as the shin extending slightly beyond perpendicular to the ground at heel strike. The analysis of this technique's effect on running performance has been in the professional literature for more than 50 years - "An athlete who runs on his heels (permits his heels to contact the ground first as he strides) is causing the center of gravity to fall behind his contact foot and thus is creating a retarding effect" (13). If you look at archival footage of early 20th century Olympic 1500 meter champions, you will see that the best runners used forefoot/midfoot technique, just as present day Olympians do. The plain and simple of the matter is that we need to run on the balls of our feet to be efficient runners. And by adopting this technique of running we will also invoke the additional shock absorptive capabilities of the exquisite arches and other force dampening features of our feet and lessen the likelihood of repetitive use injury. Both of these benefits are absent in heel strike running. Further, the simple touch and go nature of landing and pushing off of the same anatomical feature, the ball of the foot, gets us back in the air and into our next step faster. This gets you down the road faster.

Running on the balls of the feet may require wholesale changes in running technique. It is quite possible that an external coach or instructor will be necessary. As with learning weight exercises, there are number of high profile professionals that deliver running technique seminars such as Dr. Nicholas Romanov, Danny Dryer, Brian MacKenzie, among others. An advantage in the running community is that there are quite a few track coaches who have gone through the USA Track and Field coaching education system. Ask around your area as some of these coaches are quite expert and may be available to help you if their coaching duties allow it. Don't be afraid to ask for help. Don't shy away from paying for it either. If you really want to improve in any aspect of fitness, don't just Google™ it, seek out practicing and paid expert professionals who will work with you and teach you in person.

If you should choose to convert from heel striking to running on the balls of the feet, DO NOT carry over the same volume of training for the first month. Cut back in your mileage by about 40% for the first week after conversion. Then each week thereafter add ten percent back into the program. By slowly ramping up the training volume, the muscles and tendons that are now being loaded for the first time during running will have a chance to adapt and this will prevent unnecessary soreness and frustration.

With technique sorted, we can move on to the equipment of running, the shoe. Everyone wants to know what shoe is the best for running purposes. It sort of depends. If you insist on running inefficiently with a heel strike technique, then the super squishy marshmallow shoes are probably called for. But be aware that while those shoes improve comfort, they do not truly reduce risk of over-use injury and may actually increase the risk of ankle sprains (21). But really, why not just run the right way? There is enough historical and scientific evidence to strongly suggest that running on the balls of the foot is safer and produces better performance (11,12).

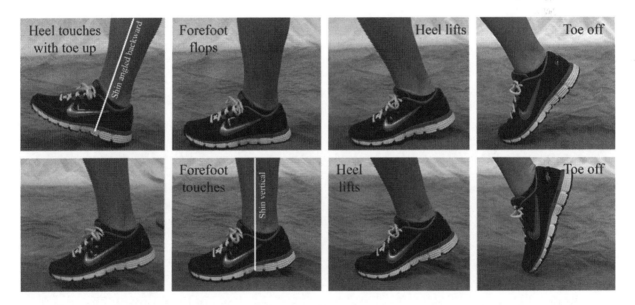

Figure 6. The common heel strike technique of running (top) provides less shock absorption, adds deceleration, and keeps the runner in contact with the ground for a longer period of time than the preferable forefoot strike technique of running (bottom).

The anatomy of the foot and its functional capacity negates the need for super padded shoes. Some will in fact say that running should be done in bare feet. We will agree that that is a mechanically and technically sound approach because you can't heel strike when barefooted. But we will always recommend some foot covering for protection from physical hazards and environmental conditions. No one can guarantee, even on a nice stretch of sandy beach or grassy park, that there are no nasty little hidden sharpies lying in wait to ambush an unsuspecting and naked foot. When the temperature is 110 degrees in Armpit, Texas or minus 20 in Insanity, North Dakota, barefoot running is also not in the cards. You can achieve all the safety and performance from running with simple racing or running flats, shoes that have good arch support but very minimal heel if any (arch support doesn't have to be from internal elements it can be delivered quite efficiently by lacing). Shoes just like nearly every champion distance racer has used during the past century.

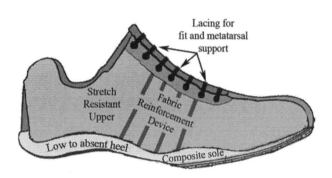

Figure 7. The elements of a running shoe are simple. A robust, minimally compressible composite rubber sole running the length of the shoe should be present. There is no need for a built up heel. A minimal heel is begrudgingly acceptable. The upper should not be made of easily stretched material as such material cannot provide support. Rather a stretch resistant material that is reinforced with stitching or fabric devices fixed over the metatarsal and tarsal area of the foot is desirable. Old fashioned lacing should be used, but if it can be microadjusted for fit and support any system can work.

FARTHER AND FASTER - THE COMMON GOALS OF ENDURANCE TRAINING

If you think about it, can we really put our finger on one single endurance goal that fits everyone? Of course not. That is why a national health initiative that puts all its eggs into one basket - the 30 minutes of low to moderate intensity activity on 3-5 days per week approach for example - is destined for failure in creating a nation of fit people. Well, it's one of the reasons. A very clear shortcoming of this type of exercise prescription is it is couched in defensive medicine (do no harm) and its only goal is to promote health - the absence of disease - and prevent premature death from disease processes. The results that are important to the National Institutes of Health, the American Heart Association, and the American College of Sports Medicine are found in lower rates of hypertension, diabetes, atherosclerosis, and death NOT in improved 10K times or other real-world measures of endurance. Fitness, as most people perceive it and as we describe it here, is not a concern and the National Institutes of Health does not even support research on how to improve fitness. While health may be an excellent by-product of exercise, here we are more interested in endurance as an element of fitness and are intent on helping trainees achieve their fitness goals to improve their functions at work and play.

Goals are important in this respect. One needs to know why more endurance is desired and should have a target in mind. Whether it is being able to do a 10 minute mile or run a marathon or being able to spend a day hauling shingles up a 16 foot ladder, we need to know what we want to accomplish in our training. The most common general endurance goal we encounter is "I want to run farther faster". If we can assign a distance to the "farther" we can then construct a training program to meet our needs. We also need to recognize which, farther or faster, has a goal priority as they are separate entities that require different strategies.

We can make this concept fairly simple by breaking endurance goals down by distance. In figure 8, running performance goals are categorized by distance, 100 yards up to 5 miles. If we want to improve our sprinting, once we have established an initial level of work capacity, there are no 30 minute bouts of moderate intensity exercise, just sprints and intervals. If we want to be able to run 5 miles quickly, we only do some moderate intensity exercise but we do many high intensity intervals with some sprints thrown in. In this simple graphic we have used the scientific principles of adaptation to create a conceptual basis for creating endurance training programs specific to individual goals ... and it was pretty easy to do. And guess what, running coaches have done things like this for decades, its just that the methodology was not explained with science just passed down in the lore of coaching from coach to disciple ... if you were lucky enough to have been mentored by a good coach.

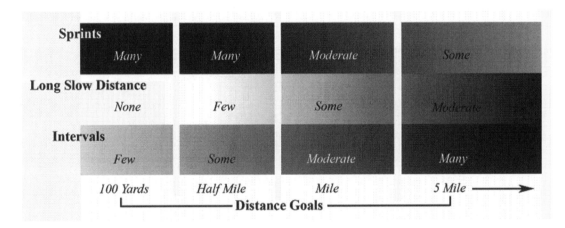

Figure 8. Individual training goals relative to endurance require different approaches to training. In the continuum above, distance goals can be found in the lower line. Above each distance goal you can find the approximate and relative amount of long slow distance, interval, or sprint training needed to achieve that goal. A sprint is any running effort that requires effort at a rate greater than VO_2max (a competitive mile requires approximately 105% of VO_2max and is the longest "sprint"). Sprints are followed by complete recovery before any subsequent work. An interval is a series of sprint efforts separated by short and incomplete recovery periods.

If we use a trainee who wants to develop their ability to run 5-10K, we can come up with a conceptual representation of what their training should look like over their training career, from beginner to advanced (figure 9). During the beginners stage of training, when the trainee has first gotten up off the couch to exercise, the traditional 30 minutes of low to moderate intensity training will work to establish an exercise base and fitness will improve from this very general stimulus. Remember that previously the body was adapted to no exercise so this very minimal stress will produce results ... for a time. By about 3 months of training, LSD is beginning to lose its potency as an adaptive stress and interval training must be added in to continue the application of adaptive stress. At about six months a small percentage of sprints is added in to apply another novel stress. Throughout the training career there is a reduction in relative percentage of continuous endurance training in favor of higher amounts of intermittent training and sprinting. It is the last two components that drive aerobic fitness. After three months of training, continuous endurance training simply helps train energy storage capacity. This is important but it is not as important to fitness as being able to utilize that stored energy as fast as possible - a capacity developed through intelligent inclusion of sprinting and intervals.

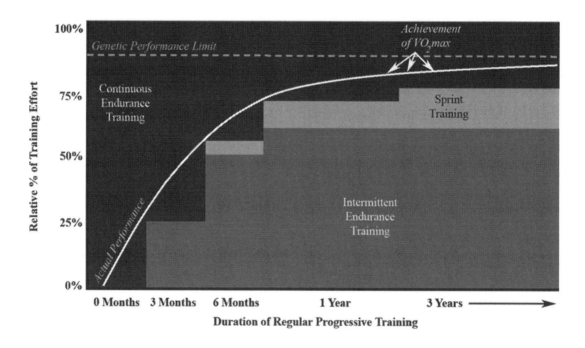

Figure 9. The relative amounts of long slow distance, interval, and sprint training for a 5-10K runner changes over the course of the training career (going from sedentary to fit). For the first three months an aerobic (LSD) base is established. Once the runner can continuously run 2 miles it is time to add in the first wave of interval training. As the runner achieves the ability to run 3 to 6 miles continuously it is time to add in the second wave of increased interval work and a small amount of sprint work. At this point the emphasis becomes employment of strategies that increase one's ability to cover the target distance faster NOT one's ability to run farther distances.

Not everyone wants to run a 5 or 10K race. Many fitness goals are satisfied with simple improvements in the ability to run the middle distances - from a quarter mile up to a mile (or the 400 to 1500 meter counterparts). This, in fact, fits much better than long slow distance into preparation for basic workplace fitness and sport fitness where it is quite uncommon to find sustained efforts from 20 minutes to an hour. Rather it is more common to find shorter, more intense efforts interspersed with lower intensity efforts or rest. Considering the basic premise presented in figure 1, along with how training experience alters the composition of training required for progress, we can develop a template of training for the entire career of a middle distance endurance trainee (figure 10). Again, as with the 5-10K runner we will find a place for LSD training. In the first few months of training it forms the basis of training. We are reaping the maximum fitness gain from the easiest training possible at the time. But within 3 months those easy gains are exhausted and it is time to add in a moderate amount of interval work specific to developing glycolytic metabolism. Some sprinting is also added in to develop high speed phoshpagenic metabolic capacity. Both of these begin developing the ability to sustain higher velocity running, an important element of middle distance running.

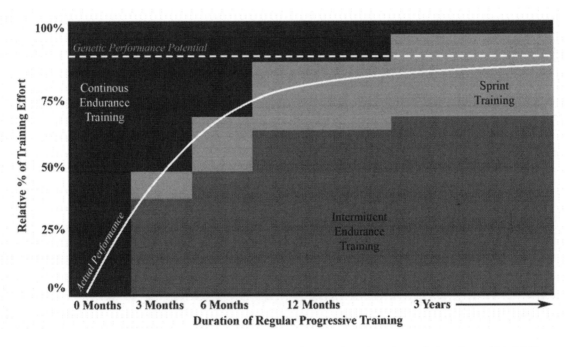

Figure 10. The relative amounts of long slow distance, interval, and sprint training for a 400-1500 meter runner changes over the course of the training career (going from sedentary to fit). For the first three months, an aerobic (LSD) base is established. Once the runner can continuously run 1.5 miles it is time to add in the first wave of interval and sprint training. As the runner achieves the ability to run 2 to 3 miles continuously it is time to add in the second wave of increased interval and sprint work. At this point the emphasis becomes employment of strategies that increase one's ability to cover the target distance faster NOT one's ability to run farther distances.

It should be apparent by now that training program composition - LSD, sprint, and interval - changes to match the demand of the nature of the endurance goal. A 10K runner's program is different than a middle distance runner's program which will be different from a sprinter's program. It sounds very logical, but there are many many "professionals" that do not approach it in this manner. When it comes to sprint, or power, performance there is a much different metabolic and anatomical demand placed on the body than that produced by the longer runs. This means that you can't train your sprinters with middle distance or long distance programs. Specifically this means that the value of LSD type training is minimal by about 6 months of regular and intelligent training and completely exhausted within 12 to 24 months. If you think about this, it makes sense as LSD is about maximizing energy storage. We don't run out of energy in the sprints, we are limited by our ability to expend energy fast enough to produce movement. Prioritizing appropriately, this means that from about 6 months into the career of a sprinter onwards, the majority of training time will be spent sprinting and in doing intervals.

Figures 8 through 11 have given us an idea of the relative percentages of training effort that should be spent sprinting, running intervals, or doing LSD over the course of a trainee's career. But most people right now simply want to know how many miles they need to include in a session of LSD when they use it. We have a handy little graphic for that (figure 12). If we have a short mileage goal, say to improve mile time, the maximum distance of an LSD run would be 2 miles. Not really that far BUT still a significant stress as it is double the goal performance distance. At the farther end of the spectrum, 13 miles or a half-marathon, the maximum single session distance is 13 miles, a one-to-one ratio. Why not a 2-to-1 ratio as in the shorter mile goal? Because by the time you are ready to tackle a half marathon you are relying on cumulative between-session stress to drive fitness AND you are controlling volume in order to avoid the negative influence of overtraining. If your LSD takes longer than two hours, it is likely more of a contributor to overtraining than to performance enhancement. This maximum mileage and time limitation carries over to any distance over 13 miles. There is very little value of logging 26.2 miles regularly, unless your goal is to damage your heart muscle (22), calcify valvular leaflets (23), or otherwise potentially cause heart anomalies (24). Distance running to excess - just like excess in any other modality of exercise - has a cost-benefit ratio that we have to consider and respect. Too much of a good thing is still too much. While lots of excessive mileage will produce cardiovascular function superior to the untrained and the diseased, it also produces maladaptations that may potentially lead to problems much later in life. It all goes back to Selye, overwhelming the body's adaptive capacity is not desirable. This concept of caution in the application of LSD is applicable to both beginner and elite alike (25).

The next likely question here is "how long are intervals supposed to be?" The easiest way to approach this is by considering the time of the interval, not the distance. For the miler they need to be from 30 seconds up to around 2 minutes in duration. For the half marathoner, they need to range from about 2 minutes up to 15 minutes in duration. And remember these are to be run at a pace that exhaustion occurs (you must slow down or stop) at the end time target. These are HARD and FAST. Intervals are not done at LSD pace, they are done as near to sprint speed as one can get over the time allotted.

How do you put these concepts together into a logical and realistic training program? Let's look at a simple running program built to help someone achieve their goal of being the best they can be as a 5K runner. As a beginner the trainee is capable of adapting to the training load between workouts. That means they go a little harder in every workout. Prototypically the beginners stage would be blocked out into three 3-month long blocks with each being constructed a little differently (table 1). The early weeks of training are a series of progressively longer duration LSD efforts moving from an initial 8 minutes of continuous running up to a target 30 minutes. An accumulated 3 minutes of training time is added each week with no planned off loads within the week or between weeks. The days off between workouts are sufficient for recovery.

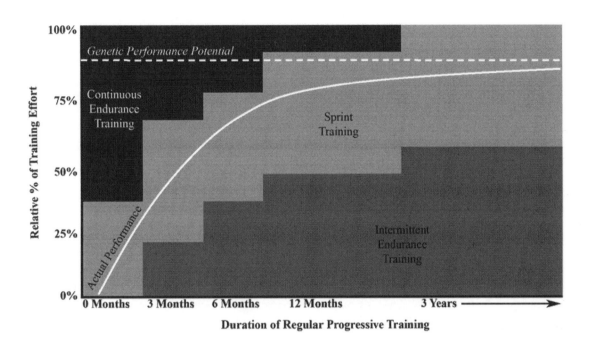

Figure 11. The relative amounts of long slow distance, interval, and sprint training for a sprinter changes over the course of the training career (going from sedentary to fit). For the first three months an aerobic (LSD) base is established and technical sprint ability is developed. Once the runner can continuously run 1 mile it is time to add in the first wave of combined interval and sprint training. As the runner achieves the ability to sprint 400-800 meters continuously it is time to add in the second wave of increased interval and sprint work. At this point the emphasis becomes employment of strategies that increase one's ability to cover the target distance faster NOT one's ability to run farther distances and LSD is removed completely in 2-3 years after beginning training.

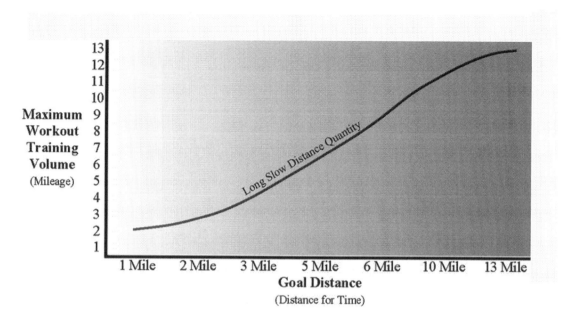

Figure 12. The total amount of long slow distance mileage included in any given training session may slightly exceed the performance goal target distance. Running a fast mile as a goal carries with it the maximal LSD distance of 1.5 to 2 miles. But as the goal distance increases the mileage excess drops. A five mile goal is associated with a 6-7 mile total mileage. A half-marathon (13 mile) or greater distance goal should not include any distance longer than the goal distance of 13 miles. There is a law of diminishing returns in operation.

In the second three month block (table 1), LSD volume is reduced by 33% and a new training stimulus is added - intervals. The intervals are performed once per week and begin with a very short distance (50 yards) and few repetitions (3) and progress over the next twelve weeks to 125 yards for 5 repetitions. The LSD volume is lower throughout the duration as there are only two LSD workouts instead of three per week. Individual workout volume does progress from 20 minutes back to the 30 minute duration targeted in the first three month block of training. It must be understood here that the goal of each LSD workout is to cover more distance than covered in the same duration workout in the first block. As is the first block, we are using simple linear progression in adding the training load in order to effectively and rapidly produce fitness adaptation. One rather variable factor to deal with is the amount of rest in between intervals. The more unfit the individual, the longer the break between repetitions should be. In general we shoot for a 1-to-1.5 work-to-rest ratio. If it takes 30 seconds for the trainee to cover the target distance, early in training it might require 45 seconds (1.5 times the work duration) of rest to recover enough to effectively complete the next repetition. Occasionally we will find that an individual that may only be capable of a 1-to-2 work-to-rest ratio and that is perfectly fine as long as there is an incomplete recovery between repetitions. The cumulative fatigue of all the repetitions is the important and active stimulus for fitness gain here. If they do not get slower over the course of the repetitions - probably about a 10% drop in running speed - and there is not a feeling of general distress and incomplete recovery at the beginning of subsequent repetitions, there is either too much rest or not enough effort being put forth. It bears repeating, *intervals are hard*. If they were easy they would not be an effective means for improving performance.

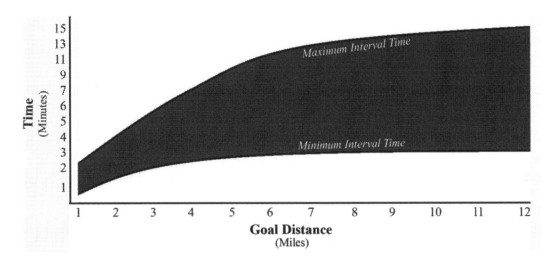

Figure 13. For any given goal distance, interval training should begin with the minimum interval times (bottom of shaded area) and progressively and gradually be increased to reach maximal interval times (top of shaded area). All intervals should be completed where each repetition is done at the maximal possible speed (you should not be able to maintain the pace any further than the end of the repetition). Initially the recovery time allowed between repetitions is approximately 90 seconds for each one minute of interval effort (1/1.5 ratio). As the goal of interval training is to cumulatively disrupt homeostasis, the trainee should not be completely recovered between efforts - the times will slow over the course of the workout. This also means that as recoverability adapts, the rest time between repetitions should be reduced (75 seconds recovery per minute of effort, 60 seconds recovery per minute of effort, etc) as trainee recovery capacity improves. The total distance of interval training should not exceed the goal performance distance. This graphic is most relevant for intermediate trainees and beyond. Beginners should begin with shorter intervals and work towards achieving the minimum duration noted by the time they become intermediates.

In the final three month block of beginners training, a new adaptive stimulus is added, sprinting. But just a small percentage of total training time is devoted to sprinting. In the example here, one sprint workout occurs about every seventh workout. Even though this is a stress separated from similar stress by about 2.5 weeks, simple linear progression remains in use and one additional 50 yard sprint is added each sprint session, moving from 5 sprints to 8 sprints over the course of the 12 weeks. It is essential to perform these efforts with complete recovery using anywhere from 2 to 5 minutes of recovery between sprints. These are not intervals where incomplete recovery is key. Sprinting with incomplete recovery diminishes the potency of this very specific adaptive stimulus. As in the second block of training, the volume of LSD training is reduced by 33%, back to 20 minutes. Then time is progressively added back into the training sessions over the 12 weeks until 30 minutes is achieved. And once again the goal of the LSD training is to cover more distance in the same time of exercise in each workout. For the interval work, the ladder used in the previous block of training is repeated but the duration of between-effort rest is shorted from 1-to-1.5 down to 1-to-1.25. It is also expected to run the interval distances in a faster time. It should be apparent that if you want to improve fitness, training never gets easier but by the time this series of workouts is complete, the trainee should be able to cover 5K in substantially less time than 30 minutes. Depending on individual anthropometry and baseline abilities, a 21 minute or less 5K time is possible.

Example of 3.2 Mile (5K) Endurance Goal
Beginner - First 3 Months

Week	Minutes of Continuous Jogging		
	Monday	Wednesday	Friday
1	8	9	10
2	10	11	12
3	12	13	14
4	14	15	16
5	16	17	18
6	18	19	20
7	20	21	22
8	22	23	24
9	24	25	26
10	26	27	28
11	28	29	30
12	30	30	Goal Distance Test

Example of 3.2 Mile (5K) Endurance Goal
Beginner - Second 3 Months

Week	Monday Minutes	Wednesday Intervals *	Friday Minutes
1	20	50 yd x 3	21
2	21	50 yd x 4	22
3	22	50 yd x 5	23
4	23	75 yd x 3	24
5	24	75 yd x 4	25
6	25	75 yd x 5	26
7	26	100 yd x 3	27
8	27	100 yd x 4	28
9	28	100 yd x 5	29
10	29	125 yd x 3	30
11	30	125 yd x 4	30
12	30	125 yd x 5	Goal Distance Test

* Work/Rest ratio of 1/1.5

Example of 3.2 Mile (5K) Endurance Goal
Late Beginner - Third 3 Months

Week	Monday Minutes	Wednesday Intervals *	Friday Minutes
1	20	50 yd x 3	21
2	21	50 yd x 4	22
3	50 yd Sprint x 5	50 yd x 5	23
4	23	75 yd x 3	24
5	24	75 yd x 4	50 yd Sprint x 6
6	25	75 yd x 5	26
7	26	100 yd x 3	27
8	50 yd Sprint x 7	100 yd x 4	28
9	28	100 yd x 5	29
10	29	125 yd x 3	50 yd Sprint x 8
11	30	125 yd x 4	30
12	30	125 yd x 5	Goal Distance Test

* Work/Rest ratio of 1/1.25

Table 1. Example progression through the beginner stage of training. By programming minutes of continuous endurance training rather than absolute distance, this program can be applied to any novice trainee. Note the steady linear progression of some endurance element through each week. At the end of each 12-week stage there is a 5K test run for time in order to measure progress and provide motivation.

By this point in a trainees running career they will be ready to move to more complex program that relies more on cumulative workloads and a longer recovery period that require a longer period between additions of training loads (see chapter 2). The trainee is ready for simple periodized training where a new and increased work load is added on a weekly basis AND where there is a variation of workloads used during the training week ranging from maximal/heavy down to light.

In weight training it is very easy to quantify heavy, medium, and light using a percentage of ones maximal lifting ability. For endurance training you can do something very similar using a percentage of your fastest time over a specific distance. However, self timing is somewhat of a barrier and determining split times and calculating percentage of your best pace during an LSD run on an unmarked trail or street. You could try to use a percentage of maximal heart rate as an indicator of intensity for use in programming training. In fact millions of people use heart rate as a programming aid, "exercise at a percentage of heart rate" is likely the most common exercise programming convention in existence. But heart rate is not a terribly consistent indicator of intensity as it is influenced by external environmental factors and this means that it is a variable measure - it does not respond in the same pattern and to the same magnitude consistently. When we program we want to USE METRICS THAT DON'T CHANGE. So it is suggested here that manipulating the volume of training is the most viable means of establishing a heavy, light, or medium day of training. Distances do not change as they are not affected by things physiological, psychological, environmental, or social. A meter is always a meter. The nut of this method is simple, you go as hard as you can for the distances prescribed for that workout, just like in the beginners programming model, but you reduce and increase the total workload by adding or subtracting distances. The amount of intensity included in training is self-calibrated by the volume of training programmed.

An early stage intermediate trainee will be ready to train four days per week. If we are intending to provide a cumulative stress to the body to drive adaptation we will have two heavy days. To facilitate recovery before the next week's addition of a higher training load we have a medium day and a light day - with the light day immediately preceding the next addition in workload. In our example here the light day is Saturday as the new higher load will be added on Monday. In the practical sense, on Monday the trainee is attempting to set a new PR at whatever distance they are scheduled to do. The two heavy days are separated by a reduced load medium day as to not overwhelm the body's adaptive capacity. The second heavy day, the trainee is attempting to match or get within 5% of their PR.

The next step in programming the intermediate endurance trainee is to refer back to figure 2. We can determine what the relative percentages of each type of training - LSD, interval, and sprint - will be for this early stage of intermediate training. In our example we assign two days to interval training, one day of sprints, and one day of LSD for each week of training. Now comes the finesse part. You are trying to approximate a 60%-25%-15% split of interval-LSD-sprint training. Not so easy to do precisely, as 4 workouts does not distribute evenly into those percentages. You could assign fractions of the different training types to the same workout but it is preferable to focus on one type at a time (KISS). This keeps the training session easy to manage, especially if there are multiple people being coached by the same person. You could also approximate, the best that could be done with a single week's schedule would be a 50%-25%-25% split and sometimes getting pretty close works, and at the intermediate level there is some squishy room for such adjustments. However, later at the advanced and elite levels of training progression this is not the case, precision is imperative. What was done here was to program the planned distribution over 5 weeks to reach the desired distribution across the three training types (table 2). There are 20 workouts in the 5 weeks; 12 sessions are assigned to intervals, 5 to LSD, and 3 to sprint work.

The next consideration is the assignment of the distances indicative of loading for each training type - what heavy, medium, and light mean in respect to intervals, LSD, and sprinting. We establish these values up front, based on trainee goals and their training history. For intervals, the previous largest volume of training was 5 repetitions at 125 yards. We need to move into at least the minimum time frame recommended for intervals (refer back to figure 6). As our target is a minimum interval duration of about minute to a minute and a half, we select a distance of 200 meters for our longest interval. Over that distance an average trainee might be able to complete the first repetition in about 30 to 40 seconds, but by the fifth repetition the time will have stretched out to the minute or more target. So on a heavy day there are 5 repetitions of 200 yards. A medium day would be 4 repetitions of 200 yards and on a light day there would be 3 repetitions of 200 yards. The rest interval used begins at the same duration as the last one used in the beginners program. As the five week cycle is repeated, a few seconds should be eliminated from the rests between intervals.

The loading for long slow distance sessions is fairly simple. A heavy day would include the longest distance indicated in figure 5. A distance goal of 5K would suggest a maximal required LSD session of 4 to 5 miles. In our example of a brand new intermediate here, we use 4 miles as a heavy LSD day. On a medium day the target distance is 3 miles, and on a light day 2 miles. Remember, LSD is only slow relative to sprinting, regardless of heavy, medium, or light, you are maintaining as fast a pace as you can relative to that distance ... you are not jogging you are running.

The final loading consideration is for sprinting. The largest previous load was eight 50 yard sprints. In this first intermediate program we assign five 100 yard sprints to a heavy day thus extending the total load on a heavy day by 100 yards. A medium sprint day requires four 100 yard sprints and a light day has three 100 yard sprints. The goal of every sprint session is to run as fast as possible. The goal of a heavy sprint day on a Monday is a new PR.

During each of the five weeks of this cycle something has been maxed out on Monday. Progression should have occurred and new and faster times should have been achieved. As long as better times are being produced, this cycle can be repeated without alteration. But as results plateau, intervals can be added, made longer, or rests reduced. Long slow distances can be inched upward towards the maximal desired. Sprints can be added or made longer. Training days can be added. Or combinations of all of the above can be made and this variability can make this a viable model of programming for a year or two, possibly more if no one gets greedy and tries to progress faster than their adaptive capacity. This is where the art and science of programming meld, every coach or trainer must be willing to experiment with even the best of their trainees or athletes in order to produce the best results in fitness gain. Every coach or trainer and trainee must also be willing to be patient and not add loads too quickly or succumb to the temptation to change programming models before the body has had an opportunity to adapt and improve in fitness level. Methodological progression and patient application of the scientific principles of endurance training are key to success.

Week	Monday Heavy (Max)	Tuesday Medium	Thursday Heavy	Saturday Light
1	Interval	Long Slow Distance	Interval	Sprint
2	Long Slow Distance	Interval	Interval	Interval
3	Sprint	Interval	Interval	Long Slow Distance
4	Long Slow Distance	Interval	Sprint	Interval
5	Interval	Long Slow Distance	Interval	Interval

Interval	
Heavy	5 Repetitions - 200 yards
Medium	4 Repetitions - 200 yards
Light	3 Repetitions - 200 yards
Long Slow Distance	
Heavy	4 miles
Medium	3 miles
Light	2 miles
Sprint	
Heavy	5 sprints - 100 yards
Medium	4 sprints - 100 yards
Light	3 sprints - 100 yards

Table 2. Example intermediate 5K running program using simple periodization. The Monday of each week a new and higher load is attempted in the scheduled training mode (faster time or reduced rest). On Thursday at least 90% of previous best is done in the scheduled training mode. This five week rotation is repeated until gains are no longer realized. At that point an increase the distance of intervals included is done along with an alteration to sprint organization. When the altered program plateaus in benefit, it is then justified to add a fifth training day. Initially added as a light day for 2-3 months, it is then increased in intensity or volume to the medium level for another 2-3 months, when it finally increased to a heavy load. When a plateau occurs after that alteration, a more complex training model is called for.

Hey! Are you sure about this?

Although the wealth of the programming concepts presented here are derived directly from the written accounts of effective programs by acknowledged experts and from scientific experimentation, the resemblance of the programs here to what is considered "normal" endurance training is remote. The seven day per week runs and the crazy big miles per week volumes are not here. Why not? As explained earlier, training is purpose driven. Doing miles and miles of exercise that can only be accomplished at submaximal velocities can only improve endurance through augmenting metabolic stores, it cannot make you run faster. In fact, empty miles as they are sometimes called are an impediment to progress and performance.

Reducing training volume has been known to enhance endurance performance for more than 20 years. It has been shown that a 70% reduction in running mileage, from 81 kilometers (50 miles) down to 24 kilometers (15 miles) per week resulted in a 9.5% increase in time to exhaustion (essentially improved ability to go a longer distance) by the third week of lower volume training (26). When elite cyclists used a smaller volume of training the results were similar between small and large training volumes, indicative that the additional miles provided no tangible benefit (27). In a 25 week long study in swimmers it was demonstrated that two one and a half hour training sessions per day provided no performance benefit over a single one and a half hour training session per day. In fact, reductions in swimming velocity were periodically experienced by the high volume trainees throughout the study duration, an undesirable effect (28). High volume training is a traditional and prominent feature of competitive endurance performance but as early as 1975 it was suggested that high volume training was ineffective in producing timely and peak endurance performance (29). Further, it is estimated that endurance athletes who utilize excessively high volume training will not reach peak performance until two to five weeks AFTER THEY COMPLETELY CEASE TRAINING (30). This goes back to the chapter 2 discussion of supercompensation. So it should be apparent that mileage is not a yardstick of a good training program nor is it an indicator of fitness. As a recent 410 pound LA marathon race finisher demonstrated, if you go slow enough anyone can go long.

REFERENCES

1. Midgley, A.W., L.R. McNaughton, and A.M. Jones. Training to enhance the physiological determinants of long-distance running performance: can valid recommendations be given to runners and coaches based on current scientific knowledge? Sports Medicine 37(10):857-880, 2007.

2. Blair, S.N., et al. Changes in physical fitness and all cause mortality: A prospective study of healthy and unhealthy men. Journal of the American Medical Association 273:1093–1098, 1995.

3. Carnethon, M.R., M. Gulati, and P. Greenland. Prevalence and cardiovascular disease correlates of low cardiorespiratory fitness in adolescents and adults. Journal of the American Medical Association 294:2981–2988, 2005.

4. Lee, D.C., et al. Mortality trends in the general population: the importance of cardiorespiratory fitness. Journal of Psychopharmacology. 24(4 Supplement):27-35, 2010.

5. Achten, J. and A.E. Jeukendrup. Relation between plasma lactate concentration and fat oxidation rates over a wide range of exercise intensities. International Journal of Sports Medicine 25(1):32-37, 2004.

6. Muoio, D.M., et al. Fatty Acid Homeostasis and Induction of Lipid Regulatory Genes in Skeletal Muscles of Peroxisome Proliferator-activated Receptor (PPAR) α Knock-out Mice: Evidence for compensatory regulation by PPARδ. Journal of Biological Chemistry 277(29):26089-26097, 2002.

7. Dudley, R. Limits to human locomotor performance: phylogenetic origins and comparative perspectives. Journal of Experimental Biology 204:3235–3240, 2001.

8. Messier, S.P. and K.J. Cirillo. Effects of a verbal and visual feedback system on running technique, perceived exertion and running economy in female novice runners. Journal of Sports Science 7(2):113-26, 1989.

9. Buist, I., et al. Incidence and risk factors of running-related injuries during preparation for a 4-mile recreational running event. British Journal of Sports Medicine 44:598-604, 2010.

10. Marti, B., et al. On the epidemiology of running injuries. The 1984 Bern Grand-Prix study. American Journal of Sports Medicine 16(3):285-94, 1988.

11. Kilgore, J.L. Running the wrong way. CrossFit Journal, March, 2010.

12. Lieberman D.E., et al. Foot strike patterns and collision forces in habitually barefoot versus shod runners. Nature 463(7280):531-535, 2010.

13. Bunn, J.W. Scientific principles of coaching. Prentice-Hall, Englewoods Cliffs, NJ, 1955.

14. Dallam, G.M., et al. Effect of a global alteration of running technique on kinematics and economy. Journal of Sports Science 23(7):757-64, 2005.

15. Brown, R.L. and J. Henderson. Fitness running. Human Kinetics, Champaign, IL, 1994.

16. Cureton, T.K. Mechanics of track running. Scholastic Coach, 4:7-10, 1935.

17. McInnis, W.P. Run anyone? .... Everyone! Canadian Family Physician, 20(4):55-57, 1974.

18. Arnold, M. How to Teach Track Events: A guide for class teachers. British Amateur Athletic Board, 1983.

19. Derse, E., J. Hansen, T. O'Rourke, and S. Stolley (editors). LA84 Foundation Track and Field Coaching Manual. LA84 Foundation, Los Angeles, CA, 2008.

20. USA Track & Field. USA Track & Field Coaching Education: Level 1 Curriculum. USA Track & Field, Inc. Colorado Springs, CO, 2005.

21. Kerr, R., et al. Shoes influence lower limb muscle activity and may predispose the wearer to lateral ankle ligament injury. Journal of Orthopedic Research 27(3):318-24, 2009.

22. Fortescue, E.B., et al. Cardiac troponin increases among runners in the Boston marathon. Annals of Emergency Medicine 49(2):137–143, 2007.

23. Schwartz J, et al. Does long term endurance running enhance or inhibit coronary artery plaque formation? A prospective multi-detector CTA study of men completing marathons for least 25 consecutive years. American College of Cardiology Conference Proceedings, Abstract 1271-330, 2010.

24. Breuckmann, F., et al. Myocardial Late Gadolinium Enhancement: Prevalence, Pattern, and Prognostic Relevance in Marathon Runners. Radiology 251:50-57, 2009.

25. Thompson, P.D., F.S. Apple and A. Wu. Marathoner's Heart (Editorial). Circulation 114:2306-2308, 2006.

26. Houmard J.A., et al. Reduced training maintains performance in distance runners. International Journal of Sports Medicine 11(1):46-52, 1990.

27. Rietjens G.J., et al. A reduction in training volume and intensity for 21 days does not impair performance in cyclists. British Journal of Sports Medicine. 35(6):431-4, 2001.

28. Costill D.L., et al. Adaptations to swimming training: influence of training volume. Medicine and Science in Sports and Exercise. 23(3):371-7, 1991.

29. Banister E.W., et al. A system model of training for athletic performance. Australian Journal of Sports Medicine. 7:170–176, 1975.

30. Hellard, P. et al. Assessing the limitations of the Banister model in monitoring training. Journal of Sports Science. 24(5):509-20, 2006.

CURRENT INFORMATION AND EQUIPMENT RESOURCES

Running Books
USA Track & Field Coaching Manual
Track & Field: The East German Textbook of Athletics - Schmolnsky
The Pose Method of Running - Romanov
Chi Running - Dryer
Power, Speed, Endurance - MacKenzie
The Lore of Running - Noakes (very dated perspective but it does have some helpful information)

Running Shoes
Nike Zoom Streak
Asics Hyper XCS
Adidas XCS Spikeless

Shoes that can be used for Running (up to 5K)
Converse All-Star (old school)

Equipment
VS Measuring Wheel (you need to know how far you are going)
Any Stopwatch

Frustration is the first step towards improvement. I have no incentive to improve if I'm content with what I can do and if I'm completely satisfied with my pace, distance and form as a runner.

John Bingam

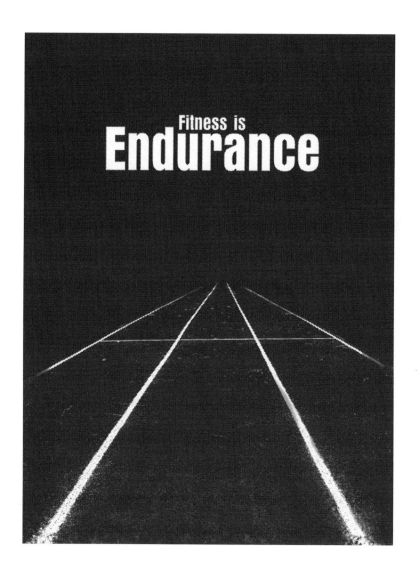

MOBILITY

Gymnastics uses every single part of your body,
every little tiny muscle that you never even knew.

Shannon Miller

Mobility is the ability to move the body and its constituent parts in a variety of directions and carry out both simple and complex motor tasks. Very simply stated, ***Mobility is Movement***. Mobility is an important - but under attended - element of fitness as stable, controlled, and coordinated movement within our occasionally unstable and frequently unpredictable home, work, and play environments is important for adequate function and survival.

Mobility is likely the most complicated element of fitness as it is a combination of joint range of motion and the motor abilities; agility, balance, and coordination. Mobility is a major component of fitness, along with strength and endurance. In essence mobility is a state of being, the possession of the required physical properties to move as needed with one's own circumstances.

Mobility varies considerably across the life span and is generally correlated with high amounts of exercise or physical activity. With increasing age mobility tends to decrease due to loss of range of motion around numerous joints (1) and also a slowly developing decrement in processing sensory information, a vital component of motor skills (2). While these decrements seem to be somewhat inevitable, a voluntary lack of exercise or physical activity, may speed these occurrences. And there is a vicious cycle put in operation, aging reduces range of motion and sensory information processing, failure to remain active in advanced age induces further reductions in mobility, and that reduced range of motion is reduced further as aging and inactivity continue. But it is not just older populations who must concern themselves with mobility, a sedentary lifestyle reduces mobility in even the youngest of populations. Only the rate of decay is different.

Here is where a problem arises. The concept of mobility is relatively complicated, not necessarily because the definition above is invalid but because of the relative lack of data and standards associated with mobility. Much of the problem stems from inadequate definitions and incorrect usage of the terms associated with mobility.

As there is presently an absence of mobility standards available for use by fitness professionals and trainees, it is nearly impossible to know how much mobility any one person should posses, other than simply being able to complete the desired activities or movements. Norms are available for some aspects of mobility but a norm is what the average person is capable of and we know that the average person is not fit (3). So norms have limited validity and utility as a reference is this application. Standards are approximations of what would be expected of performance in certain situations and as such they may summarize a desirable amount of mobility for a given task. There are, for example, standards for range of motion and synchrony of movement (coordination) for an effective golf swing (4). Striking a golf ball requires a certain magnitude of range of motion and, as anyone who has ever swung a driver will tell you, coordination. Within sport there are many similar and defined examples but for general fitness and health it is not clear how much of any component of mobility is needed. There is little scientific or clinical evidence to indicate that a person who can reach eight inches past his toes is any more fit, in the global sense, than a person who can only reach two inches past his toes. So are a prima ballerina's joints more fit than the average exerciser? Without clear definitions and standards we cannot make concrete statements one way or the other.

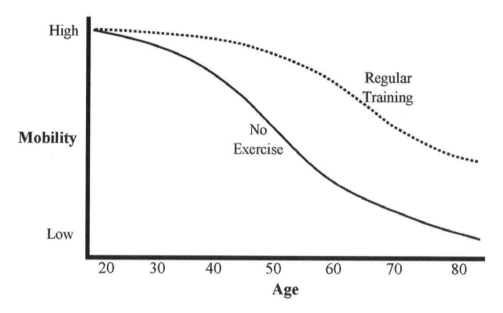

Figure 1. The decline in mobility with advancing age. Although the solid line represents total mobility, it can be accurately used to illustrate both range of motion and motor ability decline over the life span. The dotted line demonstrates the effect of regular exercise training over time, a drastically reduced decline in mobility (retention of mobility for more of the life span).

In addition to lack of useful mobility standards, in the current lexicon of exercise terms used by the fitness community, "mobility" has become synonymous with pre-habilitation, rehabilitation, and the use of various recovery modalities. While mobility does work in this context, as this is not precisely an incorrect usage of the term, there is something at odds with fitness gain here. What is out of place in this use of the term in the fitness environment is that in this context, restorative exercises and therapies are being used to return an injured or diseased joint system to health or the use of prophylactic exercises to potentially prevent injury, NOT improve fitness. The only valid uses of "prehab" and "rehab" methods, when used in conjunction with an appropriate training program, is as an aid in the restoration of lost mobility. In this application it is presumably a response to physical inactivity in beginning trainees, or for more advanced trainees who have used a training program(s) that neglected mobility as an integral feature. What is presented here is an approach to put trainees on the correct training path that addresses mobility from the onset. Range of motion, agility, balance, and coordination are all integrated into each training program contained herein. By doing this from day one, valuable training time is not wasted later due to the need to restore mobility.

RANGE OF MOTION

An essential component of training to enhance mobility is work to develop appropriate amounts of range of motion in the joint systems throughout the body. Range of motion, as we specifically define it here, is possession of ability to move a joint fully through its anatomical limits. Those limits are generally set by the bony architecture of a joint but there are other normally active anatomical limitations. Think of the elbow. At one end it is limited by the olecranon of the ulna being seated in the olecranon fossa of the humerus at complete extension. The bone on bone contact sets one limit in the range of motion. At the other end, the limitation is the contact of the surface of the forearm with the front of the upper arm when the elbow is flexed. This tissue on tissue inhibition of movement sets the second limit for elbow range of motion. Anything that prevents these two conditions from occurring, inhibits range of motion.

As bony structure is only mildly modifiable, and within this context not a significant issue, so in application, range of motion can be considered primarily the ability of the tissues surrounding a joint and the muscles that act upon a joint to contract and extend sufficiently to allow both passive or active movement completely through all joint angles between the joint's anatomical limits.

Flexibility is frequently used synonymously with range of motion. That is a fairly descent descriptor. Good flexibility, the possession of a complete range of motion around the major joints - ankles, knees, hips, shoulders, elbows, and wrists, can be beneficial to one's ability to function effectively in training, sport, work, and in daily life. A properly designed fitness program, single element or multiple-element, will increase an individual's range by intelligent incorporation of exercises that require movements through complete ranges of motion. Our reason for insistence on correct technique and why the previous chapters have described definite start and stop positions for exercises is to ensure complete range of motion is carried out with each repetition or movement.

Not everyone who starts a fitness program will posses even an average range of motion around all of the important joints. And while many of the exercises included in this text have an inherent mobility aspect within them, it may be necessary to incorporate other specialized mobility exercises to pave the way for range of motion development and future fitness gain.

IMPROVING RANGE OF MOTION

Stretching is a very familiar exercise concept to almost all people. They have done it in PE, done a semblance of it in the morning when they wake up, they have even watched their dog or cat do it. Some of humanities earliest writings, the Indian Vedas some 5000 years ago described stretching. One of Edward Muybridge's early motion pictures, the very first movies, was of a person doing a brief stretching exhibition. Athlete's pay attention to it, and ballet dancers live and die by it. So stretching is a well known and primary technique used to improve the state of one's flexibility, or in other words, to increase the range of motion of a joint or set of joints. The specific exercises used are specific to and develop only the range of motion of the muscles and joints that perform the exercise. This means that each mobility or flexibility exercise is specific to the muscles and joints recruited during that movement - and that there is no one single stretch that works for all purposes and all joints.

The degree of range of motion, or flexibility, needed around a given joint is task specific. It is purpose driven. Prior to creating a mobility training program, the body position requirements of any exercise goal or work task must be assessed, as well as the individuals ability to assume those positions. If multiple joints are involved, it is a common occurrence that an individual may demonstrate excellent flexibility in one region of the body while being poorly flexible, or stiff, in other areas. Stiff is another interesting casual term. In general stiff means "resistance to bending". So it is actually a suitable descriptor only for conditions where full flexion of a joint is not achievable, it is not suitable for use for describing an inability to completely extend a joint. Flexibility is the more comprehensive layman's term.

Most people, trainee, coaches, clinicians, and the media all assume that flexibility is an essential element of health and performance. However, the Healthy People 2020 national goals statement from the US Department of the Health and Human Services does not include a specific recommendation for inclusion of flexibility exercises (the objective was archived) as part of any exercise program. But, contained within the document the authors did note a correlational importance for stretching relative to good health. This connection between stretching and health is based on a few biological observations; (A) Movement of a joint through a full range of motion creates pressure differences within the joint capsule that drives nutrients from the synovial fluid toward the cartilage of the joint. (B) Since cartilage lacks its own blood supply, the chondrocytes (the cells that produce cartilage) depend on diffusion of oxygen and nutrients from the synovial fluid for adaptation to occur. (C) The pressure aided fluid movement enhances diffusion and more viable chondrocytes. This series of events forms the basis for the assumption that stretching correlates with joint health.

The range of motion around a joint or joints is a reflection of the extensibility and elasticity of the soft tissues at that joint and this in large part determines the extent and direction of any possible movement. A basic understanding of human anatomy is important in understanding principles of stretching and its effect on range of motion. The nature and direction of movement at a joint is determined by the shapes of the bony surfaces that articulate at the joint. There are a number of different types of joints, classified by bony structure, with certain types allowing for greater magnitudes and directions of movement than others. For example, the circular surface of the ball-and-socket joint of the hip, allows considerably more movement, including movement to the side (adduction and abduction), forward and backward (flexion and extension), rotating in and out (internal and external rotation), and circumduction (swinging the leg in a big circle). Contrast that range of motion to that of the hinge joint that we know as the knee. The knee has a much more restrictive construction that limits movement to primarily forward and backward (flexion and extension). Knowing the anatomical limits of mobility allows us to qualitatively assess range of motion.

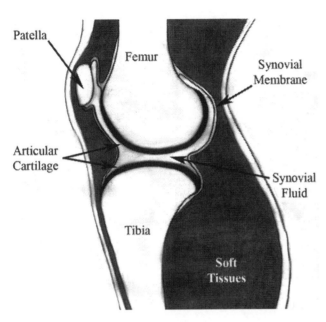

Figure 2. The basic structural elements of a joint. Note the cartilage and synovial fluid surrounding the bony structures of the bone.

The properties of connective tissue (tendons and ligaments) and muscle affect range of motion. The extent of movement available at any joint is determined not only by the bony anatomy, type, and shape of the joint, we find that the ligaments, tendons, and muscles that attach to, stabilize, or cross the joint are also factors.

Ligaments are tough and rather inelastic bands of connective tissues that connect bone to bone in order to create a joint. They provide rigidity and stability to the joint and provide a means to restrict excessive motion of the joint, as a safeguard to dislocation. Tendons are also fibrous bundles of connective tissue, however tendons connect muscle to bone, in general one muscle with a tendon at each end is attached to two different bones. Muscles are collections of specialized cells that are contractile and, important to the issue of flexibility, are also extensible and elastic. To use a rope analogy; ligaments are built like caving ropes - very little stretchability, tendons are like climbing ropes which only possess enough stretchability to add a little safety cushion in a fall, and muscles are like bungie cords that possess a great deal of stretchability. Muscles and tendons during movement are both loaded at the same time. As such when a joint is stretched, a muscle (or set of muscles) is stretched. Our primary target in efforts to improve range of motion is the muscle as it holds the greatest potential for improvement. Further, the job of the tendon is to transfer force from the muscle to the bone and if we make it more stretchable, we have decreased the ability of the tendon to transfer force.

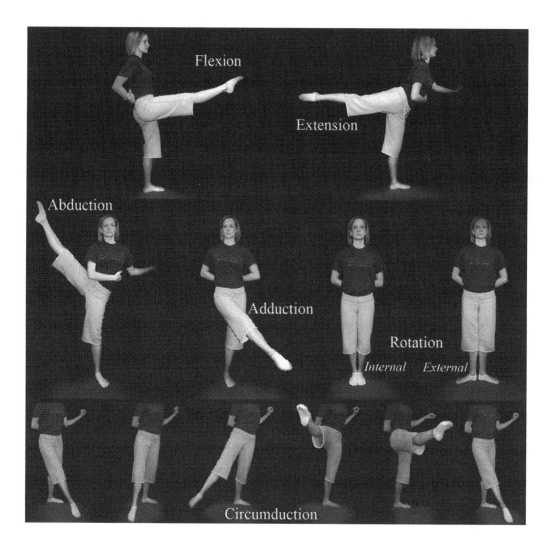

Figure 3. The hip allows for a large and varied range of motion, allowing for flexion, extension, abduction, adduction, rotation, and circumduction.

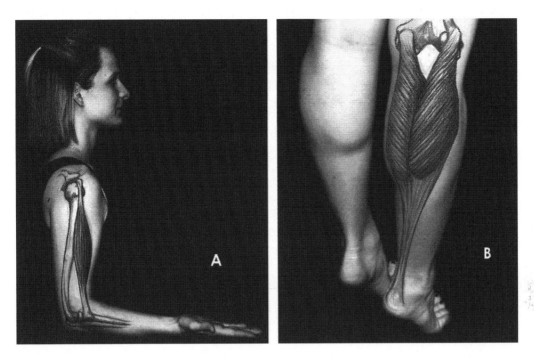

Figure 4. The tendon of a muscle attaches the muscle fibers to the bone (A - Bicep to radius and humerus, and B - Calf muscles to heel and femur) and allow transmittance of contractile forces and to allow movement to occur.

Any muscle that crosses or is adjacent to a joint - basically any muscle that acts to move or stabilize a joint - directly influences flexibility. Muscles involved with human movement generally are paired, pairs that have opposite movement actions. Given any movement, there is a muscle (or muscle group) that contracts to produce the movement. This is the agonist (Why is it not called a protagonist as in classical literature? Probably because traditionally there can only be one protagonist in a play. In the case of movement there are many primary players of equal value, so we simply use "agonist".) Opposing the agonist, often on the opposite side of the joint, is a muscle (or group of muscles) that creates the opposite movement when contracted. This is the antagonist. When an antagonist muscle is contracted with equal force to the agonist, a static equilibrium between the agonist and antagonist contractions is produced that yields no movement. It can also attempt to contract (but not actually shorten) and resist the movement driven by the agonist fractionally. In this movement the antagonist is undergoing a eccentric muscle action (generating force at the same time it is being stretched). This is one of the ways we control acceleration and deceleration during movement. This is also important in exercise as the amount of force generated to drive the movement can be either hampered or facilitated by the degree of relaxation (or non-recruitment) of the antagonist muscle(s). The more an antagonistic muscle yields, the less energy spent overcoming it's resistance to the intended movement. Stretching exercises may assist in learning how to turn of the recruitment of antagonistic muscles. Working on flexibility teaches the muscles how to turn off, or at least dampen, the reflexes that activate antagonist muscles. This is germane to range of motion as it may be limited, regardless of the amount of training invested, if the antagonistic muscles are not capable of relaxation during agonist action. There may also be a negative effect on range of motion if there is a lack of coordination between contraction of the agonist muscle and relaxation of the antagonists. It is not surprising, therefore, that individuals with poor coordination, or an inability to relax the antagonistic muscles, may have a low rate of range of motion improvement.

There are two main methods of stretching exercises used in enhancement of range of motion; static stretching and dynamic stretching.

Static stretching involves contraction of an agonist muscle or group agonistic muscle group with the aid of body weight thus causing the antagonistic muscle or muscle group to elongate (stretch) to its limit of motion. This is done to the point of mild discomfort, without excessively forcing the stretch to the point of pain, then the position is held motionless for ten to thirty seconds (for the purposes of general fitness) and released. Frequently multiple repetitions are done for each static stretch included. Static stretching can incorporate an external force such as that applied by another person, trainer, immovable object, or with a resistance band, to stretch muscle groups.

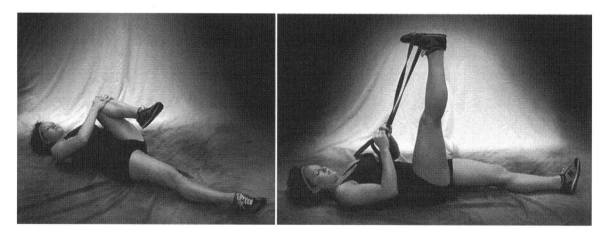

Figure 5. Examples of the most common form of stretching, static stretching.

Dynamic stretching generally is comprised of movements - thus the dynamic in the name - where a muscle or muscle group is taken through its complete range of motion in a slow and controlled manner and without the stretch being held. An example of this would be a Walking Lunge. Dynamic stretching primarily a preparatory technique whereby an individual progressively uses more of his range of motion as each subsequent repetition is done, until at the end of the exercise he is taking the targeted joint or joints through muscular contraction and relaxation cycles throughout the complete range of motion currently possessed. Using this method of stretching can be an efficient means of pre-training or pre-event preparation as aids in muscular temperature elevation, primes - to use a very casual term - the agonistic muscles to contract efficiently in training or competition, and it prepares the antagonist muscle groups to relax and yield to force production by the antagonistic muscles.

Proprioceptive neuromuscular facilitation (PNF) combines both static and dynamic flexibility and active and passive stretching. In its most basic form, PNF entails taking the muscles of a limb to their end range of motion where the limb is held immobile by a partner or trainer. The trainee then pushes (or pulls as case may be) with the target muscles while the partner/trainer prevents movement. After five to tens seconds, the muscles are relaxed and then the partner/trainer gently pushes the stretch a little deeper into the range of motion. This method of stretching often produces dramatic results, but is typically reserved for only very poorly flexible individuals. The two person nature of the technique combined with the potential for injury if the partner is not attentive and capable of applying small increments of force and directional movement makes it's broad application to all exercising populations problematic.

Flexibility can be measured a variety of ways, but most commonly it is measured as a limit of rotation or movement through a specific range of motion with a static flexibility test. Clinically there is great interest in performing static flexibility testing of areas of the body that tend to lose range of motion with age and inactivity, such as the lower back (lumbar region) or hamstring muscle group of the back of the legs. One of the most common range of motion assessments in use clinically and in commercial fitness is the sit-and-reach test to measure flexibility in the low back region is the "sit-and-reach test". The premise for such testing is a putative correlation between poor performance on the test and a higher incidence of low back pain (5, 6). Interestingly, sit-and-reach test scores are reflective of hamstring flexibility NOT lower back flexibility (think about the anatomy of the hip and the movement tested). As such published sit-and-reach norms may only be useful in identification of individuals at the extremes of inflexibility who may be at higher risk for injury. There is not enough data available to provide specific static flexibility guidance other than identification of "normal" range of motion. Fitness professionals must also remember that in measuring flexibility, attention to testing details is necessary. Static flexibility scores that are subjective like "can you touch your toes" are hugely affected by individual anatomical structure. An individual with longer arms and shorter torso will be able to accomplish the toe-touch task with a smaller range of motion than an individual with shorter arms and longer torso. There is also the psychological issue of individual differences in pain perception and tolerance during testing. Some individuals will stop at the first twinge of discomfort, others will drive deeply into their pain threshold.

The measurement of dynamic flexibility is not ordinarily done nor is it an easy and practical process. It is generally limited to research settings because of limitations related to expensive equipment, insufficient standardization, and the lack of reference data. This suggests that, in this instance, coaching experience in qualitative analysis of movement is important in dynamic flexibility assessment, more so than quantitative analysis.

One thing that must be considered and attended to is tracking range of motion improvements. There must be a means of identifying and progressing the degree of stretching stress applied. Principles of overload and progression are active here just as with any other exercise or fitness element and must be applied to a regular stretching program to both improve range of motion.

THE PHYSIOLOGY OF GETTING MORE FLEXIBLE

For range of motion to be increased, the antagonistic muscle or muscle groups must be stretched and held beyond normal resting lengths. It is important to remember a simple physical reality here, although there are many commercial exercise systems that claim to make a muscle longer, that is in fact impossible without some relatively radical surgery. Muscle A is attached to bone B and bone C. There is nothing that exercise or stretching can do to increase the distance between points B and C. This means a muscle cannot get longer in response to any exercise stimulus. What occurs is that the antagonistic muscles become more compliant, resist movement to the anatomical limit less, and range of motion is improved. This increased range of motion is erroneously assumed to be the muscle becoming longer.

When a muscle is stretched, lengthened from its resting postural state, there is a reflex, the stretch reflex that acts to resist the stretch. Nervous receptors called muscle spindles contain several small "intrafusal" muscle cells that are tucked away inside and in parallel with regular or "extrafusal" muscle cells. They provide information to the nervous system regarding muscle length. Specifically, they detect the rate of change in length and report the information to the central nervous system. When a muscle is stretched, the body attempts to retain homeostasis, in this situation, posture. These sensory receptors in the muscle-tendon system send signals to the sensory neurons (nerves that detect environmental changes), and these neurons further signal another set of neurons, motor neurons, to initiate the contractile process and shorten the muscle. Here is where proper exercise technique comes into play. If the stretching motion is applied quickly, this reflex fires, induces a counter-contraction in the stretched muscle and restricts initial efforts and progress at stretching. However, if the stretch is slowly applied and is held over time, the reflex is not strongly invoked and any vestigial reflex that does occur will subside in a few seconds and allows the muscle to be stretched more fully towards its anatomical limits. The presence of this reflex explains why it is important to slowly apply and hold a stretch for a period of 10-30 seconds. More quickly applied attempts to stretch or shorter duration stretches are limited by the opposing action of the stretch reflex and defeat progress in enhancing range of motion.

Another receptor active in muscle is the Golgi tendon organ. Golgi tendon organs (commonly referred to as GTOs) are located within the transition area where muscle cells phase out and tendons phase in where they monitor tension. High forces applied to a muscle stimulates these receptors and provides an inhibitory reflex. Although potentially active during stretching due to ballistic attempts at stretching, the normal and accepted methods of static stretching - and dynamic stretching - do not invoke this reflex. If it is, you are doing it wrong.

A slowly applied stretch of muscles creates less reflex contraction by way of action of muscle spindles. If done slowly, muscle length changes do not invoke the reflex contraction of the stretched muscle (myotactic reflex). It is likely that not all reflex activation can be avoided but as the stretch position is held, any residual stretch reflex present abates, and tension in a muscle decreases as the stretch is held over time. Most of this decrease in tension, or resistance to stretch, occurs in the first 10 seconds. And as more repetitions of the stretching exercise is done, the tension curves or how fast the resistance diminishes becomes lower. This is why not one but multiple repetitions of a stretching exercise is recommended.

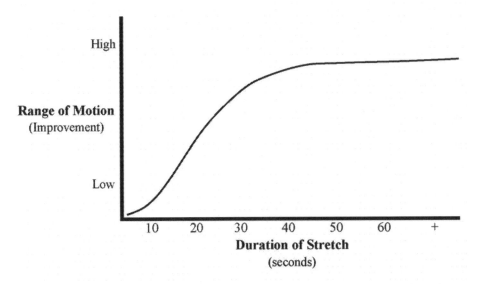

Figure 6. Benefits in range of motion begin with holds of about ten seconds and are maximized by about 30 seconds. Holding a stretch for 60 seconds or more offers minimal additional increase in range of motion over much shorter durations.

 Although there is a powerful neural component of stretching for improved range of motion, several other factors may affect range of motion and the body's response to stretching exercise. Some factors are unavoidable. Age, presence of disease, previous injury to the muscle or joint, and the presence of scar tissue are all non-alterable. There are a two extrinsic factors that are under individual control; (A) temperature - both environmental and body, and (B) muscle strength imbalances.

The former issue is an easy concept to grasp. As muscle temperature rises, elasticity increases, and the extensibility of the muscle increases thus improving range of motion at any joint around which that muscle is active. This is one of the concepts behind "hot yoga", better range of motion from being in a hot room. The opposite can also happen, as environmental and muscle temperature drops, flexibility decreases. This relationship may also explain why you feel stiffer in cold weather and why the cold has a negative influence on range of motion and response to stretching.

The second alterable factor is related to the ratio of strength between an agonist and antagonist muscle or group of muscle. The strength of the muscles on either side of the joint, or in some cases adjacent to the joint, affects its range of motion. Ideally, around each joint, the opposing muscles create a natural balance that allow the joint to move through its entire range of motion from anatomical limit to anatomical limit. It must be understood here that the natural balance referred to here *is not* a 50/50 balance between agonist and antagonist, it is simply the amount of strength required to maintain normal posture at rest, during movement, and under load. If an exercise program includes work in all relevant directions around a joint, an imbalance does not occur. If we consider the shoulder here, if we do Presses, Dips, Bench Presses, and Rows, we have placed a balanced set of directional movement stresses on the joint and have thus limited the potential of an agonist or antagonist being disproportionately stronger. But this is often not the case in the modern fitness arena. The use of machines and isolation exercises create an environment were it is easy to omit relevant musculature from a workout. This means that one muscle or set of muscles becomes weak relative to the opposing set. In this case, joint range of motion may be compromised. A common example of such an imbalance is found between the anterior and posterior shoulder muscles. Most recreational weight trainees and beginning bodybuilders tend to exercise the muscles that they can see and spend most of their exercise time doing isolation exercises requiring them to lift objects in front of their bodies. As a result, the anterior muscles become proportionally stronger than the posterior ones. The first result of this imbalance in exercise programming is a new habitually poor posture, generally seen as a hunching forward with rounded shoulders. This posture limits range of motion and provides another unwanted consequence during sport, exercise, and work, a posterior weakness driven shoulder pain. What is occurring here is that the posterior musculature is not strong enough to counter even the low level of postural muscle tension produced by the newly stronger anterior musculature. Further, the posterior musculature cannot generate enough force during stretching exercise to pull the anterior muscles through their entire range of motion. It will become a vicious downward cycle unless corrective programming is initiated. And corrective programming does not encompass prescription of isolation exercises, it is the implementation of a program utilizing large scale exercises that are resisted in multiple axes.

Considering the effect of strength on range of motion just described, it should follow that a lack of adequate muscle strength may inhibit the range of motion during virtually any exercise. Therefore, strength is an important component of range of motion and flexibility exercises. This is despite the ages old, but still active, myth that strength gains limit flexibility. But there is another myth within the strength community that substantial flexibility gains will produce negative influence upon strength. One myth proposing that training reduces range of motion, the other that improved range of motion reduces performance. There is no underlying supportive physiology for either myth. Male and female gymnasts, who are both strong and flexible, and their athletic abilities are a powerful argument against both of these myths.

While there is essentially no risk of decreased range of motion or performance with proper training, IMPROPER programming of strength, endurance, or mobility exercises could ultimately result is negative adaptations in both the trained fitness element and mobility. Further, if the exercises included in the program of exercise are not performed correctly, there is a risk of loss of mobility. Learning and performing correct exercise technique is essential in the improvement of any fitness element including mobility.

DOING A STRETCHING EXERCISE

During actual stretching exercises there is a process common to all. The correct procedure is to use the bodyweight and an agonist muscle or muscle group to move a body segment in order to develop slight tension in a target antagonist muscle or muscle group. As the end of the possible range of motion is reached, the position is held until the perception of muscle tension fades. This will occur at about ten seconds into the stretch and marks the point of stretch release for beginners. For more advance trainees, when the perception of stretch reduces at about ten seconds, a second gentle advance along the joint's range of motion is attempted and held for up to another 20 seconds. Throughout the performance of any stretching exercise, there should be a concerted effort to relax the antagonistic muscles so they will yield to the pull of the agonists, and thus a more acute angle between two body segments is achieved, *vis a vis* an advancement in stretch. This process and progression yields progressively greater range of motion over time. The key words here are gentle and slow for if too much tension is developed too quickly, the safeguard reflexes within the nervous system will be activated. It is fairly simple to determine correct stretching technique. If there is pain, uncontrolled muscle shaking, and an involuntary contraction of antagonist muscle, you are doing it wrong. Back off on the distance into the range of motion attempted, let the stretched muscles (antagonists) relax, and then proceed more carefully.

The best time to incorporate training to improve range of motion is immediately after the main body of a training session. The muscles are warm and compliant and the existing range of motion should have already been achieved through the training activities.

Stretching has become a bit of a taboo for pre-exercise and pre-competition preparation as there can be short-lived performance decrement following static stretching (7,8), although research results have been equivocal (9). One of these negative effects is potentially inhibited muscle activation, something needed during many multi-joint exercises and during any movement that requires the expression of agility. It is much more appropriate to include dynamic flexibility exercises at the beginning of the training session, especially prior to any high intensity conditioning activities.

Programming static stretching during the after a workout is much preferred as aside from the physiological favorable conditions present, stretching tends to provide a relaxing or even pleasurable sensation.

MOTOR ABILITIES

There are three main motor abilities that comprise mobility and form the foundation for exercise and sport performance; Agility, Balance, and Coordination. These abilities are important enough to have been termed the "ABCs of Athleticism".

> *Agility* refers to an ability to rapidly change the direction of body movement and to carry out multi-directional movements with ease.

> *Balance* refers to the ability to maintain control of body position at rest and while performing a given skill, be it daily life activities, work, exercise, or sport. It can be simplified into an ability not to fall over in changing conditions.

> *Coordination* is the ability to synchronize and order muscle activities so an intended movement can be performed without error.

Although these motor abilities have a substantial genetic component to them, they can be improved with repetitive training over time. This is especially true during the initial stages of an individual's training experience, when progress comes very rapidly. While these abilities are contributory to overall fitness in their role within mobility, they are generally not assigned a value in health benefit as is seen in strength, endurance, and to a lesser extent range of motion. The greatest benefit of motor ability training for a general fitness trainee is likely that it provides the foundation of mobility, in that as motor abilities increase so to does the ability to learn, refine, and perfect exercise movements. The added abilities will facilitate more efficient movements and greater application of intensity. This ultimately leads to greater improvements in fitness. Essentially, an individual who's training develops agility, balance, and coordination will be able to master skills more quickly and perform them more efficiently than someone who's training does not.

AGILITY

Movements within our home, work, and play environments are rarely controlled and predictable and usually require an individual to respond and react to different stimuli on a frequent basis. In other words work, play, and simple daily life requires a bit of what most people would simply call agility. Agility, however, can be a fairly complex entity that includes anticipation and reaction during a coordinated whole body movement in which there are movement direction changes through planned deceleration and acceleration of the body or body segments. As with so many things related to fitness, there is not a clearly authoritative definition of agility nor is their a consensus on how to improve it. A recent article on the topic by Sheppard and Young (10) suggests that "the term is applied to a broad range of sport contexts, but with such great inconsistency, it further complicates our understanding of what trainable components may enhance agility." Agility has been described as an independent component of fitness, but there are many other qualities that may be contributory to agility, including balance, speed, strength, response and reaction time, spatial awareness, rhythm, and visual processing.

Agility is frequently confused with or thought of synonymously with speed and quickness. Speed more precisely refers to linear velocity, moving in a straight line as fast as possible. Quickness is also referent to linear velocity but it is dependent on initial reaction time to a stimulus or a condition. Speed can be thought of as maximum velocity, or the top end spend in which the body or body segment can move. Quickness can be thought of as the initial velocity of a movement and the subsequent acceleration of the body or body segment in the early stages of the movement. While someone who is very agile may also exhibit great speed and quickness, it is important to understand that agility is a separate and distinct motor ability. Speed, quickness, and agility are independent phenomena, and an advanced ability in one is not always associated with the others. This means that training specifically for sprinting speed will not necessarily improve agility, or vice versa. However, in order to maximize agility it is necessary to develop both speed and quickness.

Change of direction is the unique component of agility and is ultimately what separates it from speed and quickness. Movement in a straight line is briefly interrupted by a directional change, either laterally, vertically, backwards or any permutation in the x, y, or x axes, followed by another acceleration. The movement, stopping, and starting again in a different direction is the defining characteristic of agility. There are several distinct tasks being accomplished during a change in direction during in a specific movement; initial acceleration, recognition of an external stimulus (what is being reacted to), decision making, deceleration, alteration in body position, and re-acceleration in the new direction. It should be apparent that there is a need to maintain good body control during the direction change in order to minimize the magnitude and duration of speed decrease. In a total body coordinated movement such as sprinting, acceleration refers to the period of time which proceeds the attainment of maximal running speed. Recognition of a stimulus and the resultant decision making process is always followed by a deceleration and the more acute the change in direction required the closer one gets to a full stop. A small, ten degree or so, change in running route to intercept a target does not require a full stoppage then a re-acceleration, just a slight pace adjustment during the actual change in direction. Contrast this to a 180 degree switch in direction that requires a complete stop prior to reversing direction. In sport, any situation where a defensive player attempts to guard or cover an offensive player to gain an advantage is an example of recognition, decision making, and response, in other words a display of agility. If the offensive player moves one way so too must the defensive player.

Deceleration is the period of time where the body slows down from the top speed obtained during the initial directional movement prior to and in order to change direction based on the recognition and decision making process. In any agility task or drill, the body or body segment may come to a complete, although very brief, stop prior to re-acceleration in the new movement direction. Individuals who possess and demonstrate the greatest levels of agility are those that have the ability to make this stoppage appear effortless and spend the least amount of time in deceleration and at stop prior to re-acceleration in the new different direction. For every millisecond spent decelerating and at stop is a millisecond an opposing player can have to re-adjust their movement path to further evade.

Developing agility requires the development of appropriate movement patterns and techniques along with and, perhaps more importantly, the ability to integrate movement skills efficiently with kinesthetic awareness (awareness of the body's position in space relative to other objects).

Here is where it gets tricky. We can divide movement skills into two very broad categories; (A) general movement skill like running, jumping, changing direction, and such. Then there are (B) specialized movement skills like hitting a ball with a racquet or bat, doing a snatch, shooting a free throw, etc. This can be a very gray area but it might be said that general movement skills are important for everyone and specialized movement skills are most valuable to those who use them in work or sport tasks. General movement skills encompass an understanding of how to control the body in order for efficient movements to occur. Specifically knowing how and when to change the height of the center of gravity, recognizing the value and the process of the alignment of the shoulders in relation to the hips, knees, and ankles when starting and stopping movements is important, and should be a goal of basic agility training.

Agility training is thought to aid in injury prevention in sports that require high amounts of rapid movement and changes in direction (i.e. almost all of them). The use of controlled, low stress, and repetitive drill to teach the trainee how to correctly decelerate and stabilize their body is thought to develop the necessary abilities and awareness to then transfer those abilities to the field of play. While training for agility will not prepare you for every twist, turn, stop, start, and slip that is present in sport, work, or life, understanding what needs to happen and preparing the body to withstand the events through training may be beneficial.

Although widely used in fitness and sport practice, there is in fact very limited information available on how to improve agility outside of simply performing drills that require the individual to change direction. As such, it is recommended here that specific training sessions dedicated to the development or improvement of agility should utilize guidelines similar to those of sprint training, where intensity of movement (speed at which it is performed) is of greater concern than total volume of training (amount of ground covered during the drill). Novice trainees will likely require a great deal of time spent on learning proper mechanics of general movement skills. Keeping the drills short and provision of corrective feedback is essential. It is important to develop general skills prior to advancing to specific movement skills.

Agility drills performed in training should focus on changing direction quickly and include multiple movement patterns. Two general types of drills frequently used in sport and fitness include (A) ladder drills and (B) cone drills.

Ladder drills are done using simple flexible ladders, usually made of nylon with plastic rungs spaced equally along the length of the ladder. They are placed on the ground as a framework for movement, much like a high-tech Hopscotch course. The main objective of an agility ladder drill is to perform different foot movement patterns as quickly as possible. Many footwork variations are possible, with most attempting to simulate cutting maneuvers seen on the field of play. Regardless of variant, the basic intent is to move quickly across the ladder without touching the rungs. The scale of movements included in ladder drills are very small scale with the feet moving rapidly but overall body speed along the ladder is relatively slow.

Cone drills are a fairly large group of movement drills performed using cones (like traffic cones) as a guide or target for direction of each running segment and as an indicator of where and when to change direction. The use of cones to mark a predetermined course is very common in most sports such as soccer or football in which the athletes must react to their environment.

Both types of drills, ladder and cone, are very minor components of agility training. This due to their removal of any recognition and decision making requirements, both key elements of agility. Movement of the feet and ankle during ladder drills at high speed is at best a limited precursor to acceleration and multidirectional movements that might transfer to sport and at worst they may simply be rehearsal of a rhythmic dance or complex game of Hopscotch. Similarly, the use of cone drills in training with a goal of transferring any adaptation to the field of the play presents several problems. Cones are typically very low to the ground, and as a result, the trainee must keep their head and eyes pointed toward the ground when performing the drill. Any football or basketball coach will tell you that one of the first things they teach is to ALWAYS keep their head up during play. This is especially in true in contact sports like American football where not seeing your opponent could result in severe injury. Cones drills also do not require the trainee to perform decision making when performing the drill. The course is set-up prior and the cones indicate when to stop and where to go next.

Rarely in work, sport, or life is exercise offered up in such a limited and predetermined manner. Cone and ladder drills are not completely worthless, their inclusion should be used sparingly, as an aid to agility training not the only method used. Running through these drills is not enough, there must be coaching and feedback. If the movements are performed appropriately - demanding good technique and body control - the positions and movements may very well become second nature and the body will be able to respond more quickly IF there is a recognition of need and an ability to physically change direction faster.

When adding agility training to your program, start with two or three basic drills and only introduce new or more complex drills until general movement skills or the first drills are mastered.

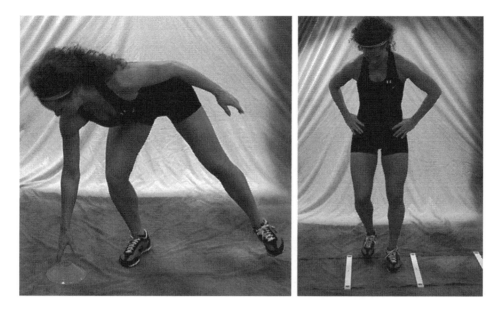

Figure 6. Commonly used agility exercises, cone drills and ladder drills.

An agility drill for a complete novice may only require one change of direction. A general template would be to start by moving forward in a straight line, quickly and efficiently decelerate into the designated stopping point, then quickly re-accelerate in a different direction. An intermediate trainee may require up to four or five changes in direction in the same drill and after each stoppage the movement may differ in direction. At the highest level of agility drill, there should be multiple changes in direction in a variety of exit angles from the change in direction, and wherever possible, predetermined route drills should be complimented with visual or audible signals to signal direction and timing. Quality is the critical for successful performance and potential improvement with any agility drill. Due to the high nervous system demand, specifically in respect to reaction time and decision making, it is important they are performed early in the training session. Keep the individual drills short and rest completely between sets. For the drills to have any transfer to sport or work activities, they must be performed at a rate of speed similar to that used in the actual and intended performance setting. Performing agility drills with a high amount of fatigue prevents performance of the movements at the prerequisite high intensity and will lead to technical errors in performance, thus preventing any progress.

A typical session of agility may consist of approximately three sets of five repetitions of a specific ladder or cone drill, with each sprint being counted as one repetition. Initially choose two or three drills that a similar to movement patterns that are perceived as important to general fitness or to sport performance, and perform then from one to three times per week. The work to rest ratio should be at least 1:5 - for every one second of exercise there should be five seconds of programmed rest. For example, a five second sprint should be followed by a twenty five second recovery period between reps. There should be at least one minute of rest, with upwards of three being acceptable, allowed between sets within a drill and in between drills.

The Bigger Picture

Improving the execution of movement is limited by simple biology and physics. To move fast we have to apply force to the body very quickly and in large amounts. If we use low muscular force, we overcome inertia and accelerate slowly. If we apply the force slowly we accelerate slowly. Simple.

A similar relationship and concept was presented in the strength chapter but it is also appropriate for inclusion here. Training for the acceleration, deceleration, and directional changes needed for agility is not so intuitive. There are two possible strategies that can be used to enhance the ability to change direction, both derived from the simple equation for power:

$$Power = Work / Time$$

Strategy A involves improving speed through the reduction of the value of the denominator in the power equation - less time taken. If a force is applied faster (smaller denominator) then power output goes up. This approach is extremely limited in how much improvement is possible. To understand this, let's divide this strategy into two concepts; nerve conduction velocity and reaction time.

Nerve conduction velocity is approximately 50 meters per second … or about 5 milliseconds per 10 inches. Some people might propose that we can improve the rate of neural conduction significantly by doing some of the drills noted above. If we approach this objectively, without exercise professional conventional wisdom, we see that this is not really productive over the long term.

Think of how close most muscles are to the vertebral column. Once a sensory nerve fires in the hip musculature, speeds to the spinal cord, then exits to the motor nerve and muscle, it takes about 20 maybe 30 milliseconds to make the trip. With weight training and sprint training (high loads and velocity) the motor end plates will adapt, and change structure as an adaptation, possibly to speed synapse. But the speed of conduction depends on the amount of myelination of the nerve axons, not really on motor end plates. And with only 20 to 30 milliseconds of total travel time, can we significantly increase nerve conduction velocity enough to actually record a movement linear velocity change with a stopwatch? Not likely.

Reaction time ranges from about 150 to 200 milliseconds (a simple stimulus yields a faster muscular response, a complex stimulus produces a slower muscular response), possibly much longer in complex, novel, and unfamiliar tasks.

We have to think consciously to make our bodies do what we want as a beginner. Think of the strength chapter reference to you learning how to ride a bicycle as a kid. But here lets look at a football (American soccer) goaltender who is facing a shot from the front of the penalty box. If the offensive player kicks the ball at 45 mph and targets a spot in the net 3 meters to the left of the goaltender, the goaltender has approximately 350 milliseconds to recognize the direction of the kick, estimate the trajectory of intercept, launch himself, and move 3 meters to block the kick. Strength is an important factor here, as it enables a rapid change in inertia of the goaltenders body towards the ball. However ALL the components of mobility are crucial to success here. Reaction time, coordination, kinesthetic awareness, and range of motion are all operating in this sport task. If you examine the physiological and skilled performance characteristics of European football players, premiere league down to the third division, the only truly significant difference between goalkeepers by division and by high success and low success is years of playing experience. The years of practice and familiarity with permutations of ball and body trajectories has rendered the learned movement or skill (blocking a kick) a simple reflex (a gross simplification).

You can improve quite a bit here, with the maximum amount of improvement being on the order of about a 50 milliseconds or so reduction in reaction time BUT there is a bottom limit for reaction time of around 150 milliseconds. Once the bottom is hit there can be no more improvement on this side of neural adaptation.

This second approach above is the most applicable neural approach to all sport movement. Improve technical efficiency through repetition and speed in that movement will increase … to a limit specific to the individual. After that the best way to improve agility (and speed in general) is to employ Strategy B – increase the numerator side of the power equation and increase force generation, i.e. work capacity – or in other words get stronger. You will gain the largest benefit from any program of agility drills if you have previously developed a solid strength base. Stronger is ALWAYS better.

Balance and Coordination

The processing of sensory information and synchronizing muscular contractions in order to adjust and stabilize body position is the basis of balance and coordination. Although they are independent motor abilities, balance and coordination are closely related components of mobility due to their reliance on the sensorimotor system; they both rely on visual, vestibular (inner ear), and proprioceptive inputs. Sensory feedback plays an important role in the control of movement. To greatly simplify a complex system, the sensorimotor system is organized so that information from the periphery (anything not the brain) is relayed to the brain or spinal cord, processed, and the resulting motor output (movement) is guided by further sensory input as it occurs.

Balance is generally defined as the ability to maintain the body's center of gravity within its base of support (the mass of the body supported over whatever parts of the body are touching the ground) and can be categorized as being either static balance or dynamic balance.

Static balance is the ability to maintain the body in static equilibrium. Note that the terms balance and equilibrium are frequently used interchangeably but we really shouldn't. So, in other words there is a distribution of the body mass to where there is no movement. All of the body's mass is spread equally a central point. Standing is an example of static balance.

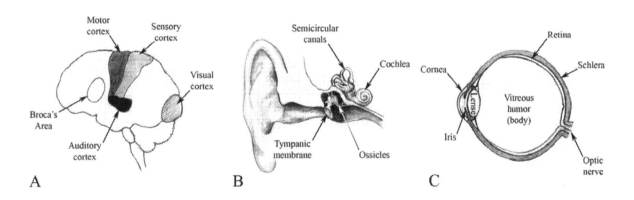

Figure 7. The basic anatomical tools of balance and coordination the brain (A), inner ear (B), and eye (C).

Dynamic balance brings something new to the table, and requires the body to maintain equilibrium during movement. This is where the definitions of balance and equilibrium are not interchangeable. When one is walking there is a forward directed disequilibrium. The center of the mass of the body is not over its base of support at times during the stride and the resulting unbalanced force (unbalanced means that it cannot be an equilibrium) drives movement. However, the body does not fall down. It maintains a dynamic balance, meaning that the movement is effectively controlled.

Both static and dynamic balance require effective multi-system integration in order to control body position. An interruption, interference, or deficit in any part of the sensorimotor system can result in a loss of balance. The most innocuous result of a loss of balance is a stumble or bobble, the most severe is injury.

Balance exerts a powerful effect on exercise technique. Poor balance is associated with reducing exercise efficiency and performance. Poor balance during exercise movements is also associated with falls or injury. So improving balance, specific to the desired exercise, is considered to be a critical component of training. Accuracy of motion and thus balance are best developed through repetitive execution of the movement intended WITH COACHING. A trainee cannot see his body in motion and an external pair of eyes can help provide feedback so the trainee can begin associating a kinesthetic sensation with effective movement.

Balance training (performing specialized exercises on unstable surfaces) has recently grown in popularity in sport and fitness professional practice. Although, balance training has proved valuable in rehabilitation settings, specifically in regards to functional ankle instability, there is virtually no compelling evidence of any kind that suggests the inclusion of training on unstable surfaces has any real and tangible effect on overall fitness. In fact, recent thesis data has demonstrated that instability training added to normal training did not enhance any element of fitness or performance (11). Nonetheless, with the aid of the media many equipment companies and fitness professionals have capitalized on this trend by promoting "balance" training (on unstable surfaces) is a crucial component of most fitness programs. Balance training implements such as stability balls (shouldn't they be called instability balls?), wobble boards, foam pads, balance discs, and even shoes, all share a common purpose. They eliminate the trainee's stable contact with solid ground. This means that the body will recruit a great deal of peripheral musculature to attempt to control balance and not fall over. Proponents of these devices suggest that this will increase the effectiveness of training and produce better balance. However, a tremendously large oversight with that logic is that unstable surfaces render the technique of whatever exercise is performed on it, non-repeatable. If you cannot create reliable and repeatable movement patterns, you cannot improve technique or worse, undesirable movement errors can be introduced.

The rehabilitation value of balance training cannot be ignored, especially in treating and ankle injuries. However, its use in training within the general population may be for naught. Balance is skill specific, and the majority of popular balance tools only work to improve static balance, which may not transfer to most real-world applications that require dynamic balance. Run the Stork Test (a test of static balance) on a bunch of athletes and a bunch of people in general and you will find very similar results between groups. However, put both groups through their paces in a sport environment and you will see the that dynamic balance is quite different, in favor of the athletes. Another major argument against balance training is that using implements that do not allow ground contact will ultimately reduce body control and the effectiveness of the exercise (12). Further, use of balance training implements does not allow for sufficient loading to induce strength gains which in many instances is the stated and primary purpose of training. It is worthwhile to note that the information labels on most stability ball packaging specifically advises against using them in weighted exercises or for any other purpose other than bodyweight support (as in stretching). There have been several high profile collegiate and professional athletes who have ended their seasons prematurely when the ball they were exercising on with weights popped from overload and induced ligament tears and fractures.

Coordination is the other piece to the agility puzzle as when present or developed, it allows a trainee to learn body movements and larger scale movement patterns and to perform them efficiently, effectively, and reliably. It is simply the ability to synchronize and order muscle activities so an intended movement can be performed without error. Coordination affects strength by allowing the muscles to fire in an efficient order to maximize force production or affect performance through precise timing of force production during a movement. We've used the example of riding a bike before, uncoordinated at first and more coordinated after practice. Another example could be the Power Snatch. This is quite a gymnastic movement requiring precise timing of a high force, high velocity, and heavy iron object. Even a slight miss-timing along the bars path can cause a miss. A gross miss-timing in moving under the bar can leave you with a knurling imprint on your forehead. A lack of coordination is evident to virtually anyone who pays attention and watches someone during any movement; lifting, running, swimming, anything. If the trainee moves in an unsynchronized manner (uncoordinated), there will be uneven flexion and extension of joints during a bilateral movement, erratic movement velocities, odd balance asymmetries, and a general lack of ease in performance.

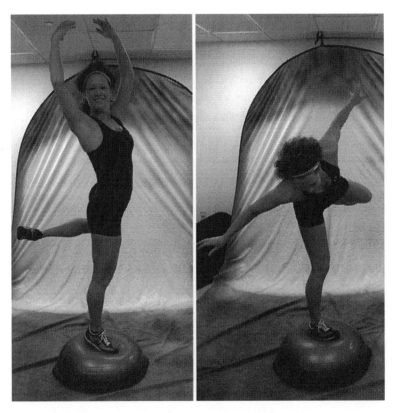

Figure 8. Balance on an unstable structure is difficult even for the most trained and graceful. Even if it is potentially difficult, the use of unstable work in a training program may not cross over and improve balance in a stable environment.

The process of learning a new movement all the way through displaying a coordinated proficiency in the movement occurs through sequential learning in which one part of a task is learned before the next. Although the process of learning is sequential, it is a quite variable process between individuals. The basic teaching/learning premise is simple and has four steps; (1) briefly explain the movement, (2) demonstrate how to do it, (3) let them do it, and (4) give feedback and repeat ad nauseum. The best results come with practice of the new exercise focusing on proper technique, then transitioning to proper technique at an acceptable rate of performance speed, and then finally practicing the movement under a significant load. Proper technique and coordination is not developed through mindless repetitions of PVC pipes, empty bars, or waving the arms and legs about in the air approximating technique. You didn't learn to drive a car by pretending, we don't learn to exercise that way either. Positive learning only occurs when the exercise environment is similar, in terms of loading, performance, tempo, and structure, to the intended movement.

There is one final aspect of coordination that we need to consider. When we train, we get tired. It is inevitable (if we train hard enough to induce fitness gain). Muscular fatigue impairs coordination (13) and we all have experienced this in some manner. This plays into the timing of training intended to improve balance and coordination. Although we strive to move in a coordinated manner in every exercise movement we do, there will be times later in our workouts where coordination will be dulled. In the untrained through intermediate trainees, this means that the best time for including exercises requiring high amounts of balance and coordination, or if learning a new exercise, is at the beginning of the workout. This ensure that the neuromuscular system is fresh and has the best chance for rapidly connecting the neural dots of good technique and avoids the deleterious effects of fatigue. Even if included early, fatigue can still occur. If it does, a rest break should be taken to dissipate the effects of fatigue on coordination. As has been stated in all previous chapters, recovery is essential to progress and this extends to adaptations leading to good coordination.

Are you mobile?

There are any number of range of motion assessments available for use. In fact, there are entire textbooks, many of them, that describe multiple and various tests for range of motion around virtually every joint present in the body (see Measurement of Joint Motion: A Guide to Goniometry, 4th Edition by Norkin & White). These *quantitative* tests are quite useful in a clinical rehabilitation environment but in fitness practice it is more common to use *qualitative* assessments such as simple assessing the ability of a trainee to assume a correct exercise position and move through the complete associated range of motion. This latter type of assessment requires the assessor to be cognizant of the anatomical reference points for the start and end points of the relevant range of motion. This is a limitation of such assessments as most coaches and trainers have not thought of or been taught exercise technique with consideration of anatomical determinants of range of motion. In the exercise description chapters later in this text, specific anatomical segment associations have been described to ensure that each exercise can objectively be evaluated for completeness of range of motion. To answer the question posed in respect to range of motion, if you can perform the exercises as described (through the complete and possible range of motion), then yes, you are mobile in one aspect.

Another aspect of mobility forwarded here is balance and coordination. Balance can be tested with simple tests such as the previously mentioned Stork Test. There are many other quantitative and general tests of static balance. However as discussed, static tests of balance do not carry over well as predictors of balance during movement. It is not something that is widely done in sport or exercise to use a static test of balance (like the Stork Test) to estimate the ability of someone to do a successful round-off or back hand-spring. The measure of the balance and coordination to do so is not found in a test, but in the successful progression through the stages of the learning how to do the gymnastic skill. This is a relevant approach to all exercise.

There is one aspect of mobility where assessment may be meaningful, change of direction. This is one of the descriptors of mobility and it is an area where improvement can be assessed using simple tests. The two most common such tests are the 20-yard-shuttle (aka, the 5-10-5 or Pro-Agility test) and the L test. In the 1950's through the 1980's the more complex Illinois Agility Test was used frequently but has been largely abandoned in favor of the shorter modern tests.

The 20-yard Shuttle

One of the reasons this test is popular is that it is part of a testing battery for the NFL Scouting Combine thus the origin of two of its alternate names, the NFL or Pro Agility Shuttle. The other alternate name, the 5-10-5 Shuttle, is the most descriptive of the test. In the test, three cones or three lines are set five yards apart along a straight line (figure 9). The trainee starts about a foot directly behind the center cone. The cone must be within easy arms reach. At the verbal start signal the trainee is given a visual cue to start running in a specific direction, right or left, towards a cone. The trainee moves to the first cone as fast as possible, touches its base (or line), changes direction, runs past the middle cone (start) to the far cone, touches its base, changes direction, and finally returns to and touches the base of the middle cone. The tester starts the stop watch upon giving the 'Go' command and stops the watch when the subject touches the middle cone. Two or three total trials are done, with the direction of start changing between trials. The fastest of trials is recorded. Performance of this test between two and four times per year can provide an estimate of improvement in the ability to change direction, a contributor to mobility. The premise here is that as agility develops, the trainee will be able to change direction more quickly than in previous tests and thus will have a lower and faster time. There are performance standards available for athletic populations. The minimum times expected of NFL players range from 4.29 seconds for a cornerback to 4.80 seconds for offensive linemen (Google^{TM} NFL football combine standards). Although there are sport specific target times for this test, the actual time is less important than being able to track improvement.

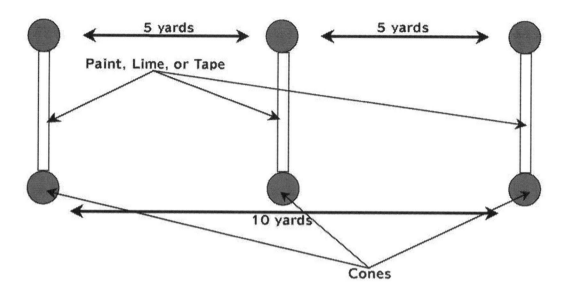

Figure 9. Course design for the 20-yard Shuttle Test.

"L" Test

The L Test is also used at the NFL scouting combine events. This assessment is more complex than the 20-yard shuttle as it includes movement from side-to-side but also from front-to-back. It accomplishes this via its course design. Two parallel lines are laid out five yards apart. At the near end of the lines, two cones are set. Cone 1 is the foot of the "L" with Cone 2 placed five yards behind it will be the point of the angle. Cone 3 is placed five yards away from Cone 2 and serves as the top of the "L" (figure 10). The test starts in a ready stance next to Cone 1. At the start signal the trainee runs as quickly as possible to Cone 2, bends down and touches the line with his right hand. He then turns and runs back to Cone 1, bends down and touches that line with his right hand. Then he changes direction and runs back to Cone 2, passes around the outside of it, weaves to the inside of Cone 3 (as if running a figure eight), cuts as tightly as possible around the outside of Cones 3 and 2, and finishes in a full sprint past Cone 1. Performance is measured by timing how fast the 30-yard course can be completed. It should be apparent that both the ability to change direction and the ability to coordinate a sequence of movements is tested here. As before there are standards for this test relevant to sport, but measuring improvement in mobility is the intended purpose here.

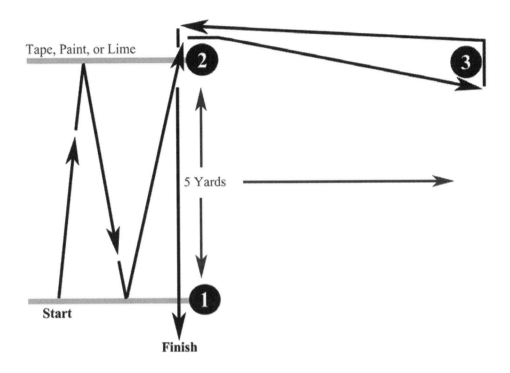

Figure 10. Course layout for the "L" Test of agility.

REFERENCES

1. Fabre, J., et al. Age-related deterioration in flexibility is associated with health-related quality of life in nonagenarians. Journal of Geriatric Physical Therapy, 30(1):16–22, 2007

2. Buchman, A.S., et al. Physical activity and motor decline in older persons. Muscle & Nerve, 35(3): 354–362, 2007.

3. US Department of Health and Human Services. Health, United States, 2010: With Special Feature on Death and Dying. DHHS Publication No. 2011-1232, Washington, DC, 2011.

4. Wells, G.D., M. Elmi, and S. Thomas. Physiological correlates of golf performance. Journal of Strength and Conditioning Research, 23(3): 741-750, 2009

5. Martin, S.B., et al. The rationale for the sit and reach test revisited. Measurement in Physical Education and Exercise Science, 2: 85-92, 1998.

6. Grenier, S.G., C. Russell, and S.M. McGill. Relationships between lumbar flexibility, sit-and-reach test, and a previous history of low back discomfort in industrial workers. Canadian Journal of Applied Physiology, 28: 165-177, 2003.

7. Behm, D.G., D.C. Button, and J.C. Butt. Factors affecting force loss with prolonged stretching. Canadian Journal of Applied Physiology, 26(3):261-272, 2001.

8. Fowles, J.R., D.G. Sale, and J.D. MacDougall. Reduced strength after passive stretch of the human plantarflexors. Journal of Applied Physiology, 89(3):1179-1188, 2000.

9. Ryan, E.D., et al. Do practical durations of stretching alter muscle strength? A dose-response study. Medicine and Science in Sports and Exercise, 40(8):1529-37, 2008.

10. Sheppard, J.M. and W.B. Young. Agility literature review: classifications, training and testing. Journal of Sports Science, 24(9): 915-28, 2006.

11. Brumbalow, J. Meta-analysis of stability ball training on fitness performance. Thesis preliminary data. Midwestern State University, Wichita Falls, Texas, 2011.

12. Behm, D.G., K. Anderson, and R.S. Curnew. Muscle force and activation under stable and unstable conditions. Journal of Strength and Conditioning Research, 16: 416–422, 2002.

13. Taylor, J.L., J.E. Butler, and S.C. Gandevia. Changes in muscle afferents, motoneurons and motor drive during muscle fatigue. European Journal of Applied Physiology, 83 (2-3): 106-115, 2000.

CURRENT INFORMATION AND EQUIPMENT RESOURCES

Books
Athletic Development - Gambetta (for it's listing of drills)
Anatomy Without a Scalpel - Kilgore (for information on joints and movements)
The Key Poses of Yoga - Long
Guide to Stretching - Fisher (presents stretches by joint area and is a 99¢ e-book)

Agility Ladders and Cones
VS Athletics
Power-Systems
Perform Better
MuscleDriver

Measuring Tape 100 feet minimum (you need to measure out courses to quantify load)
VS Athletics
Harbor Freight
Grainger

Stopwatch
Any discount store model will do

The least important things, sometimes, my dear boy, lead to the greatest discoveries.

Doctor Who (the first)

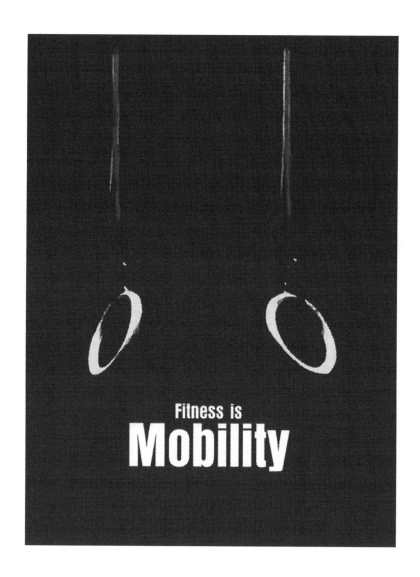

MULTI-ELEMENT FITNESS

Fitness is an expression of strength, endurance, and mobility. In order to elevate fitness, most trainees will need to devote time to all three elements in their program. Trainees will differ in that they have unique anatomical and physiological characteristics based on their genetic composition and level of training progression, but despite this individual nature the elements of fitness respond to training within the same parameters for everyone (see the first two chapters).

Multi-element training is known by many names, cross-training, circuit training, and PHA to name just a few. Any workout that combines strength and endurance elements in its structure is multi-element training. That provides us with a fairly large, diverse, and voluminous menu of training organizations.

Circuit training is the most familiar of the mixed-element training systems. Although it has been a part of fitness development for centuries, it was first described as a specific system of exercise by Morgan & Adamson in their 1962 book, *Circuit Training* (1). Circuit Training was multi-modal and sequential exercise training interjecting endurance activities between strength activities, with no programmed rest other than during movement from station to station. The first published scientific analysis of circuit training appeared in the Scandanavian journal *Ugeskr Laeger* in 1964 (2). And throughout the 60s and 70s circuit training became more broadly prescribed as a means to developing fitness to not just healthy individuals but to the elderly (3) and cardiac patients (4). Circuit training received quite a bit of attention as it produced beneficial cardiorespiratory effects along with improved strength to a small degree (5).

Roughly at the same time as the rise of circuit training another similar methodology was being popularized, Peripheral Heart Action or PHA. In the 1960s and 70s *Strength & Health* and *Muscular Development* magazines published articles by Bob Gadja (a bodybuilder) regarding a training methodology that was reported to increase both cardiac and muscular fitness. In contrast to circuit training that alternated strength and endurance exercises, PHA training was sequential weight exercises organized to distribute the work done to alternate parts of the body so the trainee could go from one weight exercise to the next with no rest between. The theory being that the continual effort, although produced by different body parts, would drive cardiac fitness adaptation.

PHA has experienced a resurgence of interest of late. Most current aficionados of the system attribute the development of PHA to Dr. Arthur Steinhaus of George Williams University in Chicago (sometime in the 1940s through the 60s depending on the source read). But Steinhaus is on record for saying that "it [lifting] does nothing for the heart and lungs; it does not increase endurance ... only strength" (6). If we truly want to understand the rise of PHA, you simply need to consider the changes occurring at the time relative to exercise. Cureton, Cooper, Noakes, Fixx, and many others had managed to create a boom in aerobic exercise and jogging.

So much so that endurance training (LSD type) was considered the only type of exercise required for health and fitness. This made the sale of weight equipment a much less lucrative market. The intent of promoting PHA in fitness magazines was to publicize a method of weight training by which York Barbell (owner of *Strength & Health* and *Muscular Development* magazines) could capitalize on the new public and clinical concern with heart health. Cooper and the ACSM had jogging, Hoffman and York Barbell had PHA. Unfortunately, circuit training and PHA both suffered a similar demise, being largely abandoned in favor of jogging for a couple decades. The only place mixed element training remained a central feature was in preparation for combative sports such as wrestling (7).

Since the late 1990s however, there has been a resurgence of interest and a dramatic increase in the number of people using multi-element training - and in the number of systems available. Everything from the CrossFit system of circuit training to a hang-on-your-door apparatus to do short-duration and high-intensity variant of PHA have garnered the attention of the public, medical community, media, and the military.

Although mixed-element training is becoming quite popular and commonplace as a training methodology, there are virtually no resources on how to perform the complex task of integrating training of the distinctly different elements of fitness into one coherent and effective program.

Likely the most cogent description of how to plan such training was authored by Greg Glassman in his 2003 article "Theoretical Template for CrossFit's Programming" (8). What was very interesting about the programming template here was that there were three basic types of training blocks serving as components of training; (A) endurance type training, (B) mobility type training, and (C) strength training. Of course the names used for each type of block were different than above, the CrossFit template uses "monostructural metabolic conditioning", "gymnastics", and "weightlifting" as the descriptors for the blocks. Each block type would be included within the training week with equal frequency. For example in the one-week duration training program he outlined, there are five training days and two recovery days (days off). During the five training days, each fitness element is represented three times.

Training Day	**Element #1**	**Element #2**	**Element #3**
Monday	Endurance		
Tuesday	Mobility	Strength	
Wednesday	Endurance	Mobility	Strength
Thursday	Endurance	Mobility	
Friday	Strength		

Also listed in the template article is a list of exercises that were to be included in the workouts for each day. There were seven exercises in the strength list, four exercises in the endurance list, and twelve in the mobility list. Exercises were selected from the list table randomly, for example on any given Monday there was an equal likelihood that the exercise to be done would be running, biking, rowing, or jumping rope. Workouts were intended to be short and intense, pushing the body's ability to operate at a high work rate, as hard and fast as possible, generally for about twenty minutes (fit individuals complete workouts faster, less fit individuals complete the workouts in a longer time).

While the CrossFit template is quite useful, it does have a weakness. Its random assignment of exercises to workouts is not satisfactory for all applications. In fact, random selection of exercises only produces desired or maximal fitness gains by chance, for in a random chance scenario we can as easily select wrong as easily as we can select right. There are other similar exercise systems for sale or use that build on the concept of circuit training and the idea of presenting the body with constantly changing physical stressors. P90X™ and its "muscle confusion" method (muscles cannot be confused, only fatigued as they do not have brains or cognitive ability) is an example. Aside from marketing and hype, multi-element training has a prominent place in creating broad spectrum fitness for the general population, athletes, and for any number of work sites. It is important then to understand why and how to structure a multi-element training program to produce the best results in the minimum amount of time.

The Importance of Strength

In the third chapter we learned that strength is the ability to generate and apply muscular force to an external resistance. It is also the fundamental capacity of physical work capacity. By increasing force production, a trainee improves their ability to move faster or move larger objects – it's the simple physics of inertia. If a trainee has used the strength development concepts presented in this text, he or she will have increased neuromuscular efficiency by developing gross motor pathway function. Additionally, they will have developed a strong and stable hip and trunk structure. This added stability enhances the ability to change direction quickly because the hip muscles can more effectively apply force to the ground. Further, the trunk muscles will not bend and wiggle when the force is applied. Consider two different potted plants; one has a trunk that is one inch in circumference while the other is five inches. If both pots are put in the back of a pick-up truck that is driving down the road at 10 mph, the thinner plant will sway and whip while the thicker trunk will not. The thick trunk is stronger and thus can better withstand the imposed force. The same concept applies to a defensive player in football who must quickly stop and change directions. It should follow here that strength contributes to mobility.

Increasing the contractility strength of muscle also has a benefit of increased density and resistance to higher injurious forces than previously tolerable. Being strong helps prevent and reduce the severity of injuries. The additional structural strength also allows the muscles and related structures to be conditioned into new activities faster and with less damage or soreness. For example, swimming is an activity that can grind the upper back and shoulder muscles in new trainees. A trainee with a developed strength base can tolerate more initial training volume than a weaker trainee. The increased ability in force application seen in a stronger trainee will allow him to maintain the same rate of work for a longer period of time and/or higher rates of work when compared to a weaker trainee. Being strong enhances the potential to develop endurance quickly and efficiently.

Hierarchy of Emphasis

Since strength augments the other physical elements, it should receive priority of attention in most, if not all, general fitness programs. The only time strength would not take precedence is when a trainee has achieved above average strength levels and aims to focus their effort on endurance or mobility. In some cases, strength can be limited by poor mobility in a trainee. An inability to move effectively through a full range of motion will hamper force production at the ends of the range of motion. Furthermore, strength training that neglects mobility and its maintenance creates a danger of introducing artificial barriers to progress and potential injury. As such, joint and muscle mobility work should be programmed in accordance with strength training. Mobility work aims to maintain the anatomical structures trained to prevent problems and won't interfere with recovery when programmed intelligently.

The limiting factor of fitness for most trainees will be their strength. This is not surprising as we are emerging from decades of a single faceted presentation of fitness equating to endurance. As late as 2006, the ACSM only devoted a total of three paragraphs to developing strength in their Guidelines to Exercise Testing and Prescription – a book used in exercise professional instruction programs around the world (9).

How do we know if a strength limitation is present and how large it is? Quantification of strength is easy through simple testing, but categorization of those results is not. Trainees can assess their level of strength in important exercises by using the age and sex-adjusted set of standards presented in the final chapter. Standards are not absolutes, they are general guidelines and there always outliers. Don't fixate on them as a means of "leveling up" as you would in a video game.

Beginning or low strength individuals will use a simple, standard strength program that progresses on a daily basis as described in the Strength chapter herein. Getting stronger in preparation for multi-element training simply requires that the major joints be worked through a full range of motion with free-standing, compound exercises. Exercises like the Squat, Bench Press, Press, and Deadlift are among the most useful. As soon as strength levels begin to increase significantly, light to medium endurance work is added into the program to improve this element of fitness. This aspect of programming cannot be over-emphasized. As force generation capacity increases over time as a result of strength training, so too will the potential for endurance improvement - since the rate that work can be done will subsequently be faster or it can be done for extended time.

Good multi-element fitness programs will take care that the endurance work included in the program, while disruptive of homeostasis, is not so stressful to interfere with the recovery from strength training. However, adding intermittent endurance training with a strength program will slightly blunt the capacity for strength increases - the tradeoff of maintaining or increasing mobility and endurance will be worth it to fitness trainees. Both intermittent endurance training and LSD training will blunt the rate of strength increase even further since adaptations to LSD are the polar opposite of strength adaptations. The inclusion of high-intensity endurance training is enough to ward off anatomical and physiological adaptations that would make someone weak and less powerful over time. Figure 1 conceptually compares the rate of strength gain with respect to emphasis of training program.

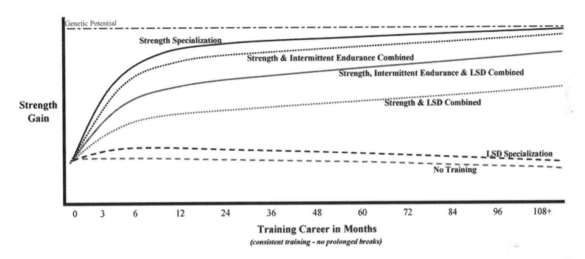

Figure 1. A comparison of rate of strength development and emphasis of training.

Strength Guidelines for a Multi-Element Program

There are a multitude of programs in the strength chapter of this book that can help achieve various strength goals. Keep in mind that the trainee's end goal will dictate their repetition scheme and intensity. This is handy, as achieving higher levels of fitness will be dependent on higher levels of strength (figure 2).

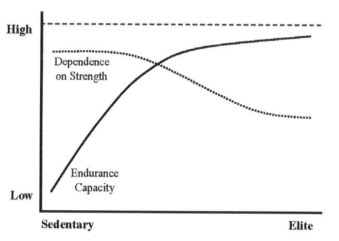

Figure 2. When development of endurance is considered over a career of training, strength is an essential element throughout. However it's relative importance and presence in training programs mildly decreases over the years.

Most trainees will initially need to increase their strength and begin developing work capacity, thus they would benefit from a repetition scheme between three and five repetitions to get adequate strength, muscular development, and increase work capacity in preparation for further and more rigorous training. The repetition and set schemes used in a mixed element fitness program should be biased towards strength development, the functional part of weight training, rather than on hypertrophy. This narrows our choices of set and repetition schemes to something similar to the following:

Repetitions	**Sets**	**Goal**
1-3	5-10	Strength with minimal mass gain
5	3-5	Strength with some mass gain

Setting up a strength program in a mixed-element environment doesn't need to be a complicated process. Using basic exercises that train the major joints through a full range of motion once or twice a week will help increase strength. In fact, doing one or two heavy (85% of maximum) workout each week has been shown to increase strength (10). As strength work will be integrated with the other fitness elements, there is a limit to how much can be done. With this in mind, the program orientation presented here distributes the training load - the exercises done - over multiple workouts rather than bundling them into a couple workouts. This distribution of work, in and of itself, can produce greater gains (11). The menu of exercises to use is relatively small and the number of times per week each exercise is done is few:

Squat – Included two times per week
Deadlift – Included once week
(***Note***: For the Deadlift only there is a single work set done)
Bench Press – Included once per week
Press – Included once per week
Pull-ups or **Chin-ups** – Included once per week
(***Note***: Sets done to failure with body weight, or additional load is added)

Using the frequencies noted above, the exercises can be assigned to training days. If using a three-day-per-week program, 2 or 3 exercises will be done. If using a five day per week program, 2 or three exercises will still be done in order to enable other specialized or potentially interfering training (interferes with strength gain) on the non-strength days.

Monday	**Wednesday**	**Friday**
Back Squat	Deadlift	Back Squat
Bench Press	Press	Bench Press
		Pull-up

The Bench Press and Press can be alternated every other workout. A Monday-Friday Bench Press and Wednesday Press week would switch to a Monday-Friday Press and Wednesday Bench Press the subsequent week. In a three day per week program, Tuesday, Thursday, and the weekend are designated as rest days. Rest is an ESSENTIAL and commonly disregarded element of training. Referring back to chapters 1 and 2, rest days allow the body to recover and adapt to the stress placed upon it by training - you gain fitness during rest days.

Most trainees who are new to strength training, and many of those who have been training according to the muscle magazines, will be skeptical at the small number of exercises in the above program here. The beauty of programming for strength is that it is simple, time efficient, and effective. Depending on the set and repetition scheme selected, there will only be 10 to 25 repetitions per exercise. If we pick a middle set and repetition scheme, there would be about 12 sets during the workout (not including warm up sets) and should take no longer than 45 minutes to complete. Any program that emphasizes lots of exercises, lots of repetitions, and lots of sets is an ill-advised program designed for people who want to add mass simply to be big and that have lots of disposable time to spend in the gym. Remember that appropriate stress followed by adequate recovery leads to adaptation and fitness. As strength is not the only fitness element we want to develop, this simple program opens the door for work on other fitness elements to be added without overwhelming adaptive capacity or being time prohibitive.

Mobility Guidelines for a Multi-Element Program

Earlier chapters have detailed the importance and mechanisms for improving mobility. There are several ways to include mobility training into multi-element workouts. Utilizing a proper dynamic warm-up prior to exercise is one way to prepare the body for training while also providing for the maintenance of the range of motion aspect of mobility. As will be noted later in this chapter, selection of exercises and the insistence on their completion through a well described range of motion will also contribute to range of motion.

For those with a range of motion limitation, static stretching can also be thought of as a corrective measure used when range of motion needs to be restored or improved. Performing stretching exercises after the cessation of a given training session is the most opportune and productive time.

Agility can also be developed as part of any multi-element training program. It could be simple as inclusion of structured 5-10-5 shuttle runs, "L" cone drills, or even systematic and repeating drills of movements related to a given task in a sport, job, or activity (in sport this could be agility ladder or cone drills).

Regardless of scenario, the idea is to help the body adapt to the desired level of work capacity and function. Non-rigorous agility work can be done prior to lifting, prior to the endurance work, or on an off day in a multi-element program. Generally the load used in such additional training is less than 70% of maximal intensity if using weighted exercise for a very few sets, a half dozen or so short repetitions of endurance related skills, and so on. Even though the loads used here are very light, they still affect recovery. They slow it. And if the volume of work is too high, it can prevent recovery and progress towards fitness. The term "recovery" ride, run, or workout is a misnomer, for as stated in previous chapters, recovery and adaptation do not occur during training but rather in the down time in between.

Endurance Guidelines for Multi-Element Training

This aspect of training is often referred to as conditioning or hardening. During this type of training there are three things occurring; (A) habituating structures to tolerate new activities, (B) improving the cardiovascular and respiratory systems ability to supply energy to the working muscles in order to sustain a task over time, and (C) developing the ability of the muscle to take up and utilize the energy delivered. As discussed in the endurance chapter, improving the latter two items has historically been attempted via long, slow distance aerobic exercise (LSD). The problem with LSD exercise is that it can only work in development of energy storage and delivery capacity, not in maximizing utilization. Further, if simultaneously or subsequently trained with strength, the adaptations produced in the muscle tend to limit the rate of strength gain. Additionally, spending more than twenty to thirty minutes on long duration, low to moderate intensity and continuous endurance activity will limit post-exercise recovery in all aspects of fitness.

Given that all three desired adaptations can be provided with shorter duration training, the model of multi-element training here minimizes the use of LSD exercise and focuses on intensity driven anaerobic exercise to drive fitness gain.

The endurance chapter discussed how reducing the saturation of oxygen in the blood (and in the muscle) is the result of a significant exercise stress. After experiencing a deficit in oxygen delivery, the body will make structural and metabolic changes so that the same level of exercise stress won't create the same level of reduction in oxygen saturation in the future. This interrelationship between the cardiovascular, respiratory, and muscular systems implies a dependence on creating a deficit of energy substrates either through exceeding the current maximum rate of supply or by creating a larger demand. The deficit is the event to which the body is not adapted. Higher levels of intensity in training forces a deficit by creating a mismatch - there is a high rate of energy substrate consumption and a slower rate of re-supply (demand exceeds delivery). Put simply, very high levels of work output require metabolic activity to proceed at such a rate it cannot be sustained for long. The body does its best to maintain the high work output for as long as possible and to recover as much as possible during any rest periods, but fatigue (a reduction in work capacity) is inevitable - and is, in fact, the desired outcome of this type of training. The aim of programming here is to implement high work rate exercises requiring high metabolic consumption, to keep the work rate as high as possible for as long as possible, and to use the shortest possible rests during the workout. Rest intervals should only enable completion of the programmed amounts of work NOT provide for complete recovery.

Although the focus of training here utilizes high intensity and high work rates, this approach improves both high and low work output activities. Practically speaking, training that consistently includes high intensity work performed for periods of four to ten minutes will improve the ability to do sustained lower intensity endurance work that lasts for twenty, thirty, and even forty minutes (12). There are physiological adaptations, increased red blood cell, increased hemoglobin concentration, and more, that occur after repeated bouts of exercise induced oxygen desaturation that benefit longer and slower exercise performance. For example, the inclusion of short sprints done on the minute for ten to twelve minutes, as given in the endurance chapter, would help someone enhance their ability to run several miles at a slow to moderate pace.

Types of Intensity

There are three useful types of training that should be included in a multi-element fitness program; (1) sprint type or maximal effort, (2) intermittent endurance or interval, and (3) sustained endurance or sustained effort.

Maximal effort training is a method where a blistering, maximal work output is sustained for as long as possible. The trainee attempts to maintain as fast and as intense level of exertion as possible until the programmed work is completed ... or until their rate of work decays below a specified performance threshold (as opposed to total fatigue requiring stopping before completion). Maximal and near maximal work outputs decline within seconds, and even with pacing, outputs will undoubtedly diminish over the course of several minutes. And that's the point. The trainee should be working at such a high rate of work that they are unable to maintain it. This is how a deficit in oxygen or energy substrates is created.

One programmatic issue that requires attention is that if the duration of the workout extends too long, rates of work diminish to the point of being rendered ineffective. By going longer you have to go so slower, and this does not provide a substantial disruption of homeostasis. To ensure that the desired homeostatic disruption occurs, the total duration of maximal effort work should consist of four to ten minutes of extremely hard work. The rationale for this range of workout times is that four minutes is long enough to cause a viable disturbance of homeostasis and ten minutes represents the longest duration where a work rate fast enough to produce the desired stress is possible. Two descriptive terms are used here to distinguish between these subtle differences:

> *Short maximal effort workouts* are those that are capped at five minutes
> *Long maximal effort workouts* are those that are capped at ten minutes

Naturally, the short maximal effort intervals will be done a higher rate of work than the long maximal efforts - but they are both still done at the body's peak ability. This distinction will be relevant in the programming section later in this chapter.

Maximal effort training can consist of a single exercise activity or a specifically assembled collection of exercise activities. The major consideration is that the exercise(s) included must facilitate a high rate of work with no intervening rest. Running a mile or rowing 1,000 meters are examples of appropriate single exercises for this purpose, as long as they are done AS FAST AS POSSIBLE. Another example could be completing 50 Burpees as fast as possible, a deceivingly difficult task. Designing this type of workout using multiple exercise activities requires creativity and experience. Creativity is needed to avoid including the same exercise in training over and over, as boredom is a barrier to participation and progress. When programming multi-element training, ***experience actually doing the exercises programmed is imperative*** as to ensure that what is being requested of a trainee is actually realistic and doable. There is no point in programming if the workout designed exceeds the trainee's ability to the point it fails to produce the desired disruption in homeostasis. If a trainee cannot do a single Pull-up, or even if they can do 20, would programming 50 one-armed Pull-ups be an appropriate workout?

Going back to the concept of circuit training, we can use multiple exercise stations to produce the desired training effect. An example of an appropriate circuit might be:

Four rounds of a circuit that includes:
3 Power Cleans
10 Kettlebell Swings
10 Box Jumps
10 Push-ups

or

Three descending repetition (20, 15, and 10) rounds that include:
Medicine Ball Throw
Kettlebell Swing
Pull-ups

Lastly, what has become known as a *Tabata workout* can be used as maximum effort training. A Tabata interval begins with 20 seconds of maximal work followed by ten seconds of rest. This is repeated six to eight times, a number derived from some of Dr. Tabata's research (12). Practitioners and coaches have found that using traditional endurance exercises like running, rowing, and cycling work best for this purpose (although almost any activity can be organized into a Tabata interval). Whether using running, rowing, or cycling, maximal effort on each 20 second interval is a must. Running Tabata's can also be easily accommodated in any facility with a treadmill that can be adjusted to an incline of 8 to 12%, and this may be the most effective means of deriving fitness gain from Tabata workouts.

Picking a target speed for a running Tabata is fairly straightforward. The first step is to set the incline to 8% for a beginner, higher for more advanced trainees. Calculating the treadmill speed is based on a target mile time. If you want to be able to run an 8:40 mile, or 6.9 mph for a mile or two, then 6.9 mph is the belt speed that should be used. The elevation of the treadmill is the key to making it hard. Target mile times should be realistic. You might want to run a sub-4-minute mile, but presently if you are clocking in at 7:28, a 7:10 goal in a Tabata workout might be more appropriate. If all eight Tabata intervals can be completed (without any danger of falling), then the next Tabata workout would be done with a slightly faster pace. The rate of progression is slow. If using miles per hour, belt speed would be increased by 0.2-0.3 mph with beginners - possibly up to 0.5 mph if the sessions feel easy. For more advanced trainees progression should be about 0.1-0.2 mph. If using minutes per mile, beginners would subtract 20 to 30 seconds off of the previous setting and more advanced trainees would subtract 10 to 20 seconds (table 1).

Minutes/Mile	Mile/Hour	Minutes/Mile	Mile/Hour
10:00	6.0	8:00	7.5
9:50	6.1	7:50	7.7
9:40	6.2	7:40	7.8
9:30	6.3	7:30	8.0
9:20	6.4	7:20	8.2
9:10	6.5	7:10	8.4
9:00	6.7	7:00	8.6
8:50	6.8	6:50	8.8
8:40	6.9	6:40	9.0
8:30	7.1	6:30	9.2
8:20	7.2	6:20	9.5
8:10	7.3	6:10	9.7
		6:00	10.0

Table 1. Miles per hour converted to minutes per mile. Both values can be used to guide progression in Tabata loading on a treadmill. This table presents 0.1 mph or 10 second reduction intervals. You can easily use smaller intervals, 0.5 mph or 5 second intervals for a slower load increase if needed.

Whether or not the workout is difficult on day one is dependent on the person. And just as in individual element training, slow and steady loading is important. Big greedy jumps are not optimal for producing gains over the long haul. Eventually workouts will become very difficult and the jumps in running speed between workouts will be small, yet these small increases will elicit an excellent training stress. With this in mind, the initial running pace may be slow and that is OK. It should be a reasonable pace, something the trainee is capable of accomplishing but still harder than they have done before.

Treadmills can pose a safety hazard if one is unaccustomed to using them. Practicing getting on and off the moving belt at low speeds is essential before doing so at training speeds. This practice will prevent any problems with mounting or dismounting the moving treadmill - one misplaced step on a treadmill when getting off or on the moving belt can upset balance and potentially cause injury (search YouTube[TM] for treadmill fails). Before doing Tabata treadmill training, or treadmill exercise in general, one should be strong enough to support the entire body weight on the hand rails. An easy litmus test for this is requiring the ability to do one body weight dip. This will ensure that the trainee is capable of supporting their entire weight if needed.

Tabata running workouts can be done outdoors, but a partner, coach, or trainer is needed as most trainees will not be able to accurately judge their pace. All Tabata methods will be more effective and safer if someone besides the trainee uses a stopwatch and paces the workout. Having someone give verbal "3, 2, 1, Go!" and "3,2,1, Stop!" at exactly the right time will pay dividends in fitness gain, gains that might go unrealized by timing errors caused by trying to accurately read and manipulate a stopwatch during highly demanding movements. An interesting twist to outdoor running Tabatas is doing them with reversed timing. Ten seconds of all out sprinting followed by twenty seconds of rest for six to eight intervals is an demanding and eye opening experience (they are done at a faster running pace). If doing reverse Tabata workout outdoors and with a group, a designated timer could simply blow a whistle as the intervals change from work to rest.

Tabata workouts on a stationary bike or a rower occur in much the same way as with treadmills. Pick a relatively easy resistance for the beginner and push as hard as possible over six to eight intervals. Exercise bikes have displays similar to treadmills and progression should be done with slow advancement with pedaling resistance (pedal cadence should always be maximal). Advancement with rowing should be done by steadily reducing the split times, increasing stroke rate, or increasing the number of meters covered in a maximal effort.

Tabata workouts can also be done with many different exercises, they just aren't as effective as the traditional endurance modalities (the larger muscle mass used the better). Calisthenic or weight based exercises could be used and in this case the trainee would go for maximal repetitions of the included exercise during each work interval. Examples of commonly used exercises are Push-ups, Bodyweight Squats, and Kettlebell Swings. Remember to ease into these workouts when including them into training for the first time. Doing six to eight intervals of maximal repetitions of these exercises will quickly accumulate volume. The involved structures – pectoralis and triceps muscles on Push-ups, quadriceps and gluteals on Squats, and hamstrings on Kettlebell Swings - can get incredibly sore from too aggressive of initial loading of Tabata intervals. Soreness is a necessity in fitness gain, but debilitating soreness is not. Use the low end of the recommended number of repetitions, or even fewer, when just starting out. Use light kettlebells to start if using them. Regardless of the type of exercise included, care should be taken when trying any Tabata workout for the first time, beginner or advanced trainee. This is the most rigorous style of intensity endurance there is - they are not for the faint of heart.

Interval training is slightly different than maximal effort training in that it has periods of high work output punctuated with periods of rest. Whereas maximal effort training produced a continuous reduction in work rate, interval training produces a reduction in work rate that accumulates over several intervals of work interspersed with periods of incomplete rest (figure 3). As alluded to earlier, it is not just work and work rate that can be manipulated, rest can also be manipulated to increase the stress of a workout or a series of workouts. There are a few simple combinations of work and rest that can be used to create a specific exercise stress (figure 4):

    Work can be increased using a constant duration of rest
    Work can be held constant and rest times can be decreased
    Work can be increased and rest can be decreased simultaneously

Interval training is dependent on high intensity, much higher than VO_2max (faster than the fastest pace you can sustain for a mile). They also must be long enough to have a cumulative stress that disrupts homeostasis. It is therefore important to program intervals that last anywhere from ten to thirty minutes.

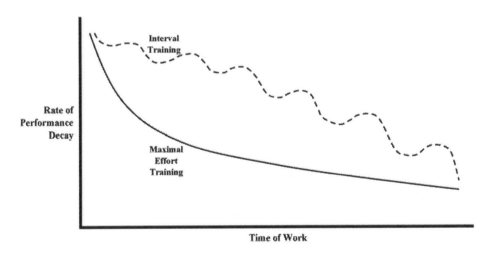

Figure 3. Patterns of fatigue in interval and maximal effort training.

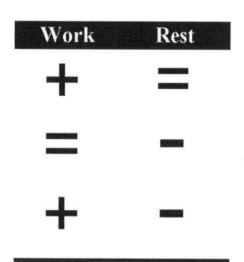

Figure 4. The possible combinations of work and rest variants one could use to drive fitness gain from interval training. + represents an increase, - represents a decrease, and = represents no alteration.

There are innumerable described interval workouts, however they all can be divided into two basic types: (1) maximal intervals and (2) goal intervals.

Maximal intervals demand, as one would expect from their name, maximal effort with each repetition included in the workout - running the fastest 400 meters possible in each repetition for example. In such a workout, the work output (or speed over the distance) may be slower as fatigue accumulates, however the goal is to push as hard as possible in each interval. This is a concept that is well described in the Russian training literature from the 1960s and 70s and is termed "relative maximum". You may not be posting a personal best time but it is the best time you are capable of at that moment. Maximal intervals provide a recovery stress as rest is allowed, but not much, and this is complimentary to maximal effort training.

Goal intervals program effort over a given distance at a specified pace - running 400 meter repeats at an 8:00 mile pace fore example. Goal intervals have a lower intensity compared to maximal intervals. Since goal intervals aren't as stressful per interval, they can include more intervals or more distance – in other words, more volume - than maximal interval training. The lower relative intensity of goal intervals can be seen as a mild form of unloading, if done on days between maximal effort training and maximal interval training. Caution must be taken not to consider this to be easy training as it is not, it is still disruptive of homeostasis but not to the magnitude of maximal training methods.

The simplest form of interval training consists of repeating a set amount of work, for a set number of times, with set periods of between effort rest. As fitness advances, intervals can be varied into ascending, descending, pyramid, or ladder organizations. Examples of these would be:

Repeated Intervals	400 meters x 4 repetitions
Ascending Intervals	100, 200, 300, 400 meters
Descending Intervals	400, 300, 200, 100 meters
Pyramid Intervals	200, 300, 400, 300, 200 meters
Ladder Intervals	100, 200, 300, 100, 200, 300 meters

A constant rest duration is used in repeated intervals. Ascending intervals may use increased rest time between efforts as the workout progresses. In the case of descending work, each interval represents a reduced volume of work so the trainee can maintain or provide an even greater effort as the intervals progress. Descending intervals typically maintain rest intervals, yet can include decreasing rest times in more advanced trainees. Pyramiding would have ascending amounts of work followed by equal descending drops that allows the later repetitions to be conducted at high levels of effort. An interval ladder has ascending distance or duration intervals followed by a repeat of the first half of the set, from shortest interval ascending to longest. Pyramid and ladder intervals will typically maintain constant rest intervals so that the changing distances provide the primary stress.

These latter variants in interval organization may appear more complicated and better than simple repeated intervals, but they are largely irrelevant for the implementation of interval training in concert with a strength program. Most trainees will make great gains through simple performance of repeated intervals of work with a fixed rest period. It is only the more advanced trainees who will reap greater benefits from more complexity of training provided with constantly changing interval variants.

Progression is as important here as it was in training specifically for strength or for endurance. In the following example, the individual interval distance is held constant however between-interval rest is reduced by 30 seconds each week. The second example holds the rest period constant yet increases the number of intervals each week. These examples show that simply running isn't enough to drive adaptation, but progressively changing the amounts of rest or work done each week can and will drive progress. Several weeks of decreasing rest times are a requisite to increasing the work interval since extraneous volume is counter-productive in lesser adapted trainees. This interval programming may seem rudimentary, but simple programming is not only easy, it is also effective. Get the most progress from simple methods before using more complex training organizations.

Example 1:

Week	Interval Distance	Between Interval Rest
1	400 meters	3:00
2	400 meters	2:30
3	400 meters	2:00
4	400 meters	1:30

Example 2:

Week	Interval Distance	Number of Intervals
1	400 meters	4
2	400 meters	5
3	400 meters	6
4	400 meters	7

Interval conditioning does not have to be restricted to simple activities like running, it can also use other modes of exercise or include more than one exercise mode. The simplest way to put together a multi-exercise interval is to use a maximal effort workout that has rounds and then rest in between those rounds. For example, a workout might have four rounds with each round consisting of Pull-ups, Kettlebell Swings, and then running 200 meters. The period of rest in between each round will have a different magnitude of restorative effect because of the differing demands of each exercise. The rest duration must be programmed to keep the perceived effort and actual work output high without being so generous to allow complete recovery between exercises and rounds. These multi-exercise interval workouts will aim to keep the work intervals between two and three minutes so that relative maximum output levels are achieved without too much fatigue. Lesser adapted trainees should rest for the same length of time as the period of work - more rest will negate the effect of substrate deficit for subsequent work intervals. The next time the trainee repeats the same workout (perhaps in the following week), they can decrease rest by 15 or 30 seconds and continue to do so each week until reaching 1:00 minute rest periods (similar to the example above).

Sustained endurance training consists of a lower rate of work that is continuous, having no breaks for rest, and is extended beyond fifteen minutes. This type of training serves the purpose of inducing structural adaptations to repetitive use activity and, as explained in the Fitness Adaptation chapter, to improve carbohydrate storage and utilization. This type of training is most useful in the event that the trainee needs to be able to perform a longer duration activity as part of a sporting activity, work, or as part of a simple personal fitness goal.

Consider an example of military personnel. An infantryman must be strong, powerful, fast, and quick as events on a battlefield do not unfold slowly. He is also required to be quite enduring, able to march twelve miles in three hours while carrying a 45 pound (20 kg) rucksack and kit and run five miles in under forty minutes. These tasks demand that his feet and supportive structures - muscles, tendons, bones, and ligaments - be conditioned in order to handle the march and run and they require metabolic preparation to complete the tasks at a sufficient pace. It should be obvious that the soldier will need to put time in carrying a rucksack and kit on the trail via sustained endurance training in order to acclimate to the task and develop sufficient energy storage capacity. But strength development cannot be ignored. If strong, the soldier can move faster and farther, thus providing his body a better platform on which to express his endurance capability.

Sustained endurance training may be a necessity for some or a leisurely pursuit for others (hiking, walking, and such). For general fitness trainees, rowing, swimming, and running are all traditional and acceptable modes of sustained endurance training. For purposeful fitness gain however, there is a specificity application that must be considered. In our example of a soldier and a loaded march, swimming, rowing, and running will provide only a partial stimulus towards improving performance. The key here is to specifically do the activity that must be prepared for, in this case carrying a rucksack and kit for miles. This concept carries over to sport, where time in weight room and on the track will contribute to competitive performance only if there is adequate practice of the sport skill. I can spend lots of time under the bar and on a cycle ergometer training for an Italian Pursuit race at the velodrome, but unless I have logged enough experiential and conditioning time actually on the track, it will be for naught. It is a delicate balance between preparing the physical basis on which fitness can be expressed and training the actual event in which it is displayed.

Structuring the Workout

The basic structure of effective intensity workouts has been described, but the actual exercises or activities have not. To get there, a few things need to be understood. Here is conditioning in a nut shell:

> Improvement in multi-element fitness (performance) requires a sufficient exercise stress
> Exercise stress is a result of substrate deficit
> Substrate deficits occur with high metabolic demands (beyond re-supply capacity)
> High metabolic activity is achieved through intense exercise

To create the conditions above, use of large-scale multi-joint movements that include a great deal of active musculature will use the most energy and are the most efficient and significant exercise stressors. Isolation exercises, like a Sit-up or Curl, only work a small amount of muscle and won't create a large enough energy demand to create a systemic stress. Using gross movement patterns that take the hips, knees, and shoulders through a full range of motion are ideal. This can be done with body weight movements or with implements - anything from barbells to rocks. Creativity and the possibility for progression with the implement are the only real limitations.

The movements chosen for inclusion need to be able to be performed fast enough to demand large amounts of energy. The rate of execution is important, as doing one Bodyweight Squat every five seconds doesn't demand as much energy as quickly as doing three squats in five seconds. Further, Bodyweight Squats are better than Walking Lunges, as the lunge is a much slower movement - more work can be done in a shorter amount of time with a set of ten squats compared to ten lunges.

Even though repetition rate (work rate) is critical, this doesn't mean that technique is forsaken in order to do faster repetitions. Correct technique produces the greatest amount of work and develops fitness throughout the complete range of motion. If only half squats are being done in order to do faster repetitions, the muscles of the knees, hips, and ankles are not being taken through a full range of motion, the amount of work is reduced and the systemic stress may be reduced to the point that the movement becomes irrelevant to its intended purpose. If a trainee is only capable of performing a poorly executed Power Clean, void of any jump or hip extension, and they are unable to manage the integrated movement of the bar and body consistently and safely in normal strength training, then they have no business incorporating this movement into their multi-element fitness training. With this latter point made, and it is an important one, technique can and will break down as fatigue encroaches, but it should not break down to the point where safety is compromised, shortcuts impose themselves, and the purpose of the movement is lost. Moving the body, the bar, or the implement from point A to B isn't the goal, creating fitness effectively and correctly is. To state this very succinctly:

Quality Work is more important than Total Work

When using implements, the load will have an inverse relationship with the number of repetitions programmed. The more consecutive *or* total repetitions that are desired to be performed in a given movement the less of a load it should have. This will prevent an undesirably large decrease in work rate during the conditioning workout. For example, if there are ten programmed consecutive repetitions but the trainee can only do two at a time with rest in between because the implement is too heavy, the slower work rate may move the exercise stress out of the metabolic target area. We do not want force production capacity as the limiting factor here; instead substrate utilization should be the limiting factor. Managing loads effectively will also prevent any unnecessary lingering localized fatigue (at the muscle) or systemic stress that may negatively affect other training days later in the week. We want to be tired and a little bit sore after training, but not debilitated for days afterward.

A simple rule of thumb is that conditioning loads should not exceed 60% of maximum and ideally will stay below 50% of maximum. Sticking to this rule will serve you well. Anything heavier can be too much to lift for consecutive repetitions and may require too long of a rest in between repetitions. Therefore, by definition, heavier loads alter the nature of the exercise to no longer qualify as a conditioning workout since the highest work output possible and desired rate is not maintained. It is important to realize that if time is going to be spent, it should not be wasted with unintentional resting. And if a trainee doesn't have the force production capabilities to move the programmed load, then there will be unintentional rest and wasted training time.

The workout should be designed to only include intended, anticipated, and programmed rest. Programmed rest may take several forms, from catching one's breath to active recovery. If rest periods are programmed properly, then the trainee won't require active recovery as they will reach the desired level of energy expenditure during the immediate work interval and simply catching their breath will satisfy the rest requirement before they move into the next work interval. However, weaker and older trainees may not be strong enough initially to create a large enough magnitude stress so active recovery becomes useful as it allows accumulation of work and elevates stress without overwhelming work and recovery capacity. Active recovery is a lower work rate activity that allows limited recuperation from the previous higher intensity portion of the workout, and does so without completely stopping all activity. Active recovery can (1) utilize slower paced exercise, (2) consist of smaller scale movements like Sit-ups, Romanian Deadlifts, or Lunges, or (3) be a lower demand continuous aerobic activity like jump roping. The total load (volume and intensity) should be no more than 33-50% of the lightest load of the week.

Including endurance activities in a strength program is fairly straightforward; one to three days of endurance work should be programmed on training days that won't interfere with the recovery for strength. Endurance conditioning shouldn't take the place of rest days. The body must be allowed appropriate recovery. Conditioning should also not be placed the day before heavy training days. In most programs, sustained endurance training should go on Saturday morning since there will be about two days of recovery before the following Monday workout.

Efficient conditioning programming targets specific muscle groups and will not use the same musculature recently trained or that will be trained in the next several days. For example, doing a lot of Bodyweight Squats on the same day as doing Squats in the weight room would be counter-productive and should not done, especially if high repetitions are used in the Bodyweight Squat. If Deadlifts or other pulling exercises are scheduled, then lots of Kettlebell Swings are not prudent as part of a multi-element training session. It is best and easiest to use movements and exercises that are not native to the strength program being used. Branching out away from Squats, Presses, and pulls and including novel exercises in the conditioning portion allows the body to improve in endurance while at the same time developing mobility and not interfering significantly with strength gain. Exercises like Kettlebell Swings, Thrusters, jumping, and agility drills force the body to adapt to new movements and are very useful in this aspect. If a trainee has specific endurance goals, then their high-intensity conditioning will reflect that. Unless otherwise noted, recommendations are based on improving general fitness.

Types of Trainees

Trainees will differ in that they have unique anatomical and physiological characteristics based on their genetic composition and recent training history (or lack thereof) and this will dictate programming for effective fitness gain. Improving an aspect of fitness that is lacking will improve total fitness. The key for all trainees is to take an honest look at their abilities, identify deficiencies in strength, endurance, or mobility, and improve upon them to elevate overall fitness. By knowing what to work on, a trainee will be able to choose and utilize effective program templates laid out later in this chapter. First, however, we need to discuss the various types of trainees, ranging from the beginner to the very experienced.

Beginners are typically those that aren't adapted to any type of training and lack both strength and endurance. The strength chapter pointed out how establishing a foundation of strength is a requisite for other adaptations, including endurance. It wouldn't benefit a beginning trainee to try and build endurance only without establishing a strength base - a strength base will substantially augment their capability to improve endurance. This means that all beginning trainees will begin some sort of linear strength progression. As pointed out earlier, the best strength tool is the barbell, but not all facilities are equipped with plates and bars, nor do all fitness trainees have access to this equipment. Some trainees may only have access to their fitness facilities machines. Others may only have dumbbells as their source of free weights. Other trainees may not be strong enough to use the barbells that are available. In any case, we'll recommend using what the trainee is capable of using and what is available. Once strength levels improve, converting over to barbells will help develop fitness optimally. Most beginning trainees will include some sort of high intensity endurance element into their training. These endurance workouts need not be violent bouts of blistering activity. Instead, the "high intensity" will be relative to what that person is used to (e.g. speed walking, described below).

As trainees progress, their strength will continue to develop as well as their relative "high intensity" in their endurance workouts. If a trainee aims for general fitness, then their program will always revolve around a proper strength program with additional high intensity endurance training. If a trainee aims to be exceptionally strong, but still conditioned to the point of being able to partake in fun activities, then they will have a focus of strength with a sprinkling of high intensity endurance. Other trainees may want to increase fitness to apply into a job or recreational activity, and their programs will reflect these necessities or goals. Let's take a closer look into these different types of trainees.

Sedentary trainees are individuals who have not had any significant exercise in at least one year. The fitness industry makes its money by preying upon the sedentary by promising quick gains and easy methods. We apologize up front; we provide no easy way. Consistent hard work over time is necessary to get fit.

When a trainee avoids activity, their body adapts to the lack of activity. New activity must be introduced carefully. These trainees will be weak with low endurance, may potentially have inflexible muscles, and poor range of motion from lack of activity. They may lack good muscle integrity and have higher body fat levels. The first order of business is to begin strength training as soon as possible, and this is best done with linear progression with *something*. As described above, trainees may have equipment limitations and should use what they have. In other cases, the trainee may have strength limitations and should use whatever equipment allows them to complete the standard repetition ranges safely through a full range of motion. If the trainee is unsure, then they should begin with machines. Refer back to the Strength chapter for various types of linear progressions with machines, dumbbells, and barbells. When in doubt, stick to the three sets of five repetitions formula.

During this linear progression, the "no longer sedentary" trainee should add *speed walking* to the end of their training days (the trainee is training for fitness as opposed to meaningless 'working out'). Sprint coach Barry Ross preps some of his sprinters for track season by having them walk 15 minutes as fast as they can (13). The trick is walking *as fast as possible* for the duration. This will act as the high intensity endurance training since it will be more intense than anything to which the sedentary trainee is currently adapted. An easy method to gauge progress over time is to begin walking and at the 7:30 minute mark, turn around and walk back. Each day the trainee should aim to walk further than the previous session. Doing this three times a week for four weeks after a normal strength workout is a very simple way to generate a baseline of endurance for future higher intensity work.

After four weeks of the machine linear progression, the trainee can either convert over to using barbells, dumbbells, or use the program in the strength chapter that integrates dumbbell work with machine work. The trainees with equipment limitations will sustain progress on whatever equipment they are using, yet they will eventually progress to the point that barbells will be necessary.

After about four weeks of speed walking, trainees will typically reach a threshold where improvement slows to a crawl or stops, at that point single activity intervals with an exercise rower or stationary bike are integrated into the program. Rowers are excellent tools for beginners because they have zero impact (the user is sitting) and the movement works the knees, hips, shoulders, and elbows through a large range of motion which uses a large amount of muscle mass. The authors have placed children and grandmothers on exercise rowers; they are accessible to everyone. The stationary bike is a distant substitute since the arms are not included in the movement. The elliptical is a terrible choice because of its limited range of motion in the body's major joints, but more specifically because it is an unnatural movement pattern which is not reflected anywhere in human movement, other than on the machine itself. A rower is the first choice here. If one isn't available, use a stationary bike. If none are available use what you have.

Begin by using the rower for intervals. These intervals can be gauged by distance (as logged on the machine's onboard computer) or time. The simplest method is to row for 100 meters or one minute. Rest for one minute and repeat. In the first session, five intervals can be completed and progressed up linearly over time to reach ten total intervals. The next progression would have the trainee aim to row five intervals with maximal or near maximal efforts, followed by an increase in distance from 100 to 250 meters. This progression will still be limited by absolute strength, but the trainee will have been training consistently for at least 3 months before successfully completing five maximal effort intervals of 250 meters on the exercise rower. At this point, the trainee can continue the progression by increasing the distance to 500 meters. After completing several workouts of maximal intervals at 500 meters, the other forms of high intensity endurance training can be introduced into the program to add variety and mobility challenges. Generally the easiest, and most common, means of accomplish this is by the introduction of calisthenic type exercises.

Improving strength throughout this progression is necessary and helpful as it will improve the baseline of endurance, visually refine musculature, and improve metabolic function. In the 12-week example below, remember that these activities are initially performed three days per week and occur along with a linear strength progression. As with any exercise progression, it is a gentle one, we pay attention to the individuals response to training sessions and to their adaptation over time.

Week	Exercise	Intervals	Duration	Distance
1 to 4	Speed Walking	1	15 minutes	As far as possible
5	Rowing	5	1 minute	100 meters
6	Rowing	7	1 minute	100 meters
7	Rowing	9	1 minute	100 meters
8	Rowing	10	1 minute	100 meters
9 and 10	Rowing	5	As fast as possible	100 meters
11 and 12	Rowing	5	As fast as possible	250 meters
13 and 14	Rowing	4	As fast as possible	500 meters

It's important to note that this progression would have been much faster and garnered a higher fitness gain had the trainee been stronger at the outset. Strength allows the trainee to push harder and create higher rates of work and also allows the trainee to endure higher amounts of work in a given week, which reduces soreness and injury. A stronger trainee is a robust trainee.

Twelve weeks is presented here, as it is an easily structured amount of time, sufficiently long to produce significant gains in fitness. For a rank novice fresh off the couch, the strength progression should consist of a linear progression. It can be ideally conducted on barbells or it can be done on machines for the first four weeks, a mixture of machines and dumbbells in the second four weeks, and then an introductory period of using barbells in the third four weeks.

Month of Training	Equipment Used	Rationale
1	Machines	Weak, lack of motor ability
2	Machines and Dumbbells	Addition of mobility element
3	Barbells	Best strength stimulus

Some sedentary trainees, especially those in their late teens and twenties may be capable of beginning barbell in their first week of training. This should be encouraged, even if they are only able to use a 15 kg (33 lb) or 20kg (44/45 lb) bar. Learning the exercises is important here as we want to make sure that the trainee is doing the lifts correctly and through a full range of motion (see later exercise description chapters). Do not get in a hurry to increase the weight on the bar. Added weight on the bar does not necessarily indicate strength increases if the target exercise started as a full range of motion squat but has devolved into a quarter squat using heavier weights. Beginning trainees will benefit more from the accumulated work of squatting, pressing, and deadlifting through the complete range of motion over time as opposed to handling too much weight too soon through a restricted range of motion.

160

Calisthenics provide a nice forward transition from relatively lower intensity intervals with traditional endurance exercise because they introduce moving through multi-directional space with body weight and gravity as the form of resistance. This develops mobility and is an excellent primer for the next progression to intervals where there is added external resistance. And this transition is necessary, if we jump directly to high intensity endurance training with implements (Kettlebell, Medicine Balls, or even various barbell movements), we do not allow the body an opportunity to adapt sufficiently. Before implements we need to condition the body with similar movements using the lighter, but still significantly heavy to the beginner, load of the body. After three months of some kind of resistance training, the trainee (male and female alike) should be capable of doing a few Push-ups and Bodyweight Squats. This means that the trainee is capable of doing a Burpee, a frequent centerpiece of calisthenic based intervals (refer to the exercise description chapters if this exercise is unfamiliar to you). For a trainee, being able to do Burpees is both good and bad. It's good because the ability to do this introductory calisthenic exercise marks progress and it is and incredibly effective tool in developing high intensity endurance. It's bad because doing them uses so much musculature and energy that it is an incredibly tiring exercise. Some people would call doing Burpees the opposite of fun. No one would argue their effectiveness.

Integration of Burpees is fairly easy. Substitute them into the program in the place of rowing intervals (or running or cycling). Start with three sets of ten repetitions. Each set of Burpees needs to be done as quickly as possible followed by ONE minute of rest. Remember that incomplete recovery is key here. Over time it is a simple approach to alternate this Burpee interval workout with an interval Rowing workout. If the trainee successfully completes all the repetitions and sets, tolerates to workload, and is not significantly sore when they come into for their next workout, increase the number of sets to four while maintaining the same one minute rest period. In most young adults after two Burpee training sessions they will be ready for this increase. After two further Burpee workouts, the load is increased to a total of five sets of ten repetitions. As progression is planned after two Burpee workouts, and those workouts are alternated between Rowing workouts, progression occurs after a week's worth of total training time. This is our rudimentary guideline for increasing the stress from high intensity endurance interval training - progress the stress by increasing total work or rate of work or decreasing rest on a weekly basis.

Basic Burpee Progression

Workout	Sets	Reps	Rest
1 & 3	3	10	1:00
5 & 7	4	10	1:00
9 & 11	5	10	1:00

(Rowing is done in the even workouts in this example)

The rate of progression doesn't have to be this fast; doing 50 Burpees in a workout is no small task and some beginners will receive quite a benefit from sticking with three sets of ten for a while, followed by progressions as small as a single repetition increase. If unsure, slow the progression, perform the workout as written, and assess physical feelings during and post-exercise. Doing sets of Burpees is not intended to feel like a day at the spa, there will be a general sensation of distress - not a fun thing, but normal. Substantial nausea during (to the point of interrupting the workout) or immediately after training is not useful. It indicates that there has been too much work done too quickly. If this is repeated frequently, we push the body towards Selye's stage three, overtraining. At the first twinges of nausea one should immediately recalculate and slow their work rate to avoid detrimental long breaks spent hunching over in a bush or in the bathroom. Being able to push ones self so hard as to induce vomiting may be a badge of honor to some, but it is not a useful means of increasing fitness or quantifying how hard you are working. It may make for interesting internet videos or conversation but it primarily smacks of poorly individualized, controlled, and implemented workouts. If it happens once, not a problem, we learn about our exercise limits and we adjust how we exercise to avoid it in the future. If we intentionally program to induce it, we are not being responsible professionals or trainees.

Other calisthenic exercises such as the Pull-up, Push-up, and Bodyweight Squats are also useful in high intensity endurance training. Push-ups and Squats are already used as part of the Burpee but can be programmed singly as part of an interval. Not every trainee will be capable of doing a single Pull-up even after the three months of strength work. Do not fret about this, it will come over time with further training and commitment. If one is capable of a bare minimum of two or three Pull-ups, then the exercise can be used in combination with Push-ups and Bodyweight Squats as the next phase of calisthenic interval transition. Grouping all three exercises together in rapid succession is a good way to work the entire body. Since the goal here is a stepwise encroachment on work capacity over time until fatigue is reached, then use of sub-maximal repetition sets. Exercises activating smaller muscle mass will use relatively fewer repetitions, those incorporating large muscle mass will use relatively higher repetitions. The importance of "sub-maximal" cannot be overstated, using maximal repetitions in a single set produces profound fatigue too soon and fails to produce the metabolic homeostatic disruption we intend. An example that might be used on a beginning young adult male could include three Pull-ups, seven Push-ups, and ten Bodyweight Squats. By repeating sets of those exercises in sequence - Pull-up/Push-up/Bodyweight Squat and repeat - a novel, whole body, and effective exercise stress will have been produced. This interval workout can be inserted into a rotation. This interval workout would be done on one day of the week, then interval Rowing would be done the next scheduled day of intervals, then, Burpee intervals would be next on the schedule.

A beginner's progression can be treated in a similar manner as with Burpee intervals, with intervals of prescribed repetitions. In the beginners progression below, 3 Pull-ups, 5 Push-ups, and 7 Bodyweight Squats are the base repetitions for each round (each individual exercise in a round is a set). The term "round" is a nebulous term that has to be specified for each workout designed. It could be as simple as one set of each exercise equals one round. Later we will find that different exercises, sets, and repetitions can be included in rounds in a workout. Here, for the beginner, there are two passes through the 3/5/7 repetition exercise organization in a round (3/5/7 Pull-up/Push-up/Bodyweight Squat followed immediately by 3/5/7 Pull-up/Push-up/Bodyweight Squat). One minute of rest follows each round, and as the exercise rounds are completed as fast as possible this rest, although providing incomplete recovery, is a necessity in order to complete the subsequent rounds at a fast enough work rate to produce fitness gain.

Calisthenic Interval Progression

Workout	Sets per Round	Rounds	Rest	Total Reps
1 & 2	2	3	1:00	120
3 & 4	2	4	1:00	160
4 & 6	2	5	1:00	200
7 & 8	Maximum repetitions in 5 minutes	1	None	Variable

A deviation in the round progression is seen in workouts 7 and 8, where the given exercises are performed for as many repeats as possible within a five minute period. Essentially the trainee is repeating the 3/5/7 repetition scheme sequentially as many times as they can in five minutes. It is important to note how many passes through are achieved as this number can be used as a benchmark for later comparison to demonstrate fitness gain. This type of workout is also a potent training stimulus. In fact, this organization, repeating exercise and repetition cycle above as many times in possible for five minutes can easily be used for beginners who possess a modicum of work capacity. However most trainees would benefit by being eased (a relative term) into this training organization by using the progression above before attempting the 5 minute session.

At this point, the trainee is "not so sedentary" and will have been strength training and participating in some kind of high intensity endurance training for four months or more. They are now ready and able to begin utilizing implements and exercises described in later chapters to creatively (but logically) structure workouts. Even though the exercises will be different, they follow the same principals and protocols of the programs presented so far. Utilizing different exercises and different organizations of maximal effort and interval training will help drive continued fitness progression.

Weak Trainees are individuals who have established endurance levels through LSD or even high-intensity methods, yet are limited in their force production capabilities. This trainee would benefit from getting stronger since strength will improve their endurance capability by having higher rates of work (increased work speed) or sustaining lower amounts of work for longer (increased duration of work) *assuming appropriately structure endurance training has been included in their program.* Even if a weak trainee merely maintained their physiological endurance yet improved their anatomical strength, they will still have a net increase in endurance due to the increase in force production. Another reason why increasing strength is important is that being weak prevents the trainee from pushing hard enough to garner a deficit in substrates and produce an adaptive stress. High intensity conditioning isn't nearly as effective when a trainee lacks a history in strength training - they can't work hard enough. But realize that this is only an inconvenience not a problem. The rate of fitness gain will just be slower until the strength deficit is treated.

Weak trainees can utilize a simple linear strength progression with additional high-intensity endurance training. In practice, walkers, joggers, cyclists, or anyone who uses old-school long-slow-distance training who begin high-intensity endurance training will see a rapid improvement in overall endurance. Furthermore, endurance trained individuals who get stronger while using high-intensity endurance training are surprised by the notable acceleration in the rate of endurance performance improvement once they are stronger.

Most weak trainees will need to develop the strength of their lumbar area, hips, and overall posterior chain (all the muscles on the backside of the body active in pushing, pulling, and stabilizing during lifting, sport, and work). Hip extension is the primary movement that makes the body move forward. At the very least, weak trainees should include, at the minimum, the fundamental strength movements described earlier for beginners. A weak trainee is always a beginner in strength training. For them, Squats, Presses, and Deadlifts done regularly will develop strength. A weak but somewhat fit individual benefits from adding Romanian Deadlifts (RDLs), a more hip centric exercise than the standard Deadlift, the RDL and Deadlifts should each be done once a week, but on opposite ends of the week so they don't interfere with each other in terms of recovery and advancement. For some reason, likely simple tradition, Deadlifts are done on Fridays and RDLs are done on Mondays. This is a good place to start but it is not a hard and fast rule.

If the weak trainee has some kind of high intensity endurance base, they can continue their high intensity endurance type workouts, but will need to shift them to follow the time guidelines indicated earlier in the chapter. They will usually need to decrease the overall frequency of high intensity work. It is not unusual to find trainees doing as many as six days' worth of high intensity endurance workouts. Attempting to maintain this frequency in the context of complete fitness training will not allow proper recovery for the newly added strength and inherent mobility training. THERE MUST BE ACTUAL REST DAYS in between training days (go back to the second chapter if this is not intuitive by now). This differs from what is commonly seen in most high intensity exercise programs where it is the norm to have several days of activity in a row. If there is additional structural and systemic stress from intensity work, and it is placed on the body as its trying to go through recovery processes (the day after strength training), full recovery will not be possible. High intensity endurance trainees must learn that not only that "more is NOT better", it is in fact detrimental to fitness gain.

If the trainee comes from a low intensity endurance background (this will be the next largest group after the sedentary), they first need to understand why LSD training will not develop the fitness they desire (explained in the endurance chapter). LSD activity is catabolic, almost muscle wasting in nature (have you ever seen a beefy distance running trainee?). Muscle is what moves us and strength is needed to make a low intensity trainee faster and more enduring. As part of a multi-element program, they would begin a strength program in the same way as someone with a high intensity endurance background, but they too will need to reduce the frequency of their workouts as not only will they add strength work but will also begin higher intensity endurance training. It is extremely common that weak trainees from a long slow distance background be resistant to reducing the frequency of LSD exercise. It is somewhat akin to an addiction. Whether addiction, ritual, physiological sensation, or subjectively positive psychological effect is the basis, many folks will not want to reduce this type of training to make room for better quality and more productive training. However, once they have spent just a few weeks in the new system and they are going faster and regularly setting personal records, they will wonder why they were ever hesitant. It can be explained like this; long slow distance is physical activity (look back at first chapter definitions) that forsakes progress for being comfortable.

The easiest method of introducing a historically low intensity trainee into high intensity work is to have them perform their regular activity for maximal intervals. Long distance runners could run 400 meter repeats as fast as possible using the weekly progression from the interval training section earlier in the chapter. This will allow them to systematically increase the stress and prepare their bodies for alternate forms of intensity exercise. They should then revert back to the sedentary trainee section above and utilize the Burpee and calisthenics progressions. Remember these trainees are naïve to this type of training and the previous programs will introduce them to high endurance exercises gradually. These latter organizations also move the joints through a full range of motion. In running and cycling, the hips go through a limited range of motion, but in a Burpee or Bodyweight Squat, they go through a full range of motion - something that is new to the trainee. This means that take care must be exercised when beginning these calisthenic-based programs and progressing through them. Full range of motion repetitions can cause significant soreness to someone whose primary activity was running or cycling, unless they are gradually indoctrinated into the exercises used.

This approach works well with endurance runners of all levels if their current training is essentially LSD focused. It's normal to reap endurance benefits when getting stronger, and adding in high intensity interval work compounds the improvement. The authors have worked with numerous trainees who have improved race times significantly by getting stronger. A recent female trainee with a LSD training background, weighing 115 pounds (52 kg) improved her strength to the point she can Deadlift 300 pounds (136 kg), do a weighted Pull-up with 45 pounds (20.5 kg) in a harness, dropped her mile time to 6:30, and qualified for the Boston Marathon. In a matter of months she went from being a jogger to being a runner. Abandonment of excessive and non-productive LSD mileage in favor of effective strength and high intensity endurance work made a huge difference. It is also important to note that her total training time per week is less than when it was composed completely of LSD training. More bang for your buck. More time for life's other fun stuff.

Strong trainees are individuals who have developed a foundation of strength, yet haven't conditioned their anatomical structures or metabolic systems to support any activity other than lifting weights (one of the authors strongly resembles this category of trainee). A strong trainee may want to develop his endurance to elevate fitness, to not feel out of breath over menial tasks, or to facilitate participation in professional or recreational activities that require endurance and mobility beyond that developed in a weight room. Some may also want to improve their endurance capacity, as small improvement in endurance may improve recovery between sets during a training session. Discussions with Dr. Mike Stone, former Head of Physiology at the USOC Training Center in Colorado Springs, lead us to suggest that as little as a 3 ml/kg/minute increase in VO_2max above average will improve recoverability between sets. This is an easy goal that can be rapidly achieved with this type of training.

Just because a strong trainee is going to begin a quality endurance training program doesn't mean that he will forgo his strength training. Having a previous specialization in strength and a high level of advancement in strength performance will mean that it will be difficult to make strength gains after adding high intensity endurance workouts. Those who are exceptionally specialized (competitive lifters or other power athletes) may even lose a bit of strength. They won't lose an alarming amount unless they completely omit training relevant to their specialization. About 2% loss maximum if wisely programmed, but as much as 10% could be lost from a strength athlete who minimizes the strength component of training (percentages from author experiences). But these losses are rapidly recovered in a matter of weeks once the desired endurance levels are reached and a focus on strength specialization is restored. And this will pave the way for future strength gains by virtue of enhanced recoverability creating the ability to work harder in the weight room.

For strong trainees doing multi-element training, it may be necessary to reduce total training volume in the program to open up recovery resources to compensate for the additional endurance work. Intensity levels in the strength training should remain at least the upper end of moderate (about 85%) to attempt to stave off strength loss. The easiest way to do that is to reduce the repetition scheme down to triples or doubles and reduce the total number of sets included in the workout relative to the program they were on at entry. As high intensity endurance training is quite taxing and may transiently interfere with strength performance, setting some realistic goals for each strength session is helpful. Essentially, a strong trainee cannot be expected to hit PRs in training sessions during the conduct of multi-element training. Expect and plan for sub-maximal weights compared to personal bests.

One type of method to try and maintain appropriate intensity levels is the ***minimum weight goal*** method. Most contemporary strength programs will use around three to five sets of five repetitions. To reduce overall volume but maintain moderate intensity, the program could shift into doing three sets of triples. However, if there is a higher frequency of endurance training, the trainee may experience a strength deficit to the point where they may not be able to maintain or increase the load every week. In such a case they should lift a minimum amount of weight to ensure they are receiving moderate intensity on a regular basis. One basic guideline is to aim for at least 80% of the 1RM for the lift trained or a use a modest 1RM prediction based on recent training lifts. If the trainee isn't feeling "great", it is suggested to do the first of three sets of triples at 80% 1RM. If the weight feels heavy, to the point they are sure they will not hit all three sets if the weight is increased even slightly, they need to stay with 80% for the remaining two triples. If the weight feels light, they could increase by the weight by 2% for the next set. If the weight is still sensed as relatively light, a further 2% is added for the third triple. If the weight is perceived to be particularly heavy (this would indicate the early symptoms of overtraining), then the trainee could reduce the load for the remaining two triples - perhaps to around 70%.

In most cases, a trainee can simply add relatively high intensity endurance workouts to his existing schedule. Most strength programs have three or four training days each week, so the trainee could add the endurance workouts to one or two days during the week and can even perform a workout on Saturday (assuming the next scheduled session is on Monday). The trainee may choose to lower the frequency of his strength training, but generally speaking it isn't necessary to have more than three high intensity endurance workouts per week. Performing four, five, and even six per week will reduce recovery rates and interfere with the strength maintenance. If the trainee is required to improve his endurance and fitness as soon as possible, then this trainee shifts into more of an "applied fitness trainee" - a designation that receives more explanation later in this chapter.

Strong trainees shouldn't rush into new activities; being strong doesn't make a trainee invulnerable. This concept of gradually conditioning the structures should be applied universally with new exercises, movements, or activities including metabolic activity. This will ensure that they don't get injured or detrimentally sore (despite the propensity of stronger trainees to give maximal effort all the time). It is easier to treat an injured ego than an injured knee or hip. If a strong trainee attempts a maximal effort, multi-exercise workout consisting of Thrusters and Push-ups, as elementary as they seem, he is in for a rather dismal few days afterwards. High repetition Thrusters will leave his quadriceps and gluteals exceptionally sore, the advanced rate metabolic activity may make him queasy during and after training, and the high ventilation rate (rate of breathing) may cause irritation of the bronchii in the lungs and cause a subtle cough for the rest of the day. Although single and multiple repetitions of calisthenic and endurance exercises are easy for the strong trainee, high levels of intensity (lots of repetitions done very fast) aren't necessary or desired. As a beginner in endurance training, a small dose of endurance stress will elicit a nice adaptation. A very large dose is tempting but after producing a huge work output in the first round, the strong trainee will have faded to a point that the subsequent work fails to produce the desired effect.

Strong trainees who lack experience with higher intensity endurance should begin with the progressions outlined earlier in this chapter: speed walking, Rowing intervals, Burpees, and calisthenics. Strong trainees are capable of pushing much harder and do a larger variety of exercise tasks than weak or sedentary trainees. This means that their rate of fitness progression will be higher. The strong trainee could spend as little as two weeks in each phase of walking, rowing, burpees, and calisthenics.

Stronger trainees are also candidates for using unconventional exercises. Things like pulling or pushing a sled (or car), flipping tires, or hitting things with a sledge hammer are frequently preferred activities. "Junkyard training" can provide an adaptive stress, but as with any training, the strong trainee should gradually introduce the movements and intensity when first using them to the workout. The authors have seen many cocky strong guys pull sled intervals for the first time and quickly get reduced to panting, sweating, quivering, functionless heaps. Reaching this level of disability so quickly is not useful and is an indicator of too much stress implemented too rapidly and too soon in the training program.

Generally speaking, when introducing a new weighted or a ballistic exercise into the program, a strong trainee should not do more than 30 repetitions in any given high intensity workout. Thrusters, Kettlebell Swings, and Box Jumps can cause exceptional soreness if carelessly performed for high repetitions. Calisthenics that haven't been normally performed as part of a trainee's previous strength program shouldn't be done for more than the maximal amount of repetitions the strong trainee could do for one set. This cap will help prevent debilitating soreness by dividing the work into several sub-maximal sets. For example, do three sets of eight repetitions of Dips instead of doing one set of 25 repetitions. This method avoids causing soreness in the proximal biceps tendon that would later reduce the effectiveness of Bench Pressing or Pressing in the next training session. It also forms the foundation for progression in endurance.

When introducing normally continuous exercises like Rowing, Sled Pulling or Pushing, or the Farmer's Walk (holding heavy implements in each hand and walking a given distance), the strong trainee should limit the number of work intervals at four. By starting with few intervals, the trainee will avoid too high of a stress, avoid high levels of soreness, and will gradually apply a stress that serves as a transition into this new activity. If using the Farmer's Walk, it should be respected and not done for maximal weight or distance until a progression has been carefully completed. This exercise imparts a tremendous stress of the trapezius, rhomboids, and levator scapulae in the shoulders, all the muscles along the vertebral column, and the tensor fascia latae in the hips. The Farmer's Walk can be done twice per week with one heavy and one light day. This controls the degree of stress and prevents overtraining and excessive soreness. After adapting to the Farmer's Walk and to Sled Pushes, a good workout can be doing a Sled Push in on direction and doing the Farmer's Walk with implements back. This is extremely functional training as both exercises are found in everyday life. Some people also think of them as good fun.

This same concept in making the body accustomed to an exercise before all-out efforts should be applied to running as well. If a strong trainee is to do sprints, or even hill sprints, but has never done them before - or has not done any running in recent history - it is wise to ramp up velocity from moderate to maximal over just a few workouts. Without first doing slower speeds of running, the stage is set for potential and profound soreness and structural failure (injury). It is strongly suggested here that when engaging in new activities and exercises, do less than you think you need to and much less than you want.

Applied fitness trainees are individuals who direct their training efforts towards improving professional performance or recreational pursuits. Applied fitness programs must reflect the unique demands/needs of the trainee's occupation or recreational goal. In all of the previous types of trainees described here, strength improvement or maintenance was an underlying point of emphasis. Endurance also had a role in each trainee type, yet it fluctuated based on the type of trainee. But the end goal was a fairly uniform improvement in all three elements of fitness. The difference between a fitness trainee and an applied fitness trainee is that a fitness trainee is simply training to become fit, an applied fitness trainee is training to improve function within a specific professional or recreational environment. There are three basic characteristics of an applied fitness program:

1. Applied fitness training is specifically intended to improve performance in a job or activity.

2. Applied fitness training program composition reflects the fitness element demands of the job or activity.

3. Applied fitness training should not interfere or hinder, physically or temporally, the job or activity.

The *professional population* of applied fitness trainees generally consists of individuals whose occupation and/or livelihood are dependent on their fitness. This includes military personnel, fire fighters, and law enforcement, but even reaches into the realm of manual laborers and factory workers. The demands of these jobs vary. Military personnel must be able to carry a heavy pack over long distances and durations and still be able to execute bursts of anaerobic activity in combat or high stress situations. Firefighters or Special Weapons and Tactics law enforcement personnel will have similar demands when performing their job. A traditional police officers may not carry a significant extra load, but they require a similar level of anaerobic capacity, as they too are called upon for periodic bouts of high to extreme exertion. These occupations demand fitness not only to perform the job well, but to protect the individual from physical insult and the environment. Applied fitness populations, the working ones, need to be fit to contend with the demands of the job itself as well as achieve certain fitness standards to keep the job. Fitness tests often consist of a baseline of running, calisthenics, and occasionally an implement carry or drag. Many such tests do not reflect the actual fitness demands of the occupation. For example the Fighter Air Crew Test of fitness used by the US Air Force does not predict success or failure in later high G-force testing nor does it physically assess readiness for physical tasks actually performed in a cockpit (14). Superficially it appears as though these personnel need to prepare for two separate tasks; specifically improve fitness for their job, and prepare to pass a potentially unrelated fitness test. This really isn't the case.

By using the principles here and preparing for mission success - relative to fitness - the ability to pass fitness tests will fall in line without special attention.

Manual laborers and factory workers also can't perform well in their job if they have a fitness deficit. Think of hanging sheet rock. Manipulating 4 foot by 8 foot sheets of ground up gypsum rock sandwiched in between layers of heavy paper and fastening them to walls and ceilings is not an easy task. A stronger individual lifts and places a sheet faster than a weak individual. An individual with endurance can put more sheets up without a break. A mobile individual can get the corners and odd sized pieces placed just right. Put all of those elements together and you have an efficient worker who gets in and out of the job site quickly and profitably. But there aren't any recognized physical fitness requirements to be a carpenter, a brick mason, or automotive factory worker. All of these jobs will be easier when the worker has at least moderate strength, mobility, and endurance levels. Now this will be a hard sell to most individuals in such professions as after an eight hour day of labor, time in the gym will not be too attractive. But, we promised bang for the buck, and by spending about three hours in the gym using this system for a few weeks, at the end of the work day there will be more gas left in the tank and less perceived fatigue. Instead of feeling beat and only desiring to plop down on the couch, watch TV, and curling a few cans, there just might be enough time to get the boat on the water for a little skiing - or what ever other fun thing there has never been enough "energy" or time to do before.

The *recreational population* of applied fitness trainees consists of individuals who want to apply their fitness towards improvement in recreational pursuits. Playing recreational sports like rugby or flag football or participating in outdoor activities like hiking, rock climbing, or mountain biking have differing demands. They can benefit from employing a very general fitness program but do require a bit of adjustment to specifically prepare for them.

Rugby, like many sports, is unpredictable; the player will move in all directions, stop and start, sprint and walk, hit or be hit. Combat has a similar unpredictability nature but with much greater ramifications attached to success or failure. Although we cannot know precisely and specifically what will happen in either environment, we do know the types, amounts, and frequencies of tasks and movements associated with both. Rugby is played on a surface that meets certain criteria and is predictable, the weather is moderately predictable in the short term, the basic movements of the game are predictable in type but not time of occurrence or frequency, the interactions with other players is not predictable but the nature of the interactions is describable. In military operations, there will be a given terrain (mountainous, sloped, flat, etc.), a given elevation with a given surface (asphalt, grass, rock, marsh, sand, etc.), and a given weight of carried equipment. So, as in sport, part of the task demand is predictable. The nature of movement within the environment changes based on opposing force actions and can range from remaining motionless for extended periods to bursts of sprinting while simultaneously operating combat equipment. The types of movement are somewhat predictable but the frequency and duration are not.

For both of these examples, the body should be prepared for any movement that can reasonably thought to occur in the given environment. The major joints of the body should have a complete range of motion. The major joints should also be prepared to tolerate stresses applied to them from outside the normal directions. For example, while side lunges are not optimal exercises for improving strength in the legs and hips, doing them periodically will prepare the hip and knees for abnormal directions of stress, something that might be seen in a rugby match. Standard lunges are not a primary strength exercise, but taking the strength built through Squats and applying it during weighted walking lunges can enhance an infantryman's readiness for carrying his ruck and equipment up a mountainside. If you think about it, what is being described here are assistance exercises, specifically *mobility assistance exercises.* These are exercises that are not intended to drive strength or endurance gain so large loads, big volumes, and rapid progressions are not desired. These exercises should be only mildly to moderately taxing and done after the strength lifts but before the high intensity endurance work. The concept is simple: add one, maybe two assistance exercises to funnel fitness gains from strength and endurance training into readiness for the job or activity. Assistance exercises are not included as part of endurance workouts since it would drop the overall intensity and diminish the adaptive stress.

Earlier in this chapter, high intensity conditioning was broken down into maximal effort training, interval training, and sustained endurance training. The applied fitness trainee will need to utilize all three types to improve and maintain their required fitness. They will also need to perform similar activities to what their job or recreational pursuit demands. For example, to get better at running, a trainee needs to run. To get better at carrying a back pack all day, they need time wearing a back pack. For the professional populations that include wearing heavy gear, they will need sustained endurance training wearing an external load. Sustained endurance training will typically be done on Saturday morning and allow appropriate recovery since regular training programs won't resume until Monday. Ruck marching and running time trials will be the standard sustained endurance training done. Trainees should take care that they ease their anatomical structures into this activity. The feet will need time to develop calluses that ward off blisters and the trunk muscles will benefit from a transition period – the concept of gradual conditioning still holds true. There is not just one such exercise solution for every job or recreational goal; there must be a variety of endurance workouts used that are still similar to the job or goal activity.

Immobile Trainees are individuals who have severe range of motion limitations at the knee, hip, trunk, or shoulder joint. Restricted range of motion around one or many joints may prevent proper exercise technique, limit progress, and potentially be debilitating. Severe problems (those that profoundly alter exercise technique) should be corrected by using the methods proposed in the mobility chapter. Progressive loading should not be attempted by those who cannot, presently, assume correct exercise positions. For those trainees with range of motion issues, but not to the extent that they cannot assume an approximation of correct exercise positions, they need to focus on pushing into correct positions with the aid of light loads (its almost like PNF). They will also need regular post-training mobility work until the issues are resolved.

Older Trainees. The term "old" is certainly a subjective term. Middle age is that age where you reach half of the current life expectancy. Presently that is about 38-39 years of age. It is not uncommon to find Olympians and world-class athletes still competing at this age. But as we round the horn on aging, we start seeing a downward slope of fitness that ends with our passage from this mortal coil. The rate of decay in fitness is dependent on the individual. If sedentary, the decay will be more rapid and there will be a profound loss of fitness and function. If exercise is part of the aging process, fitness, function, and quality of life remain elevated throughout the lifespan.

One of the first things a middle-aged and older trainee will notice is that their ability to recover from exercise is less than it once was. By the time the 40s and 50s roll around, a once elite trainee, once able to excel with 10 workouts per week will likely only be able to tolerate 5 per week. Someone of the same age but no exercise background will only be able to initially tolerate 2 or 3 workouts without edging into soreness, pain, potential injury, and no fun.

Older populations can do the same exercises that younger populations can do. The human body possesses adaptive capacity until the very end of life. So the old can get fit. It is possible to set personal bests in your 50s and 60s. The key to fitness into old age is to intelligently progress and stay consistent with fitness training. By being conservative in progression, intensity, and volume, injury can be avoided. It is injury that creates havoc in older adult fitness. By being too greedy or bull-headed and trying to train harder than your body can adapt will lead to breakdown. As age increases so does the time required for recovery from even the most minor muscle tear. An injured older trainee can lose a significant amount of fitness very rapidly, more so than a younger one.

So it is important that there is always less total work, and much more rest included in an older trainee's program. Compared to the program for a 25-year-old, there will be reduced training frequency and training volume (amount of work in a session). The older trainee still does intermittent and continuous endurance work on the rower (low impact for older joints), but will avoid doing heaps of kilometers or repeats. For each decade after 40, a guideline might be to reduce the training volume by 10% compared to a normal adult program. In the strength side, lower volume programs like Wendler's 5/3/1 work well as it controls the training stress quite well, possessing a relatively lower volume of work - nearly perfect for older populations (15).

Programming

Programs should not be rigidly structured templates that apply to everyone, a population, a sub-population, or a group. Instead, they should be thought of as tools used to force the body to make desired adaptations. There is no "one program fits all" approach, system, or equipment; anyone who claims as much is either ill informed or out to make a quick buck (think back to how many different programs and purposes we have described in the previous chapters and up to this point). Trainees should not have to struggle to comply with a given program, but instead should use a program that works *for* them to reach their goals. Good programs serve a purpose without major inconvenience and no debilitating effects. They produce fitness and they do it without misuse of the trainee's time.

The most effective way to improve one element of fitness is to focus solely on that element. This is fine for a single element goal, but that is not the case here with multi-element goals. A solution is to have a higher frequency of training sessions each week, perhaps lifting in the morning and training endurance in the afternoon to avoid interference. But most trainees have limited schedules and cannot devote more than a few hours a week to training. Figure 1 showed that strength gains - the fundamental capacity of fitness - can still exist when combining intermittent (high intensity) endurance with strength training in the same program, although the gains aren't as swift as a strength-only program. A solution to the time issue is found in that overall fitness develops very well with a strength program combined with high intensity endurance training. The gains are not as rapid as specialization but they are quite noticeable. And although they are not comprehensive gains, it is likely that such a program will satisfy the needs of many trainees. If there is adequate time in the trainee's schedule then lower intensity interval endurance work is added. Continuous endurance work is the last priority as is it is specific to augmenting metabolic stores and its inclusion diminishes the rate of gain in other elements.

As intensity-based endurance training develops fitness efficiently for most general fitness purposes we need to understand a little more about it and its programming.

Programming High Intensity Endurance Training

Note: *This section assumes the trainee has a good strength foundation and has gone through the introductory transition methods to high intensity endurance training.*

The three types of high intensity endurance training (maximal effort training, interval training, and sustained effort training) and which days to put high intensity conditioning intensity have been described earlier. Other forms of endurance training have been described as well, but there has not been a discussion about which *kind* of high intensity endurance training to use and how to integrate it into a logical program.

Just to refresh ourselves here, the types of intermittent endurance training that can be used in a multi-element fitness program are:

> ### Maximal effort training
> Short
> Long
> Tabata

Interval training
> Maximal effort interval
> Goal interval

Add *continuous endurance* to the list and you have a comprehensive list of endurance exercise types. While these train some part of endurance, the amount of stress imparted by each is subtly, or not so subtly, different (figure 5).

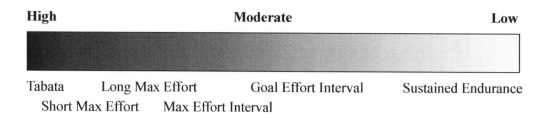

High	**Moderate**	**Low**

Tabata   Long Max Effort   Goal Effort Interval   Sustained Endurance
       Short Max Effort   Max Effort Interval

Figure 5. Relative intensity of endurance training methods.

This intensity relationship isn't surprising. The higher intensity workouts have the highest rates of work and thus provide the highest amounts of stress. Knowing this provides basic guidelines for the inclusion of intensity workouts into a program. In practice, too many of the most stressful types of intensity-based endurance workouts will promote too much structural breakdown and blunt recovery. It's also been observed that the most intense workouts - like Tabata sprints on an inclined treadmill - can only be done effectively more than once a week. The event is so stressful that it requires more time for recovery than the lower stress intensity workouts. Instead of trying to perform another Tabata workout during the week and risk inadequate recovery and moving towards overtraining, another less stressful intensity workout is chosen for inclusion (like long maximal efforts or any kind of interval).

However, intensity endurance training isn't the only mode of training in a fitness program, and we can't ignore the recovery needs of a proper strength program. Since we know how stressful each type of interval workout is, and we know how stressful each kind of strength workout is, we can determine what type of intensity workout to use based on what strength workout is done that day for an optimal combination (figure 6).

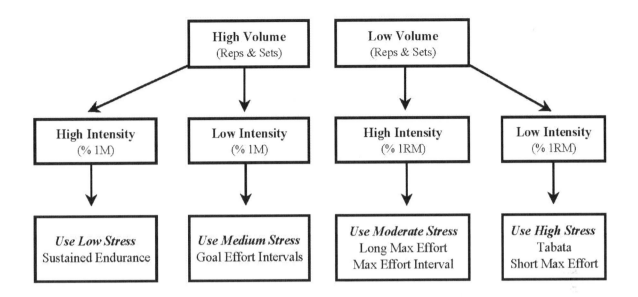

Figure 6. Decision tree for selecting appropriate level of endurance training stress relative to the preceding strength workout.

The decision tree above gives specific intensity workout suggestions based on the strength work done on that day. A high amount of volume in strength work is more disruptive than high amounts of intensity, hence the medium and moderate distinctions for high volume and high intensity days respectively. This may not seem necessary in a linear progression style strength program since all of the days have similar volume and intensity. However, consider the exercise selection on a standard linear progression. One day might have both Squat and Deadlift - this day would result in more volume than a day that only has Squats. Furthermore, a day of only Deadlifts would be considered a higher intensity, and lower volume day compared to a Squat-only day. The volume and intensity designations are relative to the current program, not absolute among all trainees.

Regardless of goal or program chosen, there should never be a question on what type of intensity endurance training to do and on what day (failing to plan is planning to fail). It should be obvious and logical that stresses applied to the body during exercise should be varied, disruption of homeostasis, recovery, and fitness improvement depend on it. The decision tree above can point the coach or trainee in the right direction.

After determining the method of high intensity endurance training to use, how do you know what exercises or activities to use? Generally speaking, the exercises used should not produce any lingering fatigue on the anatomical structures to be used in the next training session - this is the concept of not letting the intensity workouts interfere with the strength program. Let's go through workout structure for the intensity levels, from the most stressful method of intensity workouts to least stressful.

Intense Stress Level

Tabata Workouts - When properly done these are the most stressful version of high intensity workouts. Traditional endurance exercises such as running, rowing, and cycling produce the most stress. Arguably the single most stressful of these is running intervals on an incline treadmill. There is hardly any other exercise more applicable to human activities than running. It is part of most sports and some professions. A four-minute running Tabata workout will push trainees to their limit. Rowing also works well because of the large degree of muscle recruitment coupled with low impact. Cycling would be third in line because of its lower body isolation, but remains effective.

Following traditional endurance exercises in preference are calisthenics and exercises with implements. Thrusters and Deadlifts are extremely effective exercises for Tabata workouts. They do pack quite a punch and the trainee should choose less weight than they think they need (They'll know why after doing ONE such workout with too much weight). The reason they aren't ahead of the traditional endurance exercises is because there is an additional load added to the body weight, there is an eccentric component that may induce micro-ruptures in muscle cell membranes, and there is a large metabolic cost. Together these may diminish the rate of work significantly in the later rounds and alter the exercise stress away from what is intended. That is another reason proper weight selection for barbells and other implements is important - to produce the best work rate.

Not many other exercises are useful for Tabata workouts, usually because the work rate possible is too slow or the amount of muscle mass is inadequate to drive a sufficient global stress. An example of this is using Bodyweight Squats in a Tabata workout. It is quite difficult and does provide a stress, but it's more of a localized muscular beat down rather than an effective workout that creates a total body substrate deficit. A Tabata is a single four minute event designed to cause a systemic stress. Do not fall prey to the temptation to link sequential Tabata workouts using various exercises together to form one Mega-Tabata workout. This is different than a Tabata and the effectiveness in targeting the desired component of endurance metabolism is lost by doing so. Stick to running, rowing, cycling, and the implements above in a single four-minute workout. After all, it's what the original study found to be effective anyway.

Short maximal effort - Multi-exercise workouts are any combination of traditional endurance exercises, calisthenics, and exercises with implements. As opposed to Tabata's where there is a single exercise done, in short maximal efforts two, three, or four exercises from any of those groups are done. Different exercises from the same category can be included more than once to further provide variation. More than four different exercises should not be done. This is a time sensitive process and with complexity and quantity comes diminishing rates of work and longer than desired sessions. Short maximal efforts can be looked at as sub-five-minute sprints. Although it is recommended that they consist of multiple exercises, they *can* consist of a single activity repeated for five minutes. Care should be taken that a single activity workout is composed of elements that last five minutes and can be maintained at a pace as fast as possible for the duration. For most general trainees, running 800 meters or rowing 1000 meters as fast as possible would work (individual tweaking of distance up or down will be necessary).

The workouts using combinations of exercises can be organized in two ways. The first is to set a defined amount of work to be done in each exercise and attempt to complete that work as fast as possible, with a target being in five minutes or less. Keeping records of how long it takes to complete a specific amount of work can serve as comparisons to track fitness gain.

The second way to structure such a workout is to select the exercises and the repetitions and then attempt to complete a round (circuit) of the exercises in sequence as many times as possible within a five minute limit.

The first method can consist of several rounds of work that is repeated a given number of times. This is quite effective because the combination of different activities or exercises can lead to some interesting and discriminate metabolic demands, i.e. combining running, Thrusters, and Pull-ups repeatedly is very different than doing all of the running, then all of the Thrusters, then all of the Pull-ups. These rounds of work can be done with the same amount of work in each round, say for example a total of 20 repetitions per round. Alternatively, and likely more effectively, there is a *reduced work rounds* method. This approach reduces the work or repetitions in each subsequent round. The idea is when a trainee completes the first round of work as fast as possible, he won't be able to maintain that same rate of work throughout the second round if it's an equal amount of work to the first round. Reducing the work in each subsequent round allows for the rate of work to remain high until the completion of the workout. An example of this would be doing three rounds of Thrusters, Push-ups, and Kettlebell swings for 20-15-10 repetitions.

> Round 1 - 20 Thrusters then 20 Push-up then 20 Kettlebell Swings
> Round 2 - 15 Thrusters then 15 Push-up then 15 Kettlebell Swings
> Round 3 - 10 Thrusters then 10 Push-up then 10 Kettlebell Swings

The reduction in repetitions as the end of the workout approaches provides a small but beneficial motivational influence on the trainee. Being able to see the light at the end of the tunnel of hard work keeps effort elevated.

By using compound yet fast movements, lots of energy can be expended in a short amount of time. These workouts typically won't use traditional endurance exercises, unless it is running and the running is kept to less than 50 meters sprints. The rate of work possible with other traditional endurance exercises (we are talking about combined with other exercises here) are too low or the nature of some endurance exercises take too long to prepare for and perform thus

177

causing the workout to last longer than the five minute cap. Remember that loads should be light enough to allow the sets to be completed unbroken, ESPECIALLY in a short maximal effort workout since we're aiming for the HIGHEST work rate possible without doing a Tabata workout.

Moderate Stress Level

Long Maximal Effort - These will consist of the same exercises as short maximal effort workouts, however the time frame is extended to an upper limit of ten minutes. This doesn't mean they should last ten minutes - they work better if they are in the six to eight minute range - but they could extend that long if needed or desired. As before, a workout could consist of a set number of rounds completed as fast as possible, or as many rounds as possible in a specified amount of time. Anything beyond the ten minute limit will result the rate of work decaying severely.

For the same reasons that we ignored traditional endurance exercises in short maximal efforts, we can include them in long maximal effort workouts. If we add a 400 meter run or 500 meter row to our previous example, we have extended the workout to the ten minute range. We still prefer the reduced round organization so 3 rounds would look like:

Round 1 - 20 Thrusters then 20 Push-up then 20 Kettlebell Swings then 500m Row
Round 2 - 15 Thrusters then 15 Push-up then 15 Kettlebell Swings then 400m Row
Round 3 - 10 Thrusters then 10 Push-up then 10 Kettlebell Swings then 300m Row

If it took 5 minutes to do the workout prior to adding the rowing, addition of the rowing distance is a finite element. You have 5 minutes of open time for that exercise spread over three rounds. An average person who has trained regularly and is now ready for this type of training should be able to pull about a 2 minute 500 meter split on the rower. If we keep the same 500 meter distance each round, and the time it takes to go 500 meters increases, and it will, we have gone beyond the 10 minute limit. So we cut 100 meters off of the distance in each subsequent round to come in at or under the 10 minute time limit for this type of training.

As the volume of work is higher compared to previous organizations, there will be lower the average work rate making this a more moderate stress on the body.

Maximal Effort Interval - The trend of single or multi-activity workout continues but now we introduce the element of intervals. Instead of one continuous maximal effort, maximal effort intervals have periods of maximal work rate separated from the next round by complete rest. This type of organization works particularly well for running, rowing, and cycling. Maximal effort intervals of 400 meter sprints are tough, but a different kind of tough than Tabata workout tough (you don't truly comprehend this until you have experienced both - another reason we urge all trainers and coaches to do every workout they design before using it on trainees). Use varying distances of the traditional endurance exercises for a varied response, but

178

remember that the amount of distance per interval is inversely related to the number of intervals (refer back to the maximal effort interval section earlier in the chapter for some progressions of rest periods and work intervals). In a nutshell, the longer the distance, the fewer the reps.

The next option would be to use multi-exercise workouts, how to put those together has been explained above. Let's use our first exercise selection example from earlier and see how to turn it into a maximal effort interval. The first step is to select round numbers and repetitions. Here we are going to use 4 rounds of 15 repetitions per exercise. One more round than in the first example and a reduced repetition scheme is not used here (15 repetitions per exercise is done in each round) as the rest in between rounds eliminates the utility of such a reduction and facilitates another round of work to produce the desired stress.

Round 1   15 Thrusters then 15 Push-ups then 15 Kettlebell Swings – 2 minute rest
Round 2   15 Thrusters then 15 Push-ups then 15 Kettlebell Swings – 2 minute rest
Round 3   15 Thrusters then 15 Push-ups then 15 Kettlebell Swings – 2 minute rest
Round 4   15 Thrusters then 15 Push-ups then 15 Kettlebell Swings – Done

In this example the starting repetitions have been reduced, the rounds increased to four, and there are two minutes of scheduled rest in between each round. The effect is an exceptionally high rate of work offset by rest, a much different stress than doing it all in one bout, and more importantly a lower level of relative stress.

Medium Level of Stress

Goal Effort Interval - Goal effort intervals are very simple. They are the same thing as maximal effort intervals, but slower. They work best on the traditional endurance exercises. Running 400 meters at a designated sub-maximal pace is a perfect example. This relatively lower intensity allows for more total work to be done. For example, maximal effort intervals at 400 meters are stressful to the point that not many more than four or five can be done in a workout. Pacing the 400 meter runs at about 80-90% of maximal running velocity will allow the number of intervals to climb to six, eight, or even ten repetitions (higher percent pace necessitates lower interval repetitions). This approach is particularly useful when training for a military physical readiness test. The trainee would run the intervals at a pace slower than maximal effort but faster than they aim to use during the test. In this case, going faster than the "test pace" is the stress, since it's relatively higher than what will occur on the test proper.

It's difficult to quantify and precisely control pace on multi-exercise workouts (like our Thruster/Push-up/Kettlebell example above), so in practicality it's just easier to do them deliberately slower. The aim is not to completely sand bag the workout, as this wastes a workout, but the goal is also not to complete the work as fast as possible as this defeats the purpose of the workout. One way to control stress here is to lower the loads so the trainee can complete them unbroken (without rests during their execution). Further they don't need to dash to the next activity as fast as possible rather they should methodically move from exercise to exercise and round to round. Think of it as a brisk rain of exercise rather than a storm of maximal effort. A good indicator of whether the trainee pacing the work correctly is that they should feel like they are working harder than had jogging for the same amount of time.

Low Stress Level

Sustained Endurance Training - On low stress days most trainees don't even need to bother doing anything other than the strength workout. General fitness trainees are getting most of what they need for endurance development from the higher intensity endurance work. Also remember that low stress endurance matches up with high volume and high intensity strength training - and the trainee should be decently tired from a hard lifting workout. The applied fitness trainee may need to include some specific low intensity endurance exercise that helps their prepare for their job or recreational sport. This could be some marching with a full rucksack or running at a slow pace for a time consistent with the endurance chapter guidelines for mileage and distance goals. It is suggested here that this type of training occur on Saturday mornings so recovery can occur by Monday's workout. Even with this as the only activity and almost two days to recover, do not go long or fast. Follow guidelines and don't get crazy.

Program Templates

This section contains the actual programming templates to improve multi-element fitness. Please understand that this is the culmination of the information presented thus far in both this chapter and the entire book. Since it would be impossible to cover every possible scenario that could occur relative to fitness and fitness goals the program templates are organized by the types of trainees that have been described above. Each template includes the requisite strength training with added intensity-based endurance training. Specific high intensity endurance workouts aren't given, however the guidelines for constructing these were described in the previous section. Based on the stress designation in the template, the trainee can refer to the types of endurance training that apply the given stress.

Programs for Sedentary Trainees

Phase I – Machines
This program is designed for a sedentary person who is extremely limited in their physical capabilities. Some trainees may not even be able to manipulate dumbbells very well or even do one Bodyweight Squat without assistance. This program creates a strength foundation with machines before transitioning to more effective free weight exercises. The program is very elementary:

Monday	**Wednesday**	**Friday**
Leg Press	Leg Press	Leg Press
Machine Bench Press	Machine Press	Machine Bench Press
Lat Pull-Down	Machine Row	Underhand Lat Pull-Down
Back Extension	Sit-up	Back Extension
Speed Walking	Speed Walking	Speed Walking

All exercises included here - not including Back Extensions and Sit-ups - will be done initially for three sets of five repetitions for the lowest fit who will then progress up to five sets of five repetitions. More capable individuals will begin with five sets of five repetitions. This repetition scheme is used here as it is an approachable number of repetitions as to not produce excessive soreness in the unfit but is still large enough of a stress to produce a productive strength stimulus. The machine versions of the Press can be either seated or standing, it depends totally on the equipment at hand. Machine Rows will be some sort of horizontal rowing movement either bent over, seated with the chest on a support, or a seated cable apparatus and any of these are fine. Lat Pull-Downs can be done on a rigid machine or a cable machine (described in the exercises chapters). These will shift from a pronated to supinated grip between each workout. Back extensions can be done on any back extension apparatus such as a Roman Chair or a Glute/Ham Deck, or if present on a seated back extension machine. It is not uncommon for such a trainee to need to use a seated ab machine as they are too weak to perform standard Sit-ups. Sit-ups and Back Extensions will be done for three sets of ten. Since any trainee that requires beginning with machines will be too weak to tolerate or derive benefit from complex endurance training, they will begin a simple progression of speed walking at the end of each training session.

Phase II – Machine to Dumbbell Transition
As indicated in the sedentary trainee section above, four weeks are plenty of time for a solid introduction to the machines, yet machines will limit mobility and strength development. This next phase will add in dumbbell work to recoup some of the lost mobility stimulus from using machines, as stated in Chapter 3.

Week 1			**Week 2**		
Monday	*Wednesday*	*Friday*	*Monday*	*Wednesday*	*Friday*
Leg Press	Leg Press	Leg Press	Leg Press	Leg Press	Leg Press
Glute-Ham	Glute-Ham	Glute-Ham	Glute-Ham	Glute-Ham	Glute-Ham
Bench Press	Press	DB Bench	DB Press	Bench Press	Press
DB Deadlift	Cable Row	DB Deadlift	Cable Row	DB Deadlift	Cable Row

Note the addition of the Glute-Ham Raise; this exercise trains the leg and hip musculature that are neglected in the Leg Press. Not all gyms are equipped with these apparatus and if not present stick with the Back Extension. This template maintains the alternation of machine Bench Press and Press and will also cycle in the use of dumbbells for the same movements. Dumbbell Deadlifts and Rows are alternated to round out the full body workout. Continue the Speed Walking endurance progression at the end of each training session.

Phase III – Barbell Linear Progression with Endurance Training
After the transition phase of working with machines and dumbbells, the trainee will be ready for a barbell program. This program may require some trainees to find a new, better gym that allows them to perform all of the lifts, especially the Squat and Deadlift (some modifications are described in the exercises chapter).

Monday	**Wednesday**	**Friday**
Active Warm-up	Active Warm-up	Active Warm-up
Press, 3 sets of 5	Bench, 3 sets of 5	Press, 3 sets of 5
Squat, 3 sets of 5	Deadlift, 1 set of 5	Squat, 3 sets of 5
Pull-ups, 3 sets for reps		Chin-ups, 3 sets for reps
Moderate Endurance Stress	Intense Endurance Stress	Moderate Endurance Stress

This program is a simple linear progression with intensity based endurance workouts added onto it. The linear progression meets the strength training requirements with two Squat workouts, one Deadlift workout, alternating Bench Press and Press, and Pull-ups and Chin-ups. Each training day includes a short endurance workout. The choice of free weight exercises enhances mobility. The program helps weak trainees develop their strength and musculature but also allows them to establish, maintain, or build other fitness levels. A low or high intensity endurance trainee that lacks a strength training background would build quality strength on this program and their endurance ability will improve in concert with the strength increases.

The linear progression portion of this program shouldn't progress too quickly. It is better to accumulate work in Squatting, Deadlifting, and Pressing regularly with gentle increases over time instead of trying to add too much weight on the bar. Strength means more than moving more weight from point A to point B, it occurs because the anatomical structures have been conditioned to apply and withstand higher forces. The Bench Press and the Press will alternate every training session in one week then the following week there would be two Bench Press days and only one Press day. The weight should increase five to ten pounds on the Squat or Deadlift and five pounds on the Bench Press and Press. As the progression continues, smaller jumps will be necessary; 5 pounds on Squat and Deadlift and two pounds on the Presses (this is why it is important to have the essential tiny metal plates). In this template, Bench Presses and Presses are performed prior to the larger lifts. Here, it is so that the Squat or specifically the Deadlift won't induce too much fatigue for the subsequent exercises as they use the heaviest weights - that is a preference, they can easily placed on the other side of the workout order ostensibly to improve the anabolic effect.

The level of trainee should avoid any adaptive stresses on the off days (primarily Tuesday, Thursday, and Sunday). This is important and will allow the normal recovery processes to occur and culminate in readiness for the next training day.

The intensity workouts shouldn't be so stressful as to interfere with strength training. To reduce the chance of over training, the upper limit of stress for each intensity workout should be that listed with the respective lifting day (see earlier decision tree). That is, Monday's intensity workout will be capped at the "medium stress level" while Wednesday's intensity workout is capped at the "intense stress level". Any stress level lower than the cap is acceptable, but maintaining the designated upper limit will help the trainee best control the intensity of workouts throughout the week.

As far as choosing which exercises to use in the intensity workouts, the trainee may need to avoid some movements that correspond with the musculature trained earlier in the session. Acute fatigue will be dependent on how far along a trainee is in their progression; if the weight is relatively light, then fatigue may not be present, while heavier loads will induce fatigue. The trainee should also avoid exercises that place too much stress on the structures that will be used in the next training session. Below are some simple guidelines and recommendations based on what exercises occur on a training day and what exercises occur on the next training one.

Monday - Avoid movements that target the hamstrings like Kettlebell Swings since Deadlifts are on Wednesday. Keep the Squatting volume low (under 50 bodyweight repetitions) since barbell Squats were already performed. Keep Pull-up volume low since the shoulder extensors and grip will be needed for Wednesday's Deadlift. Avoid lots of Push-ups if the Bench Press is done on Wednesday. And avoid overhead work if the Press is to be done on Wednesday (remember that Bench Press and Press alternate).

It is appropriate at this point to program movements like Box Jumps, Rope Jumping, Burpees, running, and Dumbbell Hang Power Snatches. Remember to teach the movement before loading it.

The moderate stress cap will consist of long maximal efforts or maximal effort intervals with one or more exercises included. Repeating sets of 15 to 25 Burpees followed by one minute of rest is a good example of this. Goal effort intervals (part of the medium stress level workout) can also be used, especially if the trainee is tired or feels "beat down". Intensity endurance work can always be dropped from the session if the trainee is exceptionally tired. A good coach will be able to discern this from discussion with and observation of the trainee in the earlier parts of the training session.

Wednesday - Hamstring focused exercises such as Kettlebell Swings are permissible as Deadlifts were done earlier in the session, but the total volume of swings should not be so great that they interfere with Friday's Squat session.

The intense stress level assigned to this day by the decision tree would indicate Tabata workouts or short maximal efforts using the treadmill, rowing, or cycling are desirable. For those who require a larger volume of work, a five minute circuit of calisthenics (Pull-ups, Push-ups, and Bodyweight Squats) could precede the Tabata work.

Friday - This is the most fun day of the week for a program designer. There is free reign on what movements can be included into the workout since there are over two days of recovery until the Monday session. Total training volume still should stay in check, as it always will in properly programmed intensity workouts that use the decision tree. It is permissible in trainees that are ready to increase the total workout time up to 15 or even 20 minutes (if the trainee really has the motivation to do so). Remember: the longer the duration, the less intensity and the less of an adaptive stress there is. Getting sweaty or having the sensation of fatigue isn't an indicator of quality work, but a quantity of work. Any stress equal to or lower than the moderate stress level is acceptable on this day.

If there is a specific need for sustained endurance work, or a trainee simply wants to include some sustained endurance training (some people just want to run because they like to), then this work should be shifted onto Saturday morning and on Friday the intensity based endurance workout should shift back into a sub-ten-minute effort.

Programs for Weak(er) Trainees

Barbell Linear Progression with Endurance Training - Remember that weak trainees typically will have some kind of endurance base and are aiming to get stronger to elevate their fitness. The linear progression immediately preceding this section will be a good starting point and can serve its purpose for at least six months for many trainees. Weak trainees, even those who compete at a high level in endurance sports, usually make the mistake of thinking that they should do a single cycle (meaning 4-8 weeks) of a strength focused program and call it good for the year. This is definitely not the case as strength should be a regular and repeating aspect of every training week of their career. The frequency of strength training may vary but the need does not.

Some weak trainees simply do not train because they have been conditioned by society or sport to want to avoid muscle gain. Contrary to popular belief, the addition of muscle mass, even 20 pounds of it, will not slow an athlete if the majority of that weight gain is in the appropriate force producing muscles. Getting stronger will increase speed while maintaining the endurance that will allow that speed to be maintained longer. The following linear progression (derived from the strength chapter) includes lower repetition ranges to increase strength without adding large amounts of muscle.

Week 1

Monday		Wednesday		Friday	
Squat	2	Front Squat	2	Squat	2
Bench Press	2	Press	2	Bench Press	2
Row	5	Pull-up	5	Row	5
Weighted Sit-up	5	Romanian Deadlift	5	Weighted Sit-up	5

Week 2

Monday		Wednesday		Friday	
Front Squat	2	Squat	2	Front Squat	2
Press	2	Bench Press	2	Press	2
Pull-up	5	Row	5	Pull-up	5
Romanian Deadlift	5	Weighted Sit-up	5	Romanian Deadlift	5

This linear progression varies slightly from the strength chapter in that the chosen exercises are not exactly the same. The Back Squat and Front Squat, Bench Press and Press, Row and Pull-up, and weighted Sit-up and Romanian Deadlift are alternated continuously to vary the stress and to create well rounded hips, knees, and shoulder musculature - having been trained in all the axes of movement. Notice that the standard Deadlift isn't included in the above template. We are limiting stress here for the weak trainee. But it's easy, and should be done at some point, to add Deadlifts to this program. Simply replace the second Romanian Deadlift workout in week two with standard Deadlifts. To keep with the doubles theme, the Deadlift can be done for three doubles. Notice this would have the trainee Deadlifting every other week and doing Romanian Deadlifts every week.

The intensity based endurance workouts are done at the end of the training sessions, and will shift in intensity throughout the week so that the trainee does not overwork themselves. On days that include the standard Deadlift, the trainee should cap the intensity workout at the medium stress level. On any other day, the trainee can cap all workouts at the moderate level while allowing one intense stress level workout each week. A basic set up would include one each of the intense, moderate, and medium level workouts. By maintaining this fluctuation, the trainee gets a varied endurance stress while avoiding the structural break and persistent fatigue that mark the descent into overtraining.

S&C Program – After some time with the previous training template, it is time to transition to the next, more rigorous template. This basic template has been widely used online as well as in a structured gym setting by the authors and numerous other coaches and trainers. It received the name "Strength and Conditioning Program" since it was a basic strength program that included high intensity "conditioning" work and the name was simply shorted to the S&C Program (it has also been referred to as the CFWF program). It's a very good fitness template that can be tweaked in various ways.

FIT

Monday	Tuesday	Wednesday	Thursday	Friday
Press	Power Clean	OFF	Bench Press	Deadlift
3 sets of 5	5 sets of 2	or skill practice	3 sets of 5	1 set of 5
Squat			Squat	Chin-ups
3 sets of 5			3 sets of 5	3 sets as many as possible
	Intensity based			Intensity based
	endurance			endurance

This program essentially stretches two days of a normal linear progression out over four days. This is not a specialization training session so this works just fine in terms of producing fitness advancement. It includes two days of Squatting, one day each of Bench Pressing and Pressing, Power Cleans, Chin-ups, and Deadlifts, all of the fundamental strength exercises. A trainee with an endurance background may consider this to have too few intensity workouts, but this is not the case. There have been hundreds, possibly thousands, of trainees who have improved their overall fitness with this basic template. It is not uncommon to see well over 20% improvement in fitness levels within a year of training.

As mentioned earlier, this template can be tweaked, even if the trainee is using it for the first time. Power Cleans can be done on Monday and the Deadlift can be done on Friday. This would leave Tuesday and Friday for exclusive high intensity endurance training. In fact, this was the original template until it was noted that some trainees neglected to technically complete their pulling movements satisfactorily on Monday and Thursday. The two lifts were moved over to the following day to ensure trainees completed them, and it worked well and the revision became the standard. Dips can also be added into the program on Monday and/or Thursday. Dips, Pull-ups, and Chin-ups should be progressed with bodyweight initially, but later can be weighted to a resistance that allows the trainee to complete three sets of five repetitions.

Squat and Deadlift weight progressions will begin with ten pounds and will eventually taper off to five pound progressions. Press and Bench Press weight progressions will begin with consistent five pound increases, but will later require smaller increments for proper progression (as will all lifts eventually). At some point doing a single work set of five repetitions in the Deadlift will be difficult to recover from or will be unrecoverable. It is prudent to switch to triples in this case to continue progress. Triples subtly reduce Deadlift training volume (it's surprising how much this helps) while still allowing heavier loads to be handled for an extended strength gain progression.

If the OFF day is not taken, the resulting skill day is typically associated with practicing sport, running, or agility technical work. For sport and running practice, no significant intensity or volume should be accumulated, this is time set aside for developing movement patterns not disrupting homeostasis. Agility work that is included should also be low intensity and low volume but even these small amounts will help ready the anatomical structures as joint loading will generally occur a way not typical to a normal training session. For those who don't want an off day but also don't want a formal training day, this is the day where you can do physical activity (go back to the first chapter and review the definitions). So fun activities like mountain biking or walking the dog (who will need it anyway) or any activity that won't constitute an adaptive stress is fine. Whatever occurs, it should not provide a stress that interferes with Thursday's Squats.

As fitness progresses, an additional intensity based endurance workout can be done on Saturday. In such a case, the trainee would vary the stress level of the workouts. In general, only one intense stress level workout should be done each week. That can be done on Saturday but that means that the remaining intensity based endurance workouts during the week could be no higher than the moderate stress level (always refer back to the decision tree). Do not add superfluous amounts of intensity based endurance workouts to this or any template, doing so extends the time needed for recovery, blunts the rate of strength progression, and diminishes fitness improvement.

Programs for Strong Trainees

The S&C Program Part II -The S&C Program can also be used for strong trainees who want to improve their endurance frequency, yet still include a minimum amount of strength work. The progression may be equal or slower compared with other linear progressions - it just depends on what program has preceded it. An intermediate squatting approach could be applied to this template. The first Squat session could consist of a medium lifting stress (e.g. three sets of five repetitions) while the second Squat session could consist of fewer reps and sets with more weight to constitute a heavy lifting stress. Technical work on Wednesday will be beneficial to improve movement efficiency, and the Saturday morning option can be utilized for an additional higher intensity workout.

The first obvious change that a stronger trainee can make in order to elevate fitness is to sprinkle relatively high intensity workouts into their existing programs. However, most strong trainees have developed their strength to a point where any additional work will limit progress in their training week. In this case, a strong trainee who is still receiving a benefit from a linear progression can use one of the programs above – the standard linear progression or S&C program. A trainee who has exhausted a daily linear progression or uses a weekly periodized progression may opt to utilize some of the concepts described in the "Intermediates" section in the strength chapter. Two different loading possibilities are present for a Monday-Wednesday-Friday schedule:

1. Medium-Light-Heavy
2. Heavy-Medium-Light

Intensity based endurance workouts will have an inverse relationship with the lifting stress. Heavy lifting days will include only low intensity endurance efforts while light lifting days can consist of higher levels of endurance stress. Maintaining this fundamental relationship in endurance programming prevents too much stress occurring throughout the week to the point of poor recovery.

Triples to Maintain Strength - This program template was alluded to in the "Strong Trainees" section earlier in the chapter and discussed the "minimum weight goal" method to try and maintain strength.

Monday	**Wednesday**	**Friday**
Press	Bench Press	Dips
Squat	Row	Deadlift
Pull-ups	Calisthenics	Chin-ups
Medium stress endurance	Intense stress endurance	Moderate stress endurance

The big lifts (Squat, Deadlift, Press, and Bench Press) are all done for three triples, with and goal to lift more than 80% of pre-endurance training 1RMs. Although 80% marks the minimum weight target, trainees may do more and use ascending sets to get there. To be clear here the work sets do not begin until the weight has reached 80%, so one might do 80% x 3, 82.5% x 3, and 85% to complete their work sets. All three sets at the same weight, sets across, is the normal approach as long as that 80% or greater is achieved on each set. Unfortunately this method isn't quantified and relies on subjectivity, but when a trainee has a specialization in strength and desires to improve total fitness, something has to give, the body does not have a limitless adaptive capacity. This method is generally reserved for experienced strength trainees who have a better grasp of their capabilities and limits than a normal trainee. Once into the system for a time, they may find is that the weight used in each lift increases on a weekly basis as they adapt to additional endurance stress and develop endurance recoverability.

If this template is used for an extended period of time (three or more months) then an additional Squat workout should be added on Friday. Squatting only once a week will usually result in a slow Squat strength loss over time compared to a program that includes more frequent squatting. This is to be added in after time is spent using the template as written, not added in from the beginning.

As one would expect, the stress level from the intensity based endurance workouts should be planned to fluctuate throughout the training week and there is a need to consider which exercises to include and not include. Monday's workout does not generally include Push-ups (since the Bench Press follows on Wednesday), but Monday is an excellent place to add more variety of movements in the endurance segment, as it is capped at the medium stress level. Wednesday is ideal for performance of a Tabata workout or short maximal effort workout. Friday is open for a variety of exercises (since the weekend will allow substantial recovery) as long as they do not breach the moderate stress cap for endurance. This program can be a transitional program to the "Get Conditioned Fast" program described in the coming "Programs for Applied Fitness Trainees" section.

Programs for Applied Fitness Trainees

As described earlier in the chapter, applied fitness trainees consist of professional or recreational populations that must prepare specifically. This section includes programs that funnel into the trainee's obligatory or desired goal.

Get Conditioned Fast - This program is aimed at stronger trainees who want to get conditioned very quickly. The concept of "one lift a day" is obviously a minimalist approach to strength training, and that's the point. The trainee will accept the fact that they will be unable to gain new strength or even maintain the absolute pinnacle of strength as they will expend significant physiological resources recovering from a higher endurance frequency AND are not presented with large-scale strength stimuli. This type of program done for four weeks has produced an improvement of over two minutes in mile time (in two separate unpublished studies, mile time went from mid 9 minutes to low 7 minutes) in elite level masters strength athletes. This significant result is somewhat offset by a drop in overall body strength by about 10%. At the other end of the spectrum, weak trainees are able to get decently strong on this program as they are far from their genetic potential. One representative such trainee began by Squatting 95 pounds (43 kg) for three sets of five (his limit at the time) and five months later was able to Squat 275 pounds (125 kg) for three sets of five. This means that this template has differential effects on different training populations and can be used to develop the weak points of a variety of trainees effectively.

Monday	Tuesday	Wednesday	Thursday	Friday
Squat	Press	Deadlift	Bench Press	
Intensity based Endurance	Intensity based endurance	Intensity based endurance	Intensity based endruance	Intensity based endurance

The strength scheme is moderate in repetitions, sets, and overall volume. Three to five sets of five repetitions work well to accumulate enough work in a specific lift once a week with heavy enough of a load to help stave off strength loss in the strong trainee and to develop it in the weak. As mentioned previously, the Deadlift is a stressful lift and is only done for one set of five. More sets might cause too much structural and systemic stress that may outstrip recuperative capacity. The intensity based endurance workouts that occur on a strength training day will be short and intense. A cap of 10 minutes is placed on these workouts. On Friday there is no strength training done and two days of recovery to follow so the intensity based endurance session can be longer, working up to 20 minutes if desired or if needed to accomplish an applied fitness purpose. Again, the longer the workout is the lower inherent intensity. Do not try to force maximal intensity training into a longer or sustained framework. For recovery and improvement, the stress intensity of the endurance work should be varied and in general more than two high stress level workouts should not be included in any given week. An example of the five intensity based endurance inclusions could be:

	Monday	**Tuesday**	**Wednesday**	**Thursday**	**Friday**
Lifting Stress	High volume	Light %1RM	Heavy %1RM	Light %1RM	
Endurance Stress	Medium	Intense	Moderate	Intense	Low
Example	Goal effort interval	Tabata workout	Long max effort or Max effort interval	Short max effort	Sustained effort

Going back to the basic concept presented by Selye, some individuals will not be able to recover from repeated episodes of high intensity exercise in that the catabolic hormone cortisol may be persistently elevated and overwhelm the recuperative effects of the anabolic hormone testosterone. The variations presented here help prevent the onset of overtraining while being aggressive enough to produce fitness gain.

S&C Variation for Military (or other similar occupations) - Earlier in the chapter we discussed the unique demands of being a soldier. A soldier/sailor/aviator/marine must satisfy traditionally non-specific endurance assessments (e.g. physical fitness tests that include running and calisthenics) and in some cases job specific endurance assessments (3 mile road march while carrying a 45 pound rucksack for example). Combat itself is predictably highly anaerobic, but its physical demands can occur at any time, in varied states of recovery, in general fatigue, or directly following a sustained effort activity. For example, the landing zone for helicopter is never directly on the objective. In any case, a strong, agile, and enduring soldier is needed to meet the requirements of the modern battlefield.

Here the standard S&C template has been modified to incorporate a broader spectrum of physical demands:

Monday	**Tuesday**	**Wednesday**	**Thursday**	**Friday**	**Saturday**
Press 3 x 5 reps	Power Clean 5 x 2 reps	Mobility	Bench Press 3 x 5 reps	Deadlit 1 x 5 reps	Continuous endurance
Squats 3 x 5 reps	Pull-ups 3 x reps to max	Squats 3 x 5 reps	Chin-ups 3 x reps to max		(ruck or time trial)
Dips 3 x reps to max	Running (400m intervals)		Dips 3 x reps to max	Multi-exercise Endurance	

The strength work remains from the original S&C Program, however Dips are made a regular part of the program. Tuesday's endurance work consists of four to eight intervals of running

400 meters. The number of intervals is inversely related to the intensity; max effort intervals will stay in the four to six range while goal effort intervals will be done for six to eight intervals. This workout will provide the baseline fitness level needed for doing well on the running portion of the physical fitness tests (the distance changes with branch of service). Wednesday's technical work consists of mobility work like ladder drills, cone drills, and abnormal movement drills (movements not normally encountered - but definitely not silly or non-applicable ones). This is the day of the week that the body can be prepared for those weird, random forces to which the body may be subjected. This could alternatively be time spent on a mat for combatives training. Friday's endurance work should be a multi-exercise workout using mostly implements along with a traditional endurance exercise and/or calisthenics. By using implements in the exercises, the trainee will receive a stress that is different than the traditional body weight military physical training to which he is normally subjected. Saturday morning will be the day the trainee puts in his time with a ruck. This maintains the structural conditioning related to the wearing a rucksack and can help tender feet adapt to load, mileage, and footwear. Loads should not exceed 50 pounds in training nor should the trainee run with a pack - this destructive exertion should be reserved for deployments or selection processes. Every third week the trainee could perform a running time trial. This acclimates the training to running the tested distance (potentially at the same location), but also helps prepare them for longer efforts (like a five mile run in 40 minutes). By working strength throughout the week, running on Tuesday, doing mobility work on Wednesday, getting an implement stress on Friday, and undergoing longer duration efforts on Saturday, the soldier adequately prepares his body for his job.

As short as they are, Tabata workouts are excellent for preparing individuals for running tests. However, they shouldn't be used more than once a week. They can be inserted on Tuesday or Friday, but the be weary of adding high intensity endurance training on any more than the few days than indicated here. Overtraining is not consistent with mission readiness.

Dips and Pull-ups are done twice a week as they will help contribute to higher scores on the Push-up and/or Pull-up portions of a fitness test. However, these movements should be weighted as soon as the trainee's strength allows it. It is more important to have Dip strength than to have Dip endurance. Early on in the template's use, the first session of Dips and Pull-ups of the week can be weighted while the second session of the week would done with just body weight. The goal is to progress the weighted movements with three sets of five repetitions and progressively add weight. Later, they should use an organization attributed to Bill Starr that is recommended for Dips, but is also effective with Pull-ups. It follows a basic three week cycle:

Week 1	Eight repetitions with as much weight as can be done for eight repetitions
Week 2	Five repetitions with as much weight as can be done for five repetitions
	Subtract 50 pounds from the weight used and do as many repetitions as possible
Week 3	Three repetitions with as much weight as can be done for three repetitions
	Subtract 50 pounds from the weight used and do as many repetitions as possible

Push-ups and Sit-ups can be added to the template. Sit-ups will work well on Monday and Push-ups on Thursday. These can be done in virtually any repetition and set organization as long as it is a complete range of motion and the added load is more rigorous than required by the fitness test standards (note load is not intended to be endless repetitions here).

Programs for Older Trainees

5/3/1 - In the strength chapter it was stated that "one lift a day" programs generally blunt strength progress in most trainees because of the lack of systemic stress supplied. However, older trainees can benefit from an overall reduction in training stress as their recuperative capacity is very much challenged in a multi-element training program. As mentioned earlier, a strength program that lends itself well to this population and application is Wendler's 5/3/1 program (15). Reviewed in the strength chapter the basic scheme of the program is:

Week	Repetitions	Sets	Intensity
1	5	3	85
2	3	3	90
3	5-3-1	3	95
4	5	3	60

As written, each of the last sets of the workouts are done for as many repetitions as possible to get a near repetition maximum with the weight used. For older populations, cutting the set off by a repetition or two will prevent technical breakdown due to fatigue, contain workload to a recoverable amount, and may help prevent muscle strains. Basically the trainee should stop the last set when they think they have just one repetition left before failure. A typical 5/3/1 program has four days of training that focus on the Squat, Bench Press, Press, and Deadlift along with designated assistance exercises. For the older populations discussed here, the assistance exercises from the original program are not done as the additional stresses from the endurance exercises require recuperative capacity that additional strength work would dampen.

Because of its inherent reduced volume and high exertion level on the last sets, many trainees above the age of 35 or 40 enjoy this program. It allows them to push hard without feeling too beat down. Specifically for our purposes, it allows them to push hard on the fundamental strength lifts, yet still allows enough "energy" to be devoted to endurance training.

Older trainees can do their intensity based endurance workouts on training days, but care must be taken to limit their exposure throughout the week. Four days training is plenty for strength and endurance work - rest is an older trainee's greatest ally. A typical 5/3/1 week will include a day devoted to Squat, Bench Press, Deadlift, and Press. An older trainee should cap their intensity workout stress based on the lift done as follows:

Exercise	Complimentary Endurance Intensity
Squat	Medium
Bench Press	Intense
Deadlift	Moderate
Press	Moderate

The intense stress workout could also be done on the Press day as both the Bench Press and Press are relatively low stresses. This set up differs from the "Get Conditioned Fast" program in that it limits the intense stress workout to only one per week instead of two. One is enough for this population. If an older trainee is feeling extremely sore or fatigued, or appears to be struggling with completing a workout, for any reason - not sleeping, work stress, hangover, or even if there is no explanation for the reduced capacity - then the intensity workout should be dropped one level of intensity (high to moderate, moderate to medium, medium to low, low to rest). Do not be afraid to forfeit a day of training to prevent overtraining and the potential loss of many future days of training and a resulting loss of fitness that goes along with it.

Tying It All Together

The programs above are organized from sedentary, to weak, to strong, and to applied fitness trainees - similar to how a trainee could progress over time. This doesn't mean that a given program can't be done by a different trainee type, they can be. But the trainee, or trainer doing the programming, should keep in mind that the program won't be optimal for populations other than those designated in the text. Anyone can create their own template, but they should consider the guidelines presented in this chapter and throughout this book. Good fitness programs will have a foundation of strength training, additional intensity based endurance workouts, and consideration for mobility applications. Any program that neglects one or more of these elements for a significant amount of time has lost sight of what improves fitness in the short and long term.

REFERENCES

1. Morgan, R.E. and G.T. Adamson. Circuit Training. Bell and Sons, London, 1962.

2. Johansen, P.E. "Circuit" training of normal persons. Effects measured by a cycloergometer. Ugeskr Laeger 126:1238-41, 1964.

3. Kavanagh T. A conditioning program for the elderly. Canadian Family Physician. 17(7):31-3, 1971.

4. Morgans C.M. and W.M. Buston. Supervised circuit training after myocardial infarction. Physiotherapy 58(10):340-3, 1972.

5. Wilmore, J.H. et al. Physiological alterations consequent to circuit weight training. Medicine and Science in Sports 10(2):79-84, 1978.

6. Gannon, R. Science or Supermen. Popular Science 182(5): 62, 1963

7. Jesse, J. Wrestling Physical Conditioning Encyclopedia. Athletic Press, Pasadena, CA. 416pp. 1963.

8. Glassman, G. A theoretical template for CrossFit's programming. CrossFit Journal 6:1-5, 2003.

9. American College of Sports Medicine. ACSM'S Guidelines for Exercise Prescription. 2006.

10. Baker, D. The effects of an in-season of concurrent training on the maintenance of maximal strength and power in professional and college-aged rugby league football players. Journal of Strength and Conditioning Research 15(2):172-177, 2001.

11. McLester, J.R., P. Bishop, and M. Gulliams. Comparison of 1 day and 3 days per week of equal-volume resistance training in experienced subjects. Journal of Strength and Conditioning Research 14(3):273-281, 2000.

12. Tabata, I. et al. Effects of moderate-intensity endurance and high-intensity intermittent training on anaerobic capacity and VO_2max. Medicine in Science Sports and Exercise 28(10):1327-1330, 1996.

13. Ross, B. Underground secrets for running faster: Breakthough training for breakaway running. BearPowered.com, Bellevue, WA, 2005.

14. Maulsby, W. Predictive capacity of the USAF Fighter Air Crew Test. Thesis preliminary data. Midwestern State University, Wichita Falls, TX, 2011.

15. Wendler, J. 5/3/1: The Simplest and Most Effective Training System to Increase Raw Strength. Jim Wendler, Columbus, OH, 2009.

STRENGTH EXERCISES

Strength is best developed through the use of programmed weight training as described in chapter 3. Any exercise where there can be virtually unlimited and small incremental addition to the resistance to movement can produce an increase in strength. As such an effort to list all of the possible weight exercises is prohibitive. The following are descriptions of some of the most useful weight exercises that, when used progressively over time, will increase strength.

Press	French Press	Weighted Sit-up
Dumbbell Press	Lat Pull Down	Back Squat
Push Press	Curl	Front Squat
Push Jerk	Dip	Leg Press
Jerk	Shrug	Romanian Deadlift
Bench Press	Row	Deadlift
Dumbbell Bench Press	Goodmorning	Power Clean
Pull-up	Back Extension	Power Snatch
		Calf Raise

PRESS

This is likely the best overall upper body exercise done with a barbell. It holistically trains the musculature of the shoulders and elbows. It is also quite effective at providing an isometric training stimulus for the entire body below the shoulders as everything between the floor and the shoulders is involved in stabilizing body position.

In the start position for the Press, the feet are placed directly under the hips (figure 1A) - a more narrow stance than used in squatting. Having the hips over the feet puts the thigh and calf in nearly vertical line making it a very efficient supportive position. Depending on the individual, the heels will be about 6-10" apart and the toes will be pointed out slightly. At the other end of the system, the bar will be resting across the shoulders as in the front squat. The only difference is that the elbows will be close to directly underneath the bar (figure 1B). This position allows for more efficient force application to the bar as it eliminates detracting levers. Given that there are anatomical differences in limb lengths between individuals there will need to be some fidgeting, in regards to elbow position forward and laterally, to get the best position for an individual.

The start and the execution of the press is simple but tricky. Simple in that all you need to do is press (push up) the bar from touching the shoulders to full extension (where the elbows are locked) at the top. Tricky in that the mind and the body want to cheat on this exercise, almost involuntarily. When the weight gets a little heavy or the muscles become a little fatigued, a universal pair of technical errors will appear. The first is knee kick. Everyone, EVERYONE, will bend their knees an inch or more and quickly extend them to get the bar started on something they think is at their limit. It's a confidence thing. The strategy is that the momentum combined with muscle contraction will carry the bar up past the sticking point (where the upper arm is parallel to the floor - peak mechanical disadvantage). Lots of people do this and don't even know they are doing it. You have to make a concerted effort not to kick. The second cheat is to cut the press short and not lock out the elbows. Both of these cheats are to be avoided. A true press uses only the musculature of the shoulders and arms to begin and complete every repetition ... of course this is a purist position. There are times when the above rules don't necessarily apply, but of course we also have enough variants of the press to choose from to accommodate any needed variation so that strict execution of the press when used should not be an issue.

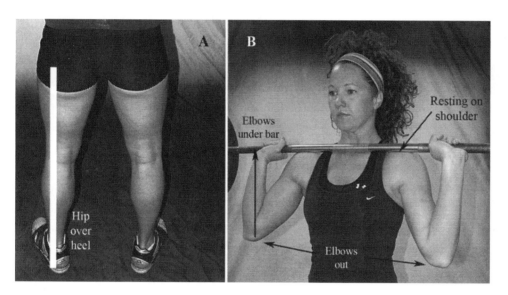

Figure 1. Starting position for the Press.

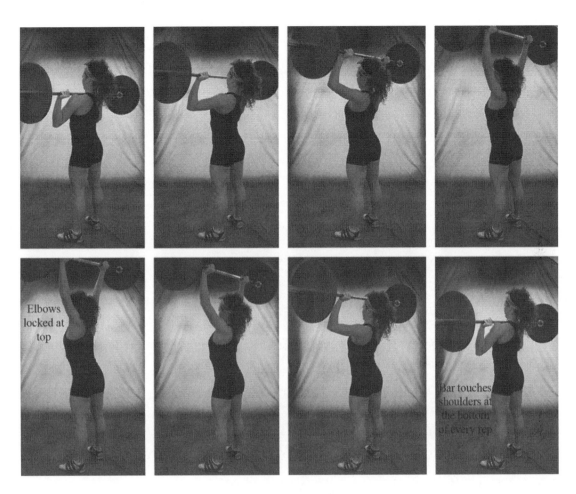

Figure 2. The Press.

DUMBBELL PRESS

The Dumbbell Press is a pretty hard exercise that not only develops strength but develops independent hand control during loaded movement. It combines strength development with enhancing the coordination element of mobility.

The start position for the Dumbbell Press has the dumbbells at the shoulders. One end of each dumbbell should be touching the shoulder - this gives us an objective landmark for teaching and quantifying complete repetitions (figure 1A). The other end of the dumbbells can either be directly lateral (straight our to the side) or be slightly forward (at a forward angle). Since we are mimicking the Press with a barbell, the straight orientation is desired, but occasionally flexibility issues require the angled start position. Each repetition starts and ends in the same location - the dumbbell touching the shoulder and the elbows directly under the dumbbell handle.

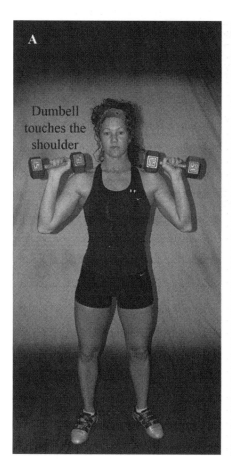
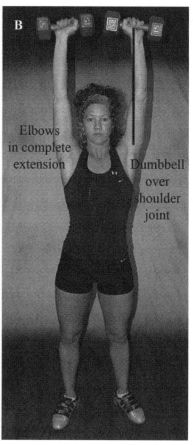

Figure 1. The start and top positions in the Dumbbell Press.

The top position of the Dumbbell Press has the arms overhead with the elbows completely extended (figure 1B). The dumbbells are oriented straight - from left to right - just like they were one bar. Each dumbbell will also be supported directly over their respective shoulders.

It is the movement in between the start and top position that provides us the unique mobility stimulus from this exercise. A novice with dumbbells will find it difficult to make both arms extend at the same rate, they will have a hard time keeping the dumbbells moving up and down along a slightly angled (in) straight line over the shoulders, and that makes slow and steady progress imperative. Staying in control is crucial in dumbbell work. Control of progressively heavier weight is a marker of training success, a marker as important as simple progression in weight lifted.

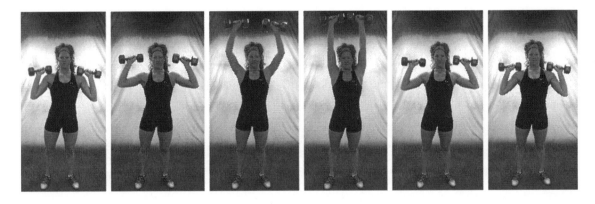

Figure 2. The Dumbbell Press.

PUSH PRESS

This is the exercise that people frequently do when they actually intend on doing the Press. In the Push Press, the knees and hips get flexed and extended very quickly to impart momentum to the bar and assist in moving the weight overhead. The hips and knees PUSH and then the shoulders and elbows PRESS. In that sequence. You can Push Press more than you can Press by virtue of the ballistic hip and knee push. With a velocity component and a strength component, the Push Press is a combination strength and power exercise. It is also a good systemic stressor, as all of the major movers and all of the stabilizing musculature from feet to hand are invoked during the exercise.

The start position in the Push Press is nearly the same as in the Press. The stance is the same as in the Press (figure 1A) however the elbows are more forward in order to keep the bar stable during the early part of the movement (figure 1B). Frequently the descending portion of the hip and knee contribution of the push is called the "dip". The upwards portion is called the "drive". This is a fairly useful pair of terms. A dip is different from any full squat variant. A dip is a very shallow squat, maybe six inches at most (figure 1A). A dip is also quick. The transition from dip to drive is on the order of milliseconds. At the bottom of the dip there is an instantaneous (as instantaneous as possible) change in direction from down to up. The drive portion is aggressive and fast. At the top of hip and knee extension, the knees lock out and the hips move into normal erect posture (figure 2) and then the shoulders and elbow musculature begin pressing as fast as possible. Note that even though the drive is very quick, the feet remain on the floor. In some ways the Push Press shares a movement pattern similarity to the free throw.

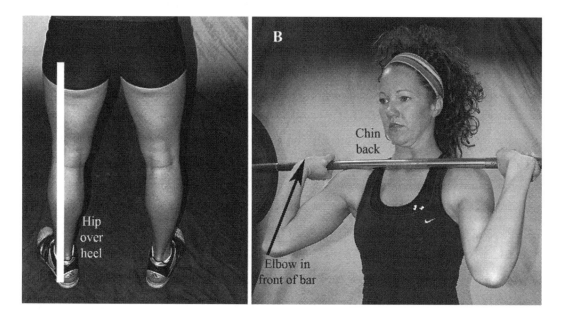

Figure 1. Start position for the Push Press.

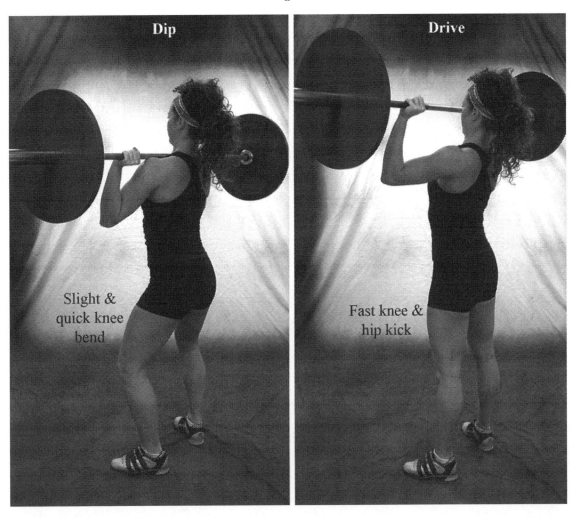

Figure 2. The "dip" and "drive".

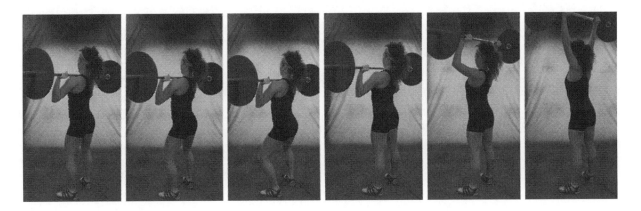

Figure 3. The Push Press.

PUSH JERK

This is a very useful pressing variant that adds a small gymnastic element to the Push Press. By adding a jumping component, a dynamic body movement under load, and a mild balance component, all performed at a high velocity, the Push Jerk creates a potent fitness adaptation stimulus.

The start position in the Push Jerk is exactly the same as in the Press and Push Press (figure 1A). The stance is also the same. As in the Push Press, the descending portion of the hip and knee contribution of the push is called the "dip". The upward directed portion is called the "drive". The dip is again very shallow squat, maybe six inches at most (figure 1B) and is also very quick. At the bottom of the dip there is an instantaneous (as instantaneous as possible) change in direction from the bar moving down to moving up. The drive portion is aggressive and fast. At the top of hip and knee extension is where the exercise differs from the Push Press. Here at the top of the drive, the knees and hips extend completely and there is an actual jump off of the floor (figure 1C). While the body is in the air, the knees and hips slightly re-bend and the feet move laterally up to a few inches (some people will replace their feet in exactly the same spot). This occurs as the shoulders and elbow musculature begin pressing as fast as possible. This produces an effect similar to pushing yourself under the bar. The body mass will drop under the bar into an arms-extended catch position (figure 1D). Simply standing up with the bar supported overhead completes the repetition (figure 1E).

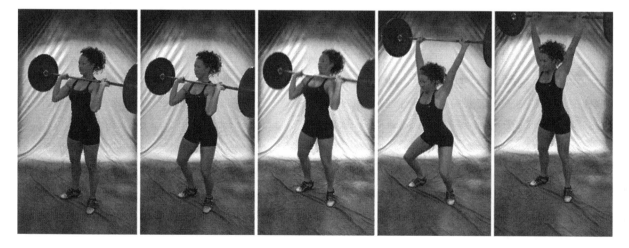

Figure 1. The start position, dip, drive, catch, and finish positions for the Push Jerk.

JERK

The Jerk is not just a strength and power exercise, it ratchets of the gymnastic and dynamic loaded movement elements seen in the Push Jerk and takes it up a notch. So along with the strength stimulus the Jerk produces a profound mobility adaptive stimulus.

The Jerk shares the same initial set up as the Press, Push Press, and Push Jerk. The dip and drive segment of the lift is also the same (figure 1A, 1B, 1C)). It is critical however that maximum upwards velocity is produced during the drive as the movement executed while the body is in the air is more complex. At the top of the drive, the knees and hips extend completely and again there is an actual jump off of the floor. While the body is in the air, instead of skipping to the side as in the Push Jerk, one foot moves forward and one foot moves backward (figure 1D). The distance the feet move is much greater than in the previous exercises. When the feet touch down, the front foot should land directly in front of its hip and the foot will be slightly angled inwards a couple degrees (pigeon toed). The shin should be vertical and the knee angle should be between 90 and 120 degrees. The rear foot should be directly behind its hip with the ball of the foot planted and the heel up. The trailing knee should be slightly bent. The bends in both knees are important for getting the depth needed to get under the bar. The bend in the rear knee allows the vertebral column to be maintained in normal extension. Straightening the rear leg forces the assumption of an exaggerated lordotic curve position (low back is arched excessively). Keeping the rear knee bent also enables better overall control of the body-barbell system. When the feet touch down, they should hit simultaneously and they should not be in line one in front of the other (tight-roping). They should be directly in front of and behind the hip joints (figure 2). The body should not make any net movement forward or backward. It should be fairly easy to see why this exercise is considered a mobility enhancing exercise as it creates a balance and coordination stress.

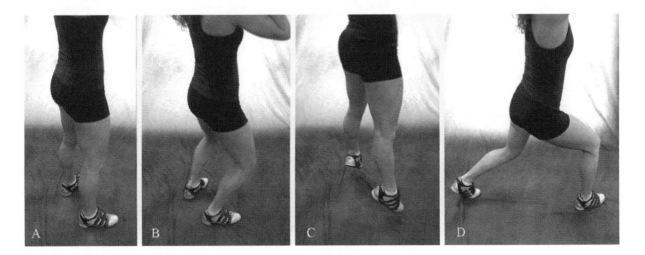

Figure 1. Critical positions of the Jerk.

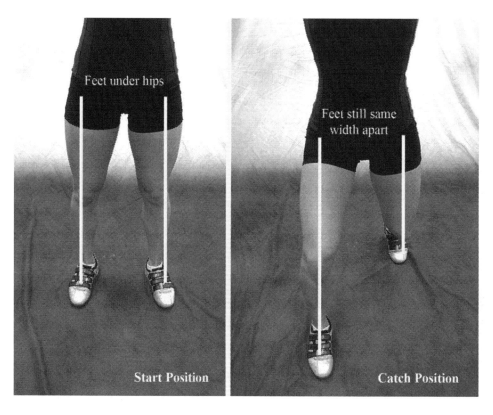

Figure 2. The feet move directly forward and backward to get into the catch position.

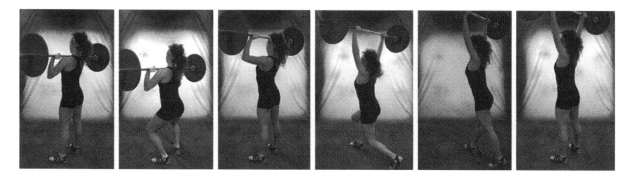

Figure 3. The Jerk.

BENCH PRESS

The Bench Press is seemingly everyone's favorite exercise. "How much can you bench" is typical alpha-male gym conversational fodder. This is way too high of a status for this exercise, although it is an important exercise for developing the chest and shoulder's ability to produce force along the anterior-posterior axis. The start position of the Bench Press is lying down on a flat bench. The feet should be flat on the floor and point slightly out (figure 1A). Contact between a solid surface and the feet is important as this is where body stability comes from during the exercise. If you are a healthy individual with no low back issues, keep your feet on the ground. The knees should be directly over the ankles. If you are looking at angles, the ankle and the knee should both be at approximate 90 degree angles. The low back should be in an arched position, a normal postural arch, and one should be able to slide at least a flat hand under the low back without resistance. The shoulders should be tensed by squeezing the shoulder blades together. The bar should be gripped in a double overhand grip with the *thumbs wrapped around the bar* (figure 1B). About 12 people die each year from Bench Press accidents - don't use a thumbless grip and risk becoming a statistic. There is no performance advantage to using a thumbless grip. The hands should be on the bar at the width of the out spread elbows (figure 1C). In this position, at the bottom of the bench press the forearms will be vertical, making for a more efficient force transfer and a more complete range of motion exercise than any other grip width.

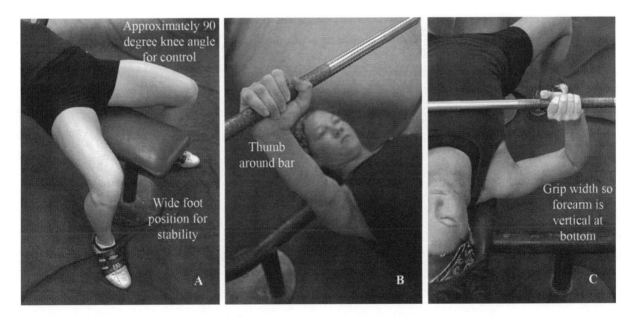

Figure 1. Essential positions in the Bench Press.

More weight can be lifted with a wide grip and a longer bar travel is found with a narrow grip, both which can be used to achieve specific goals, but development of the complete shoulder and elbow range of motion is our goal and is best achieved with the elbow width grip. Aside from vertical forearms, the bottom position of the Bench Press is also described by a chest touch point at mid-sternum. This is best achieved by using an elbows out position. Each repetition of the Bench Press starts at the top with elbows extended, is lowered to make gentle physical contact with the chest at mid-sternum, then is pressed back up to full elbow extension. Throughout the movement the bar should follow a straight line between the top and bottom position.

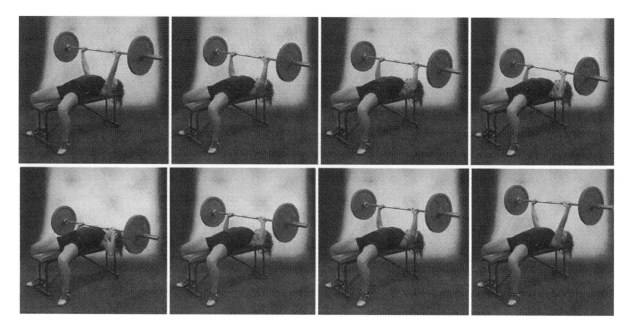

Figure 2. The Bench Press.

DUMBBELL BENCH PRESS

The Dumbbell Bench Press is, as is the Dumbbell Press, a pretty hard exercise that not only develops strength but develops independent hand control during loaded movement. It combines strength development with enhancing the coordination element of mobility.

Getting into the correct starting position for the Dumbbell Bench Press takes either a partner to hand you the dumbbells while you are on the bench or it takes a small bit of planning and coordination. We will describe the latter here.

Grab the dumbbells you have placed on the floor at the end of the flat bench will lie down on and stand up with them. Place one end of each dumbbell against each thigh. Place your feet in your squat stance and sit down, the dumbbells will be sitting on end on top of your thighs. Pull the dumbbells close to you chest as you lie back on the bench. Keeping the dumbbells tight to the chest, adjust your back and feet into the same orientation used in the Bench Press. Now rotate the dumbbells to where the handles are oriented across the chest with one end of each dumbbell touching each shoulder, this is the start position (figure 1A). In order to control the dumbbells safely, they are maintained in a position close to a vertical line through the shoulder joints throughout the movement. At the top the dumbbells do move from out to in slightly as the elbows fully extend (figure 1B). This is seen as the hands being just outside the shoulders at the bottom and directly over the shoulders at the top.

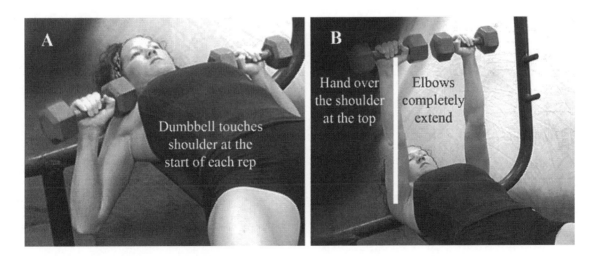

Figure 1. The start and top positions of the Dumbbell Bench Press.

To exit the exercise after the last repetition, the reverse process of lying down is used. Move the dumbbells tight to the body and near the hips and sit up. You can lift a leg (or two) and use them to establish momentum to aid in sitting up. Once sitting, place the dumbbells back on the floor (figure 2).

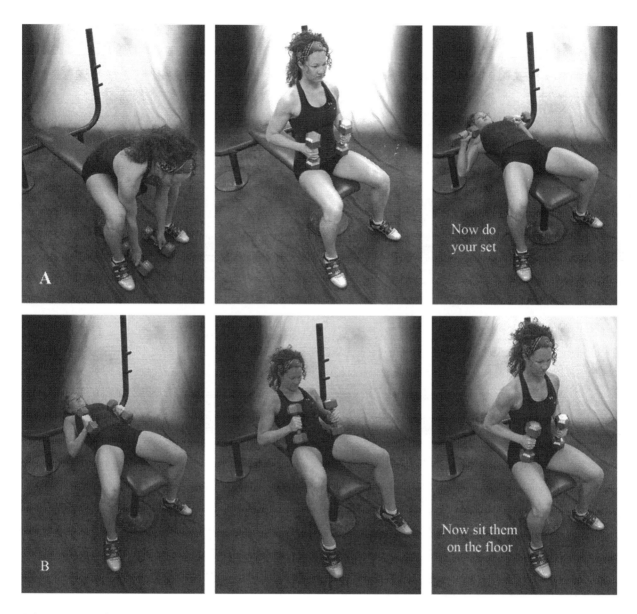

Figure 2. Getting down for the first repetition (A) and getting up after the last (B). As heavier weights are used it will become increasingly necessary to move one dumbbell at a time to and from the hips.

PULL-UP

The Pull-up is an elementary gymnastic skill and can be used as a strength or a local muscular endurance adaptive stimulus. It is a valuable exercise as it represents the "up" component of an "up and over" obstacle. Being good at Pull-ups translates well to being able to overcome elevated physical obstacles in the work place and in sport.

To get into the start position for the Pull-up, you have to jump up to a high bar or grasp a bar and lift your feet to the rear by flexing your knees. The important thing is that the body must be completely suspended with no contact to the ground (figure 1A). The width of the double overhand grip on the bar should be slightly wider than the shoulders. This width provides the best fitness results. A narrower grip provides a longer range of motion but adds a mechanical disadvantage. A wide grip makes for a shorter distance of exercise travel, but we want complete range of motion development. As in all exercises involving the arm, the elbows are completely extended in the start position for every repetition. The up position occurs when the shoulder and elbow joints work to raise the body to the bar. The up position is attained when the complete jaw line is above the bar (figure 1B). This gives us two absolute anatomical reference points to both teach and quantify Push-up execution.

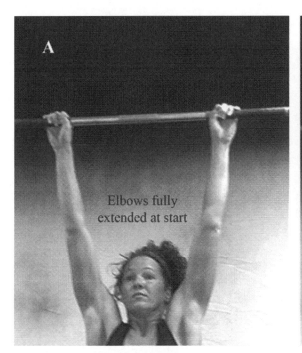
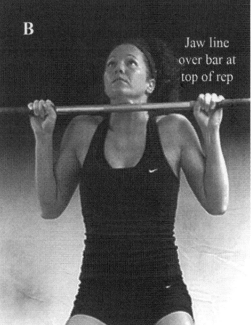

Figure 1. The start and up position for the Pull-up.

Pull-ups can be used in the development of upper body endurance if only bodyweight and high repetitions are used. However, with a hip harness additional weight can be added to the system and strength can progressively be developed.

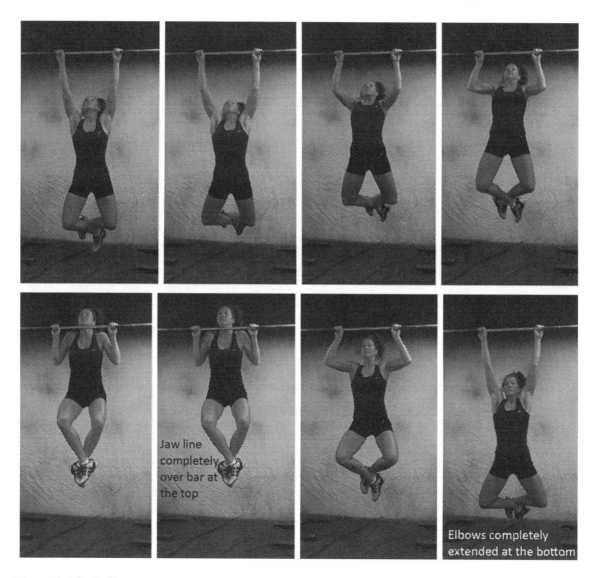

Figure 2. The Pull-up.

The Chin-up is a variant of the Pull-up where the grip is changed. All key elements of the exercise are the same except the grip used is an underhand grip instead of an overhand grip.

Another variant of the Pull-up is the Kipping Pull-up. The Kipping pull-up is a coordinated full-body movement that can help increase the rate of work compared to dead hang Pull-ups. It originates from basic gymnastics in which a gymnast would use the momentum from an efficient swing of the legs and hips to help "kip" up onto a bar or rings. There is misconception that the Kipping Pull-up is a strength movement or that it can help develop a dead hang Pull-up or chin-up. The Kipping Pull-up is no more a strength movement than the Burpee or

Bodyweight Squat, and a weaker trainee should increase strength to develop a dead hang Pull-up. Trainees with existing shoulder pathology or tightness should avoid this exercise. The exercise is described here as it can be useful in multi-element fitness training.

To perform a Kipping Pull-up, the trainee will first hang from a bar (as in figure 1A). They will then push their hips and trunk forward while the legs are extended behind them to initiate a body swing. The resulting body position will be a half-moon crescent with the limbs posterior to shoulders and hips (a forward arc). Prior to executing the first rep, weaker trainees may need to perform several swings to generate momentum (a stronger trainee will not require this). After pushing the hips forward, the trainee will push the hips back and push the appendages forward - the knees extended forward and slight extension of the shoulder (arms in front of shoulder). The result will be a half-moon crescent that is opposite to the initial swing (a backward arc). The trainee will again push the hips forward with the limbs back and at this point the trainee will forcefully flex the hips up and extend the shoulders to generate momentum that will carry the center of mass back and up. While in motion, the elbows are flexed and chest is pulled to the bar. In ordered to perform a subsequent repetition, the trainee must return along the same path in which they ascended. This is accomplished by pushing the bar away horizontally, much like a bench press. The result is the center of mass traveling back and down – the exact, yet opposite arc that occurred on the ascent. On the descent, the trainee will allow their center of mass to push forward and return to forward arc position and immediately utilize the stretch reflex in the anterior shoulder girdle, hips, and abdominal region to forcefully contract for the next rep.

FRENCH PRESS

This is not a coffee maker. It is an ages old modification of the press that creates a focused stress around the elbow, working the elbow extensors - the triceps being one such muscle group. The French Press is built around doing a movement from a quite mechanically disadvantageous position. And because of the relatively small muscle mass involved and the mechanical limitations imposed by the exercise positions, the amount of weight used is a fraction of what can be Pressed.

The start position, contrary to much popular opinion, is standing with the elbows directly vertical over the shoulders. The bar is held in the hands in a narrow double overhand grip (thumbs around the bar) with the bar touching the back of the neck at about the level of the 7th cervical vertebrae (bottom of the back of the neck) and the elbows as high as possible (figure 1A). In this position the triceps are maximally stretched. The finish position is with the bar, elbows, and shoulder joints in a nearly vertical line (figure 1B). The elbows are completely extended overhead. During the movement from start to finish, the upper arm - shoulder to elbow - stays near vertical, only the forearm and weight rotate around the elbow. This is why the weight used is relatively low, even in the most advantageous position there is still mechanical and anatomical limitation imposed. And that is not a bad thing, it helps us accomplish our purpose.

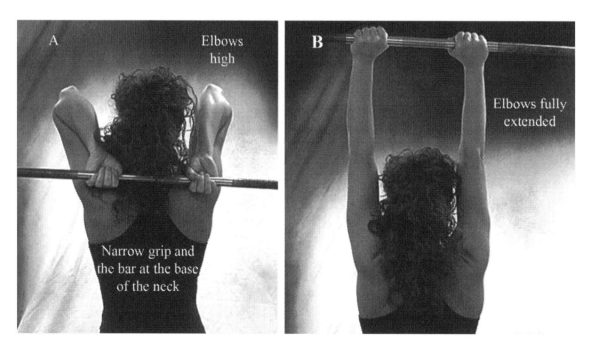

Figure 1. The start and finish positions of the French Press.

There is a Bench French Press also known as Triceps Extensions or of more recent nomenclature, "Skull Crushers", obviously re-named to make lifting sound more manly. You don't really need to do the bench version since it removes some of the range of motion required of the triceps from the exercise. The overhead version is superior.

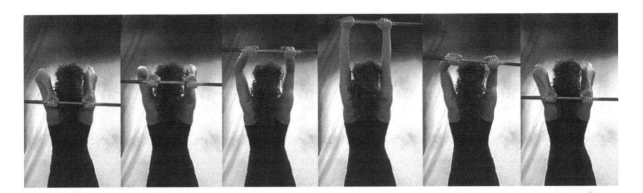

Figure 2. The French Press.

LAT PULL DOWN

The Lat Pull Down is aptly named as it uses the latissimus dorsi muscle of the back (along with many other muscles) to pull an overhead suspended load down to the body. Although this is a machine-based exercise, it does have a degree of utility in establishing initial latissimus strength in order to support progress towards Pull-up achievement in fitness trainees (it does NOT substitute for Pull-ups). As it utilizes a fairly large mass of muscle it can also produce a fairly decent amount of homeostatic disruption to aid in fitness gain. This favorability as an exercise resides only with the cable-machine versions of the exercise and does not extend to lever-based machines that remove the motor control element of the exercise. There are literally dozens and dozens of makes and models of Lat Pull Down machines, the most valuable are the cable-based versions. And with every such machine there is a large menu of bars and gizmos that can be attached to the cable. You only need one, a straight bar. The straight bar attachment provides the best grip orientation to develop the goal musculature.

The grip for the Lat Pull Down is fairly wide, the best descriptor being the humerus of each arm angled up and out at a 45 degree angle to the floor (or suspended bar)(figure 1A). A double overhand grip is used. As the exercise is completed when seated, sit erect with normal vertebral extension from the tailbone to the skull. This is a shoulder joint exercise along a vertical plane so the bar moves up and down only (figure 1B). You will see lots of people forcefully extending their hips (leaning back as they pull down) but this diminishes the value of this exercise as it changes the orientation of the exercise more along a pseudo-horizontal plane. It in effects comes to resemble a Row. Rows move along a horizonal plane and are quite effective at development in this plane, much more so than a mutated Lat Pull Down. Do not give up valuable functional development just because you can lift more weight by throwing your upper body backwards during the Lat Pull Down. At the bottom of the exercise, the bar touches the collar bones (figure 1C).

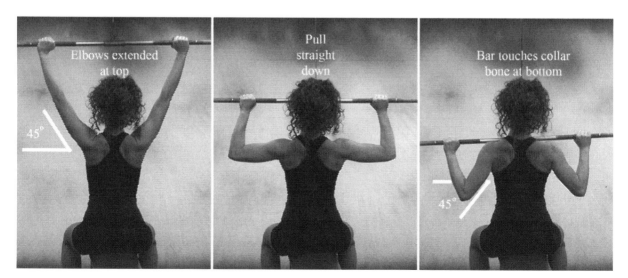

Figure 1. Basic positions of the Lat Pull Down.

When this occurs, the humerus of each arm will be angled down and out at about 45 degrees to the floor (or bar). The bar touch at the bottom, and the complete elbow extension at the top, is important for developing the complete range of motion and quantifying successful repetitions.

CURL

This is probably the least utilitarian exercise listed in this book (or anywhere). But we understand that the concept of the Curl as symbolic of a developing sense of masculinity and as such we know that many people will do them anyway. The Curl does develop the elbow flexors - all of them, not just the biceps. There are two ways to do them, the standard way that most people do them, and then there is the best way where the biceps are worked through their complete range of motion.

Both techniques start in the exact same position. The barbell is held at arms length with a double underhand grip. The bar is resting on the top of the thighs and the elbows are *completely extended* (figure 1A). The stance is of minimal importance but a Front Squat foot position is recommended. Phase one of the curl has the elbows held in close proximity to the hips and the upper arm stays vertical as the barbell is rotated up and around the elbows until movement is inhibited by the forearm touching the biceps (figure 1B). This is generally the where most people stop. But if we want to more completely exercise both segments of the biceps, the elbows are now rotated forward about four inches and the barbell is pushed up to the level of the chin at the same time (figure 1C). The barbell is then lowered back to the start position - all the way down to completely extended elbows - in exactly the reverse process.

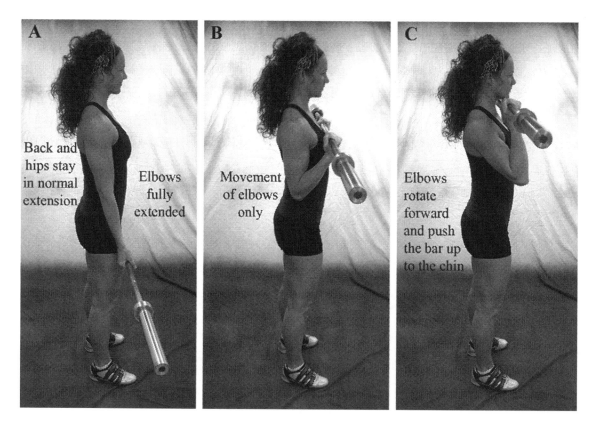

Figure 1. Important exercise positions for the Curl.

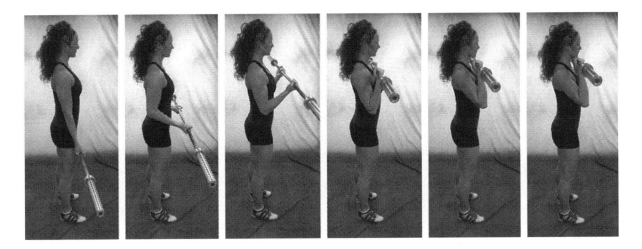

Figure 2. The Curl.

DIP

The Dip is another basic gymnastic exercise representing the top part of the "up" in the "up and over" in clearing an obstacle. It is a good developer of the shoulder and elbow primary movers but it also statically loads the thoracic and shoulder postural muscles. An excellent ancillary benefit.

The Dip requires an apparatus, a set of parallel bars, a parallette, or something as simple as two dining room chairs oriented back to back (with enough space between them for the body to fit). Ideally the hands on the apparatus will be nearly directly under the shoulders or a couple inches wider than the hips.

The start position for the Dip is assumed by stepping up into the apparatus, or in the case of chairs, lowering onto them. Ensure that the thumbs are wrapped around the bars or around the back of the chair. This will prevent slippage and precipitous falls. When the grip is assumed and the shoulders are over the hands, the feet are lifted so the entire bodyweight is supported on the extended arms (figure 1A). This is the start position. The shoulders should be held rigid and the line of shoulder joints should cross near the base of the neck not the base of the skull - think of pushing them down. The elbows should also be completely extended. The bottom position is where the body has been lowered to a point where the shoulders are lower than the elbows (figure 1B). Completion of the repetition is the return to the start position with elbows completely extended.

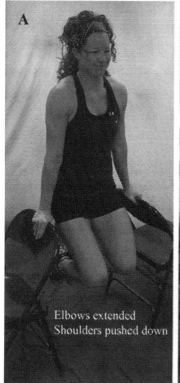
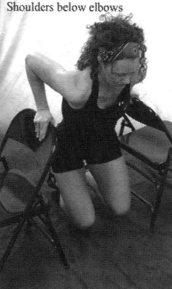

Figure 1. The start and down position of the Dip.

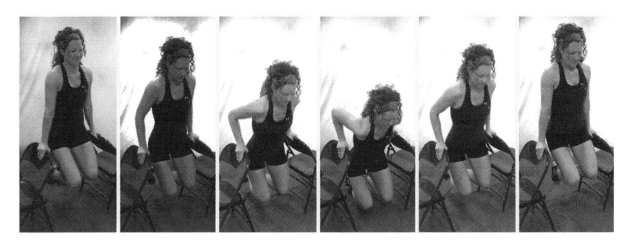

Figure 2. The Dip.

SHRUG

The shrug is likely on of the easiest exercises to do. It is a simple, short range of motion exercise that specifically develops the large trapezius muscle that elevates (lifts up) both scapula. It also develops, through loaded isometric contraction, the stabilizing musculature around the shoulder joints and along the length of the vertebral column.

A proper shrug begins with the bar held in a double overhand grip. The weight is carried at arms length, hanging and touching the upper thigh (figure 1A). The overall posture is erect but with the neck and head in normal extension or slightly tilted forward. This latter point is a nuance but it is of practical importance. Looking up pre-shortens the cervical portion of the trapezius and limits maximal force production and range of motion (figure 2). As this is already a very limited range of motion exercise and heavy weights must be used in order to produce an adaptive stress reducing active range of motion and active muscle mass needs to be avoided. Looking up interferes with our ability to load effectively throughout the complete range of motion. When standing with weights, it is normal for the shoulders to be pulled down lower than in relaxed standing BUT they should not be allowed to roll forward. At the top we squeeze as high as we can, we do not squeeze backwards. We are developing our strength along the inferior-superior axis not along an anterior-posterior axis (we have better exercises for that).

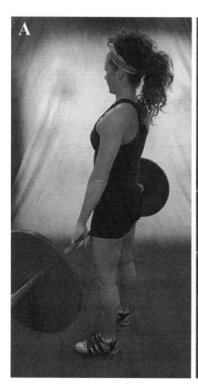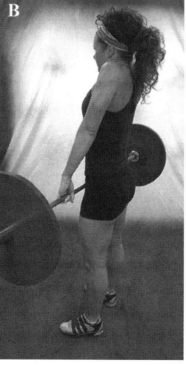

Figure 1. The start (A) and finish (B) positions for the shrug.

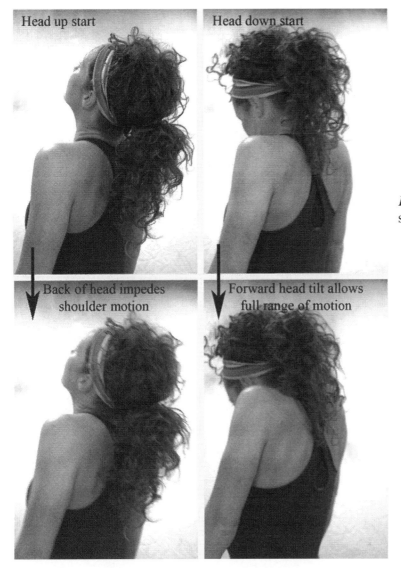

Head up start

Head down start

Back of head impedes shoulder motion

Forward head tilt allows full range of motion

Figure 2. Head position affects shrug range of motion.

To execute the lift just raise the shoulders as high as possible - try to touch your ears with the shoulders (figure 1B). The movement should be straight up and straight down. As heavy weights are generally used with this exercise it is difficult to move very quickly BUT one should attempt to shrug as fast and as completely as possible with every repetition. For general fitness trainees, there should be no other body movements aside from the shrug. For power athletes and lifters it is acceptable to provide an inch or two of quick hip extension to overcome initial inertial resistance in order to facilitate a higher velocity exercise using larger weights. This is a sport specific variation - use it if it contributes directly to performance. Use the strict shrug for all other functional goals.

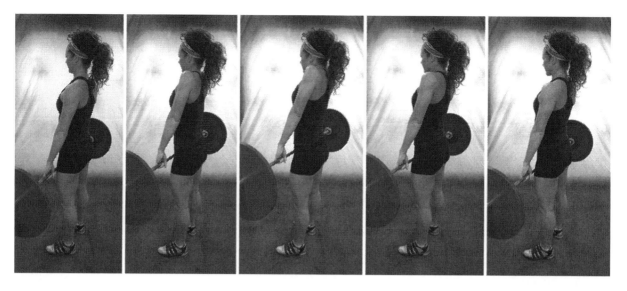

Figure 2. The strict Shrug.

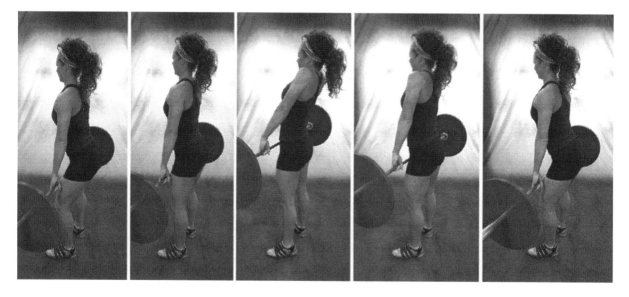

Figure 3. The hip assisted Shrug.

ROW

More correctly called the Bent Row because the exercise is performed while bending over at the hips, this is a strong developer of the latissimus dorsi and the other muscles that pull the arm to the rear. It can even help you build biceps.

The start position for the row is much like the bottom position of the Romanian Deadlift except there is more knee bend that allows gripping the bar while it is on the floor (figure 1A). In this position the back is very close to parallel to the floor. Each repetition of the row begins and ends with the barbell on the floor. At the start the bar is on the floor and the elbows are completely straight - we are working the complete range of motion. At the top, the elbows are pulled to the rear and move behind the most posterior aspect of the torso (figure 1B). Incomplete extension to the floor or not getting the elbows far enough back means the weight is too heavy, that you aren't getting good feedback from your coach or trainer, or that you are training "lazy".

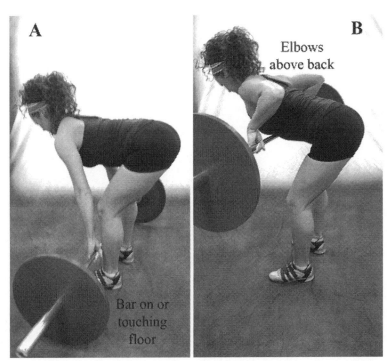

Figure 1. Starting and top position of the row.

For purists, in the row there is no joint movement in the knees, hips, or any other part of the body - thus enhancing the ability of the worked muscles to generate force from a dead stop. There is some inevitable elevation of the back around the hips in this movement due to momentum at the top, BUT this does not mean that this is a defining movement. The hips and knees should be as motionless as possible. There is a variant that does utilize this movement though. For those that want to handle larger loads or work at higher velocities, it is permissible to give a few inches of hard hip extension (a little kick with the hips to generate initial momentum) immediately off of the floor.

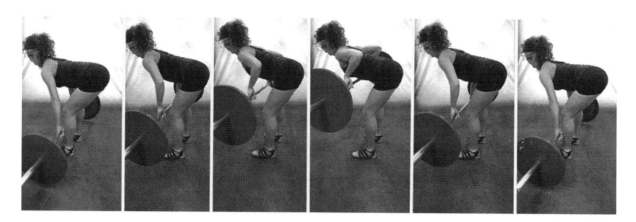

Figure 2. The row.

GOODMORNING

The Goodmorning is a fairly old school back and hip exercise. It is simply bending over with a weight on your shoulders and then raising back up.

The start position is very much like setting up for the squat (figure 1A) - preferentially the low bar squat as this gives the weight a fairly stable support when the upper body is tilted forward. A high bar position can be used but this may be a bit uncomfortable for some as the bar may work its way up and press directly on the cervical vertebral spines. Once the bar is positioned on the shoulders, the knees are unlocked and the torso is tilted forward by moving only the hips. The back retains a normal arch throughout the exercise. The bottom of the Goodmorning is where the back is low back is nearly parallel or precisely parallel to the floor (figure 1B). Going lower produces an obvious problem relative to keeping the weight on the shoulders. The angle at the hips should be about 45 degrees at the bottom.

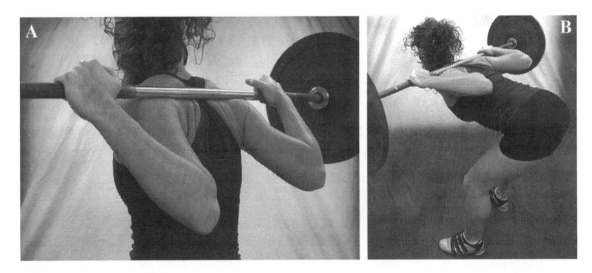

Figure 1. The basic positions of the Goodmorning.

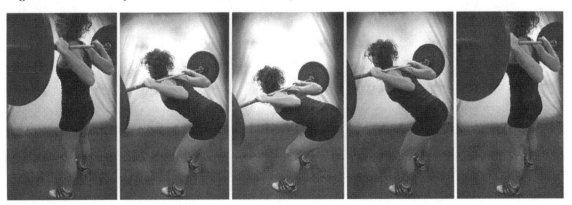

Figure 2. The Goodmorning.

BACK EXTENSION

The Back Extension exercise is often called - quite inappropriately - "hyperextensions". This little nomenclature issue needs to be clarified immediately. A hyperextension is the extension of a joint beyond its anatomical limits, i.e., it is injurious. This is not an injurious exercise and it does not go beyond anatomically possible range of motion - so it is not a hyperextension! The BACK EXTENSION can be used to develop both strength and local muscular endurance of the lower back and hip extensors. Achievement of this actually helps reduce the risk of developing low back pain from occupational, recreational, or sporting stress.

This exercise is performed on a Roman Chair apparatus (see apparatus in figure 1), an inexpensive piece of equipment costing as low as $70. The design of the apparatus varies by manufacturer but they are all used in the same manner.

The start position for the Back Extension has the top of the thighs resting across the hip pad, the back of the ankle (Achilles tendon above the heel) underneath ankle roller pads, and the torso declined to near -90 degrees (head down) (figure 1A). The normal placement of the hands is fingers interlaced behind the base of the neck. For low fit individuals, the arms can be crossed in front of the chest to reduce the distance of resistance to the point of hip rotation in order to create a lighter load. During the exercise the torso is raised until the torso angle exceeds 45 degrees above parallel to the floor (figure 1B) and then is lowered back to the start position. Although this is frequently considered a "back" exercise, it should be apparent that it is not the intervertebral joints creating most of the movement, it is the posterior hip extensors moving the torso around the hip joint. In fact, the primary job of the posterior vertebral muscles is postural and static. It is only in the last few degrees of the movement that the lumbar vertebral joints move beyond postural lordotic extension.

Higher repetitions of the Back Extension is a means towards developing local muscular endurance. However, the exercise can be adapted readily as a strength developing exercise by adding weight. Initially a single barbell plate is held in the hands during the execution of the movement to add the external load. There are two appropriate ways to hold the plate; (1) held in the arms firmly against the chest and (2) resting across the upper trapezius while being stabilized with the hands. Again these positional variations change the degree of difficulty of the movement by altering where the load is placed along the lever arm. The weight-held-on-chest position places the load closer to the point of rotation and reduces the torque (think of it as reducing the resistance to movement). The weight-resting-on-shoulder position moves the load out to the end of the lever arm and provides maximal torque, making this the most difficult of the two load carrying positions.

Progression with weight simply means methodically using the next bigger plate as called for in your program. This works very well with denominations from 2.5 pounds to 45 pounds (1.25 kg to 20 kg), and this may satisfy the needs of most trainees, but after 45 pounds one would need to use a loaded barbell to enable systematic and low increment additions of weight. At this point the weight-held-on-chest position is no longer viable and the weight should only be held on the shoulders.

In the Back Extension when using heavier weights, it is common, necessary, and quite acceptable to use a range of motion of about minus 40-45 degrees at the bottom and 35-45 degrees at the top. This modification of angles makes it easier to keep the bar safely immobilized on the shoulders.

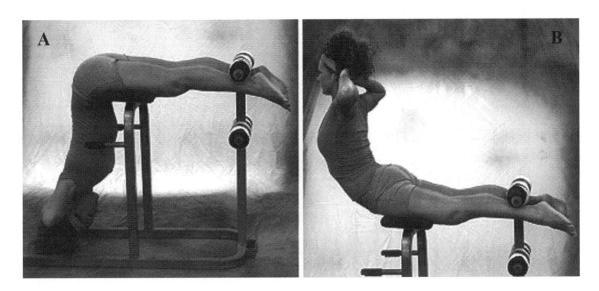

Figure 1. The start position (A) and top position (B) of the Back Extension.

WEIGHTED SIT-UP

Yes we do Sit-ups. We don't do crunches. There are ZERO reasons to do crunches and there is ZERO actual clinical or scientific data demonstrating that any type of Sit-up has produced any harm to any healthy human EVER. Crunches provide a fraction of the adaptive stimulus, only work a fraction of the range of motion, and provide a nightmare for quantification. We do Sit-ups. We also do weighted Sit-ups for the same reason we do Bench Presses to get strong rather than use simple body weight Push-ups. The Bench Press allows us to add load in a way that the Push-up cannot. Unlike the Push-up, in the Sit-up, our hands are free and we can easily hold weights in them to add load. Once you can do 20 Sit-ups with no weight, its time to start adding weight.

The start position for the weighted Sit-up has the feet flat and anchored, either by having a training partner hold them or by wedging the toes under something that is heavy enough not to move if you lift your toes (figure 1A1). The knees are bent to no less than a 90 degree angle (a bigger angle is OK). The torso and head are resting on the floor. The weight is held in both hands at the level of the shoulders with the elbows completely extended (figure 1A2). The arms are perpendicular to the floor. This is the start and end position. Do not let the weight be used as a momentum aid, keep it as close to directly over the shoulders as possible throughout each rep this keeps the lever arm long and provides the greatest resistance.

The up position has the hip joint, the shoulder joint, and the weight - fully extended and supported overhead - all in line (figure 1B).

Using contact with the floor and the anatomical alignment shown in figure 1B provides us a means of consistent teaching and quantification of the work done. It also provides for a uniform training stimulus throughout the complete range of motion.

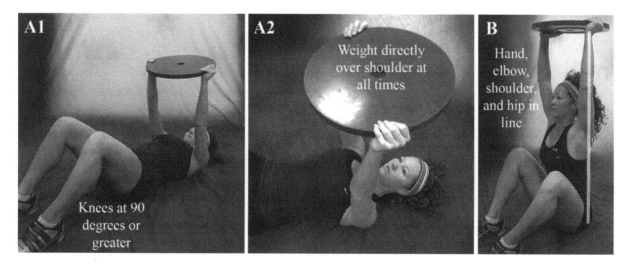

Figure 1. Key positions of the weighted Sit-up.

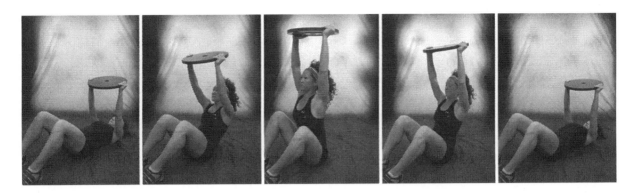

Figure 2. The weighted Sit-up.

BACK SQUAT

There are two basic variants of the back squat, low bar and high bar. Both are quite useful in lower body strength development. There is considerable debate regarding the superiority of one over the other, and indeed they do produce mildly different joint loading patterns. The low bar variant produces greater hip development than the high bar squat and the high bar variant produces greater quadricep development. But both variants do not neglect developing the total assemblage of lower body joints. Weightlifters historically use the high bar squat variant and powerlifters use the low bar variant. This is related to the assumed specificity of each variant to the respective sports. It would likely be wise training to systematically include both into training as this would provide a more comprehensive adaptive stress than using only a single variant endlessly.

In the low bar variant the bar is carried across the back at the level just above or directly on the scapular spines (the hard diagonal bones just under the trapezius) (figure 1A). A moderately wide grip is needed here in order to make the trainee comfortable with the stretch in the anterior shoulder caused by assuming the low bar position. In the low bar squat the trunk will have a noticeable forward tilt during the descent and during standing up out of the bottom. In the high bar variant the bar is carried on top of the traps at the base of the neck (figure 1B). To make this position more comfortable it is recommended to grip the bar as close to the shoulders as possible. This contracts the trapezius and makes a little shelf of muscle on which the bar rests - rather than pressing down uncomfortably on the cervical vertebral spines if a wide grip is used. With this bar placement the torso will be much more upright than in the low bar variant.

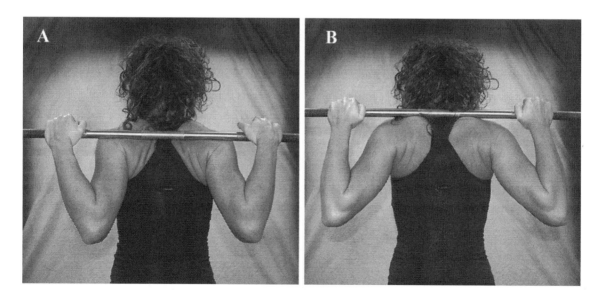

Figure 1. The two basic bar positions of the back squat: (A) low bar and (B) high bar.

The feet should be placed where the outside surface of the shoe heel is directly under the outside surface of the deltoid (figure 2). The feet should also be pointed out at about a 30 degree angle. There is a little variation on both stance width and foot angle, but every effort should be made to conform to this convention.

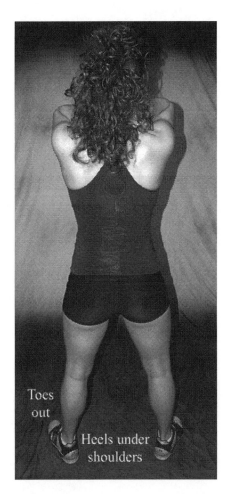

Figure 2. Squat stance.

The bottom position of the squat is also a hotly debated topic. How deep to squat? Half squat? Quarter squat? Ninety degree knee flexion? Line of the femur parallel to the floor? Top of the thigh parallel to the floor? Hip below knee? Ass to grass? There are two acceptable depths for healthy people who want to become fit. The first is the same depth that has been used in judging powerlifting contests for decades - the inguinal fold (where the skin creases when you flex your hip) drops below the top of the patella (figure 3A). This depth has many advantages, primary of which is that it provides a visible anatomical standard that allows a basis of coaching and performance consistency. The other acceptable depth is anywhere lower than the previously described position, in other words squatting through the complete range of motion (figure 3B). And this latter point is the advantage, developing the complete range of motion around a set of joints.

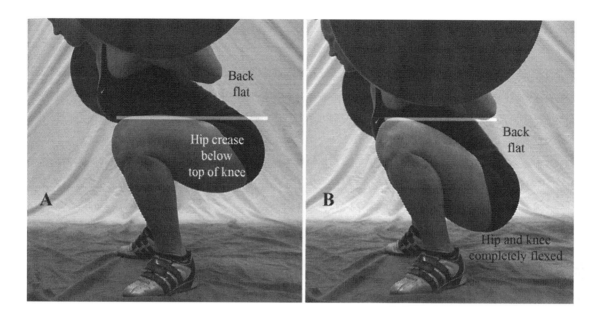

Figure 3. The two acceptable depths for squatting: (A) inguinal fold below the top of the patella and (B) complete range of motion (rock bottom, ass-to-grass, etc.).

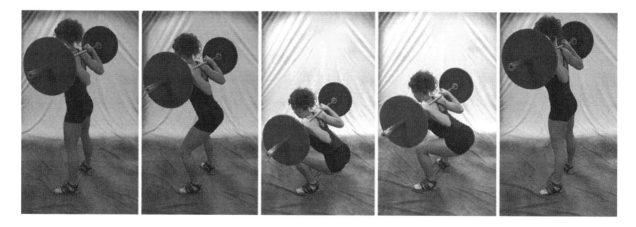

Figure 4. The low bar back squat.

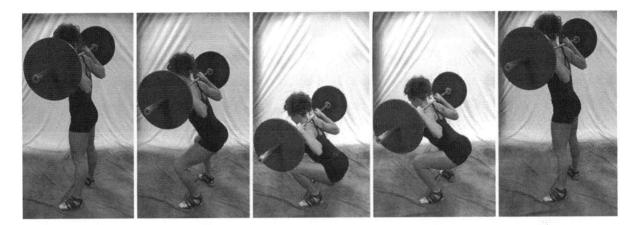

Figure 5. The high bar back squat.

FRONT SQUAT

Although the front squat is a simple variant of the back squat, it is different enough that it warrants separate treatment. The major difference here is that the bar is rested across the deltoids and clavicles (across the front of the shoulders)(figure 1A). Arm position is fairly important in setting up for the front squat. The elbows should be sticking out to the front of the body and should be mildly pointed outwards to the side (figure 1B). The bar should rest in the hands which are on the outside of the shoulders and are in relaxed open position (figure 1C). The hands however do not support the bar, the shoulders do. There is a lot of squishy room here. Ideally the bar would be across the palms, but individual flexibility issues may require the bar to cross the fingers or finger tips. Any orientation that allows the bar to be supported on the shoulders NOT held in a deathgrip in the hands is operable.

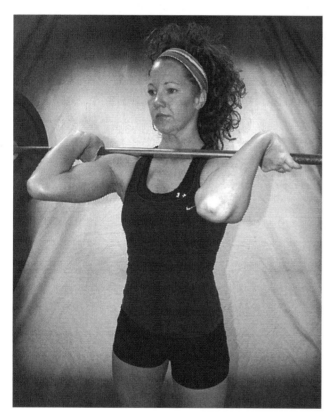

Figure 1. The bar position relative to the shoulder.

The placement of the bar to the front of the body changes the center of mass of the system and produces a very upright torso position. Although the front squat still develops the complete assemblage of lower body joints, there is a bias in stress towards knee and ankle loading more so than either of the back squat variants.

The bottom position of the front squat follows the same rules as the back squat with only two acceptable depths. The look at the bottom will be different from the back squat, either variant, as the knees have to be more forward to accommodate the vertical torso which brings the hips closer to the heels than in the back squat (figure 2).

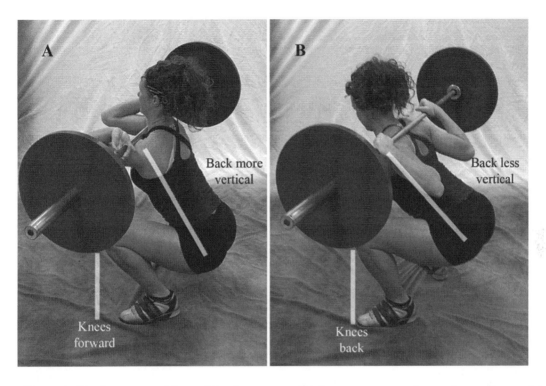

Figure 2. The bottom position of the front squat (A) is more erect and more knees forward than the back squat (B).

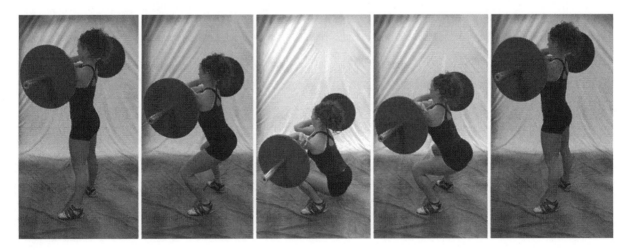

Figure 3. The front squat.

LEG PRESS

The Leg Press exercise is a useful exercise for use in developing leg strength in individuals who are not strong enough to do weighted squats or bodyweight squats. They are also useful for delivering lower body work to individuals who cannot, for some reason, carry a weight on the shoulders for squatting. Leg presses are not a substitute for squats as the kinetic chains involved are quite different.

There are any number of Leg Press machines, the simplest and most useful is the leg sled. In a leg sled you sit down onto the seat, the back of which is inclined about 35 degrees from the floor. You then put your feet up onto the foot deck/weight carriage with your knees fully extended (figure 1A). The feet are placed at front squat stance width with the toes pointed out. This will often be problematic based on the make and model of the machine. Ergonomics and anatomical efficiency do not seem to be part of the manufacture process with many equipment companies.

As the weight carriage is lowered down the angled guides, the knees are pushed out as they bend (figure 1B). The line of the femur should parallel the line of the foot, heel to toe. This will allow the thighs to move to the sides of the abdomen an allow full hip flexion. The goal on the Leg Press is to get as complete of a range of motion in action as allowed by the machine, you are attempting, although in an inverted position, to get the knees higher than the inguinal fold as in the squat (figure 1C).

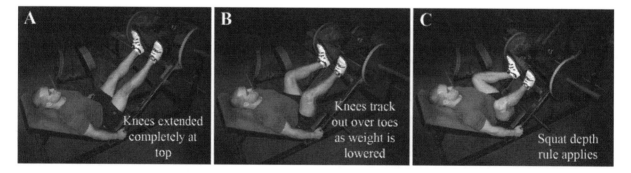

Figure 1. Basic positions of the Leg Press.

ROMANIAN DEADLIFT

The Romanian Deadlift, depending on how you look at it, is actually a variant of the stiff-legged deadlift or the goodmorning, or maybe a fusion of both. Regardless of its derivation it is a useful exercise in developing the hip and low back musculature. It strongly develops the extensors of the hip - the glutes and hamstrings - along with isometrically stengthening the low back. The RDL moves at only one joint, the hip.

The Romanian Deadlift starts in the standing position with an overhand grip on the bar. It is best to load the bar in a power rack and step back with it at that level. Or load the bar while it rests on low blocks and then lift it to the standing position. We then unlock the knees slightly, but no more than about 5-10 degrees. This is the start position, and each rep begins and ends here (figure 1). It is important to maintain this knee position throughout the entire set. There is no knee movement in the Romanian Deadlift.

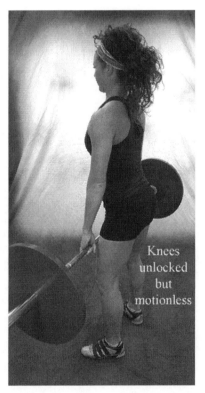

Figure 1. Getting into the starting position for the Romanian Deadlift.

To do the lift, bend forward, only at the hips, and steadily lower the bar down the front of the thighs towards the floor until you feel a moderate stretch in your hamstrings (figure 2). This is most effectively done by keeping your lower back arched throughout the exercise, moving ONLY at the HIPS. This forces the glutes and hamstrings to do the work. It is important that the bar stay in contact with your legs the entire trip down (and up). Return to the start position in a quick but controlled manner.

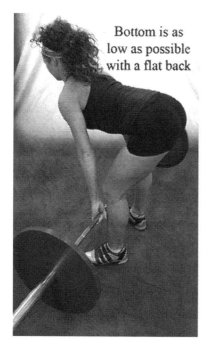

Bottom is as
low as possible
with a flat back

Figure 2. The bottom position of the Romanian Deadlift. Over time, and as flexibility improves from doing the exercise, the bottom position will become lower naturally. So if you can't get below the knee the first day, this is not a problem.

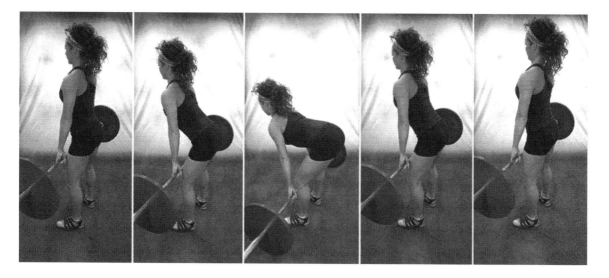

Figure 3. The Romanian Deadlift.

When done correctly the Romanian Deadlift more directly and efficiently loads and develops the hip extensors than other free weight exercise. Accessory to this is that by holding the arch in the back, the spinal erector muscles are statically loaded and get very strong. And by squeezing the bar back to contact the thigh throughout the complete range of motion, the lats also get a fair amount of isometric developmental work.

DEADLIFT

The concept of the deadlift is simple, grab a barbell and stand up with it. A simple concept with quite a bit of controversy on how to do it. Note that here we are deadlifting for fitness, which means complete development - trying to become as strong as possible through the normal range of motion. We are not trying to lift the maximum amount of weight through the shortest range of motion possible. This point gives us some direction into how we will set up at the beginning of the lift. As with the squat there are multiple variations in use and multiple reasons for using them. We focus here on the most important of them, the standard deadlift.

We propose a very simple starting position that is set by simple anatomical geometry of the body. By identifying simple and visible anatomical landmarks and orienting them relative to the bar on the floor we can very *reliably and consistently teach and perform* an exercise skill. By doing this, the start position achieved will be individualized to be appropriate for the anatomy of the trainee.

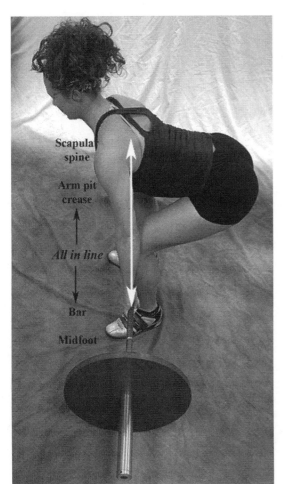

The feet must be under the bar (figure 1A). Preferentially directly over the navicular bone of the foot - about one inch in front of the ankle. The shoulder is placed over the bar as the bar is grasped (figure 1B). Specifically, the axillary crease - the fold where the arm meets the torso - is set above the bar. This correlates to the most medial and inferior point of the scapular spine, and this is where the bar will always be suspended under. Visually just look for the bottom of the armpit to be over the bar as you look from the side. Once these two landmarks are in line with the bar in between - navicular, bar, and axillary crease in a vertical line - the bar can now be lifted. Note that the hips are set higher than lower (figure 1B). This is desirable, as from this starting position, the bar will be lifted in a straight line from the floor to the fully erect finish position. The most efficient movement possible.

Figure 1. The start position for the deadlift.

Inevitably a trainee will want to start with the bar farther away from the shin and toward the toes as this seems more comfortable to them. As long as the bar stays well behind the ball of the foot (metacarpophalangeal joints), it is marginally OK. Moving the bar forward over the foot adds a lever arm that detracts from efficiency and adds unnecessary torque around the low back. Besides, within the first six inches of lifting the bar off the floor, the body-barbell system auto-corrects and the bar swings backwards until it is over the appropriate position over the foot. But really, why not just start in the body's anatomically preferred position?

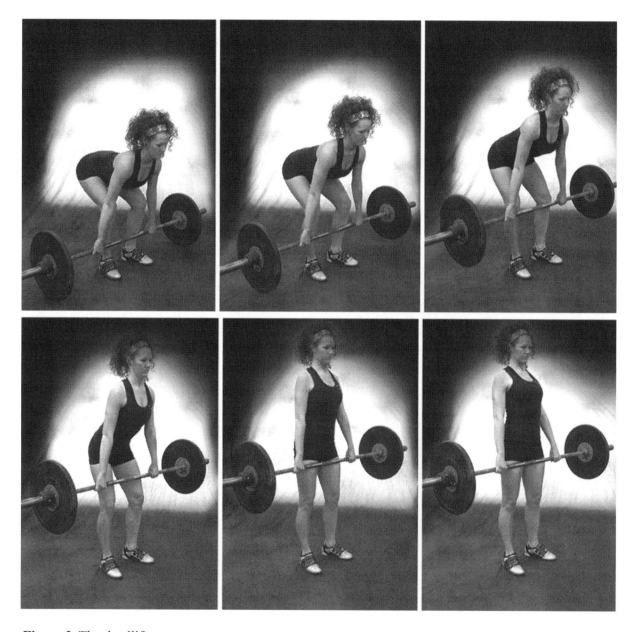

Figure 2. The deadlift.

POWER CLEAN

This is one of the most valuable functional and high speed exercises around. It is actually fairly easy to learn if you simply think about jumping and catching.

The start position for the Power Clean is with the barbell on the floor. The stance and set up is exactly the same as described in the Deadlift. And this is the contentious part. Coaches with Olympic lifting backgrounds will say that the bar needs to be forward over the balls of the feet or toes. The logic being that when the bar breaks contact with the floor, the swing it makes back under the scapula in the first few inches helps produce more vertical acceleration and helps keep the bar close to the body during the execution of the lift. Even if that logic is sound - and there is great debate about this - we do not use this little "trick" in general fitness or other sport applications. We want to be able to teach and have the trainee perform the lift in a very measured and repeatable manner. Adding an inconsistent element that also decreases movement efficiency - even if it might work in a few elite weightlifters - is not what we want to do for fitness or sports performance trainees. These populations need to be able to use consistent, effective, and efficient technique. So, unless you are a weightlifter and believe in the concept of a rolling dynamic start, you set up exactly like in the deadlift (figure 1A). Once the bar is over the area of the navicular and the armpit is over the bar, the knees begin their extension. The back remains at very close to the same angle as it was at the floor while the knees extend (figure 1B). Once the bar passes the knee an interesting and natural thing occurs, the knees re-bend slightly as the back becomes more vertical. The end of the body repositioning is complete at the last moment the shoulders are over the bar (figure 1C). This is the position where you jump violently with the bar (figure 1D). It is important in this action that the elbows remain straight as bending them will reduce force and reduce the amount of weight that can be lifted. When the body has completely extended at the top there is an instantaneous change in body direction. Gravity and a little tugging on the bar begins to move the body under the bar. This is a mobility aspect of the lift. During this phase of the lift, the feet move to the side. You are essentially moving them from Deadlift start width to Squat start width. Moving them out like this makes it easier to lower the body into the catch position on the shoulders. At the catch, the bar is caught on the shoulders with the elbows well forward. At the bottom of the lift the knees are bent but to no more than 90 degrees (if you go lower, it's called a Clean). At the catch there is an impact. The impact is cushioned by bending your knees NOT by catching the bar's load with the hands, elbows, and shoulders. After the impact the bar and the body squat down a little by necessity, this is the body accepting and cushioning the impact. This is why we do not catch Power Cleans on stiff legs. If we do, tons of things get jarred. After the bar is firmly on the shoulders, you stand up and the repetition is complete.

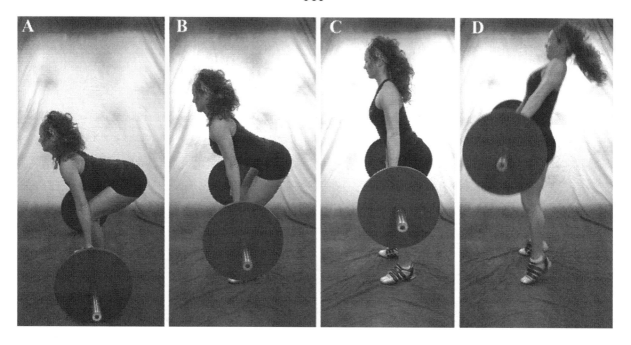

Figure 1. Critical positions of the Power Clean.

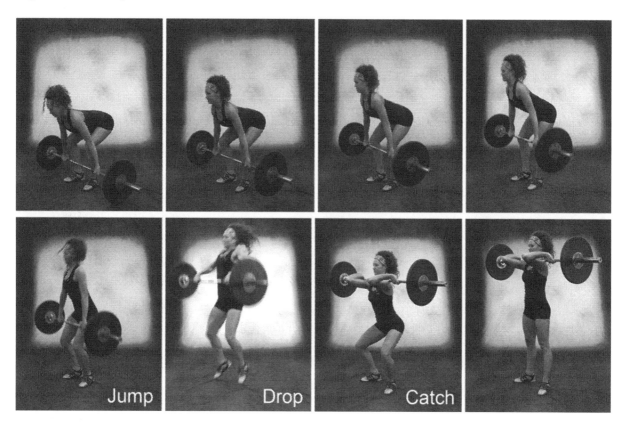

Figure 2. The Power Clean.

POWER SNATCH

The Power Snatch is a bit more difficult of a movement because in requires a little more of a gymnastic effort over a longer range of motion than the Power Clean. However, both the Power Clean and Power Snatch are conceptually the same; pull, jump, drop, and catch. Simple. The difference is that the Power Snatch requires the bar to be caught overhead on completely extended arms. This means a higher critical bar velocity is needed which translates to less weight used compared to the Power Clean. As you will learn often in your training career, less weight does not always translate to less hard.

There is a preparatory step prior to setting up for the Power Snatch. You have to determine how wide to grip the bar. Grip width is an important determinant of two things; (1) how effectively the bar gets pulled to the correct jumping position and (2) how much clearance over the head there is at the top of the exercise. A wide grip is intended to get the bar very high on the thighs at the jump and to provide about four to six inches of clearance of the bar over the head. This latter point provides for a shorter pulling distance compared to a narrow grip. So to determine the grip width for an individual's unique anatomy, simply Deadlift the bar to the standing position, then methodically widen the grip until the bar has moved up and is resting across the inguinal fold (hip crease) (figure 1A,B,C). Now, without changing grip, put the bar up over the head to ensure that it will clear the top of the head when the arms are fully extended overhead. If both conditions are satisfied, that's the correct grip for that individual.

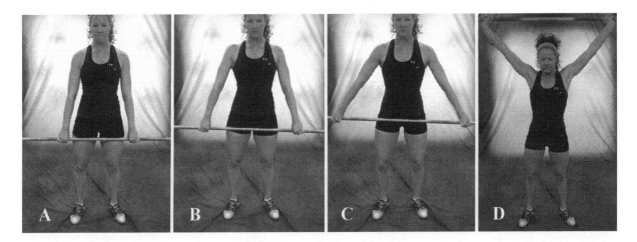

Figure 1. Selecting the correct grip width by moving the hands wider to bring the bar up to the inguinal fold (A,B,C) and then verifying clearance (D).

The floor set up for the Power Snatch is the same as all pulling exercises described so far - with one exception. The grip width will change what the starting position looks like. It does not change, however, the rules. The stance is the same, the bar position over the foot is the same, and the scapular position over the bar is the same. We can't change physics by changing grip.

Once the bar is over the area of the navicular and the armpit is over the bar, the knees begin their extension. The back remains at very close to the same angle as it was at the floor while the knees extend. Once the bar passes the knees, the knees re-bend slightly as the back becomes more vertical. The end of the body repositioning is complete at the last moment the shoulders are over the bar. In the Snatch, this position is slightly more vertical as the bar rides higher up on the thigh than in the Power Clean. With the shoulder still over the bar, you jump. As in all pulling motions, is important that the elbows remain straight as bending them will reduce force and reduce the amount of weight that can be lifted. When the body has completely extended at the top there is an instantaneous change in body direction from moving the bar up to moving the body down under the bar. During this phase of the lift, the feet move to the side. Moving them out like this makes it easier to lower the body into the catch position. At the catch, the bar is caught on the completely extended arms - with the elbows completely locked for support. At the bottom of the lift the arms have the weight overhead and the knees are bent to no more than 90 degrees (if you go lower, it's called a Snatch). At the catch there is an impact. The impact is cushioned by bending your knees NOT by catching the bar's load with bent arms and soft shoulders. After the impact the bar and the body squat down a little by necessity, this is the body accepting and cushioning the impact. After the bar is firmly on overhead, you stand up and the repetition is complete.

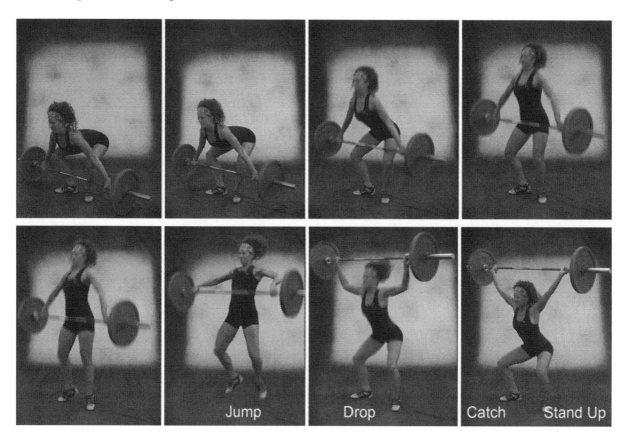

Figure 2. The Power Snatch.

CALF RAISE

Although the calves get lots of work during Squats, Deadlifts, Cleans, and Jerks, they have a high work capacity owing to their dual postural and prime mover roles. As such some people can benefit from additional calf work. Bodybuilders primarily fall into this category.

The start position for the Calf Raise is the stance is the same in set up as the front squat and the same shoulder set up as for the high bar squat or low bar squat (figure 1A). During the Calf Raise, on the way up and on the way down, the center of pressure should remain on the balls of the feet (you should feel your weight on the balls of your feet). Keeping the pressure localized prevents unnecessary and inefficient body sway. This means the body will have a very slight forward lean from the start. When your ankles are extended at the top position (figure 1C), the barbell and bodyweight are supported on a very small surface, and excess sway from poor body control prevents full extension and maximal fitness benefit. One repetition of the Calf Raise goes from heels on the floor to heels lifted as high as possible then back down to heels down on the floor. If you have to lean forward to get the weight moving up or you can only raise the heels an inch or so, the weight is too heavy. Remember general fitness is best developed with full range of motion exercise.

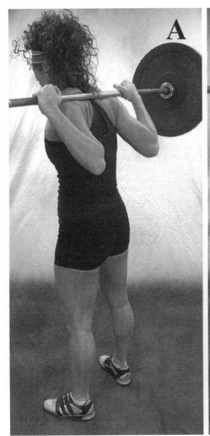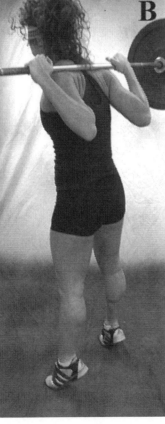

Figure 1. Key positions for the Calf Raise.

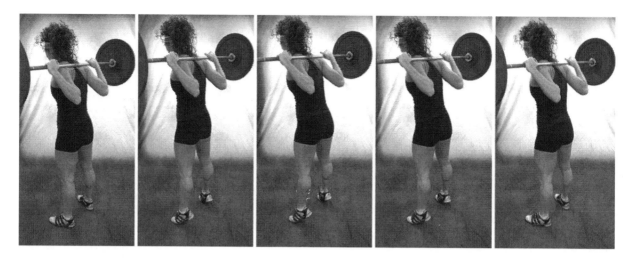

Figure 2. The Calf Raise.

Scientific progress is dead without a willingness to embark
upon at least a few carefully calculated ridiculous ideas.

Carl Sagan (a comic book version)
in *Atomic Robo Vol. 3 #4 by Brian Clevinger*

ENDURANCE EXERCISES

Running, as described in chapter 4, is the most common form of endurance exercise undertaken in modern times. However, any exercise can become an endurance exercise if continued for a long duration or done intermittently with incomplete recovery in between repetitions. For example, an ascending ramp of repetitions of Power Cleans done "on the minute" (1 rep at the beginning of minute 1, 2 reps on minute 2, 3 reps on minute 3, etc,) until failure makes a potent power exercise an intermittent endurance exercise. What follows are descriptions of useful exercises that lend themselves to developing continuous or intermittent endurance.

Rowing	Kettlebell Swing	Thrusters
Push-up	Burpee	Medicine Ball Throw
Sit-up	Dumbbell Hang Power Snatch	Box Jumps
	Bodyweight Squat	

CONCEPT II ROWER

Rowing on a rowing ergometer is an excellent and physically demanding training modality. With proper technique, a nearly whole-body training stress can be modified in intensity and volume to target any metabolic development goal - intermittent endurance or continuous endurance, even sprinting although this is less commonly done. While mechanical rowers have been part of gym inventories for more than a century, it was not until the creation of the Concept II rower by the Dreissigacker brothers that a machine could closely mimic the motions and metabolic demands of actually rowing a scull (two oars per person - sculling) or a shell (single oar per person - sweep rowing). The widespread use of these machines (Model A introduced in 1981, Model E introduced in 2006) by crews across the globe made indoor rowing a viable exercise modality. The lack of impact and the amount of body mass used during the rowing motion make it arguably the best endurance fitness apparatus available. While the Concept II does not mimic the total mobility training stimulus of a scull or shell (these are very narrow and unstable boats requiring a great deal of developed balance and coordination), the amount of joint movement included is quite large and assists nicely with developing range of motion in most trainees.

To set up the start position for a bout of rowing, sit down on the rolling seat and strap your feet snugly onto the foot plate. The straps should cross your foot behind the ball of the foot. Once the feet are set, reach forward and grasp the handle with a double overhand grip at a width just a little narrower than shoulder width. Make sure the hands are equidistant to the right and left of the chain. To finish the set up for the first pull, roll your hips (on the seat) forward until the knees are high (shins vertical or very close to vertical to the ground). While holding the handle at arms length directly in front of the body at the level of the chain at the wheel, lean forward bringing your chin towards or over your knees, depending of body segment lengths (figure 1A). In this position, the low back will be a little rounded, but not excessively, keeping close to normal vertebral extension is a goal. Skinny people with be able to keep their knees close together in this position, more robust individuals will need to open up the knees (laterally) to let the torso move into close to normal vertebral extension. This will also aid in breathing. At this point you are ready to pull.

In the start position you are in essentially an awkward half squat position, this means that the very strong hip and knee extensors are in a position to produce a lot of force, and that is what happens first, the knees extend and starts the body's movement backwards. Knee push drives the first half of the movement (figure 1B). As the knee nears extension, at about 130-140 degrees, the hips start forcefully opening up and the body begins its backwards lean (figure 1C). Within milliseconds after the hips kick in and move the torso behind perpendicular, the arms begin contributing. The forearms, which are still close to parallel to the ground and in line with the chain, are pulled to the rear until the handle touches the chest along the rib cage at a point lower than the sternum (figure 1D). The order of contribution to movement is knees, then hips, and finally arms. How an individual looks during each stage will vary based on body segment lengths, but the basic premise is to maintain a straight line of pull along the chain. Just as in the Deadlift, pulling along a straight line produces the best force production, the best workout, and the best fitness results.

After the pull there is a return to start, where the arms extend, then the hips and knees flex to bring the body back towards the feet and the handle back towards the wheel. The order of movement is simply reversed from that of the pull.

The stroke cadence is important here. For long slow distance type work, a stroke rate of around 30 strokes per minute is operable. Lower fit individuals will use slightly fewer, more fit trainees will use slightly more. The key is to use a stroke rate that can be sustained over the target time or distance. For interval work stroke rates of 40 per minute or more are desired.

One consideration that should be made when training on a rower is that due to the nature of the movement, breathing becomes linked to the stroke rate. Frequently trainees will adopt an exhale on the pull and inhale on the return to start position breathing pattern. If training at low exertional levels or doing very short sprints, this is not an issue BUT if working near VO_2max, doing high intensity intervals, or during longer sprints, the body will want to breathe at a rate of about 60-75 breaths per minute. If the stroke rate associated with the high intensity work is 50 strokes per minute, there is a mismatch in rates. The trainee will need to create a breathing strategy that allows adequate ventilation, through deeper inhalations or attempting to double up on breaths on the return to start position during alternate strokes. If unattended the mismatch will prematurely induce fatigue.

For a more detailed equipment tutorial visit the Concept II website.

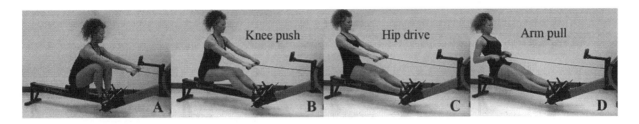

Figure 1. Key positions of the rowing stroke.

PUSH-UP

The Push-up has been a mainstay of physical conditioning programs for centuries. It's utility in developing upper body fitness has never been questioned. Although it is good for developing initial strength in beginners and is best for developing local muscular endurance in experienced trainees (two different purposes for two different populations).

The start position for the Push-up is dependent on the initial fitness of the trainee. If they are low fit, the start is lying face down on the floor, a modification of the down position. If the trainee has the ability to maintain normal vertebral posture (no sagging) when they support their bodyweight on their hands and balls of their feet, the up position is the starting position.

The down position has the trainee's hands placed palm down on the floor about one thumb length lateral to the shoulder at the level of the armpit (figure 1A). In this position the forearms should be close to vertical. The shoulders are below the elbows. This position gives us an anatomical relationship to teach and quantify correct exercise execution. The length of the body is held in normal postural extension, no sagging down or arching up in the middle, and no touching the floor with anything other than the hands and feet. The other key position in the Push-up is the up position. In this position, the shoulders and elbows have done their work and elevated the body. The elbows are completely extended and the body remains in normal postural extension (figure 1B). One repetition of the Push-up for a beginner starts in the down position, moves to the up position, and finishes in the down position. All other trainees start and finish in the up position.

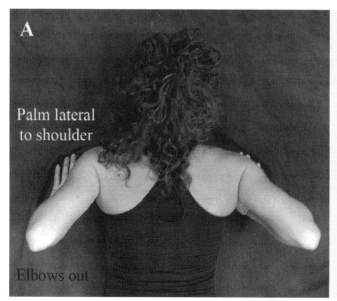
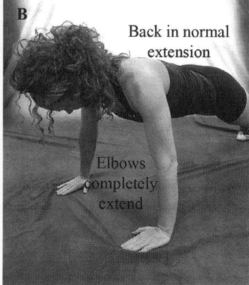

Figure 1. The down and up position of the Push-up.

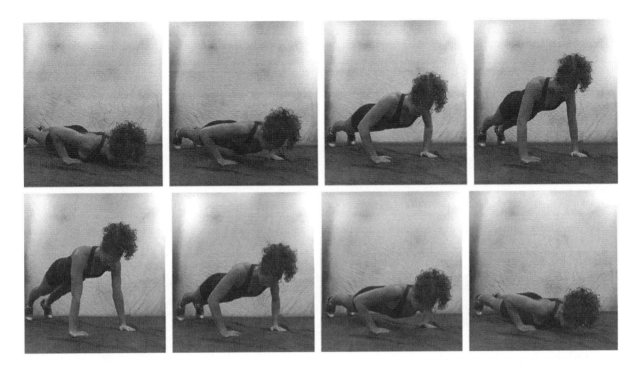

Figure 2. The Push-up.

If you can do ONE Push-up there is never a need to do any modification of the Push-up, the on-your-knees variation being the most common. If you simply add a set of singles (do a normal Push-up, rest, then do another one) each Push-up session, and do this progressively until you can do 10 singles, you can then begin doing multiple repetition sets of normal Push-ups. If you cannot do one Push-up as described, a wider hand placement can be used. If that solution still does not allow completion of one repetition, then using the knees-on-the-floor start position is appropriate.

SIT-UP

To do a simple Sit-up, all the same positions are used as in the previously described Weighted Sit-up except there is no weight held in the hands. The hands are either placed behind the base of the neck (fingers interlaced) or, for a lower resistance, the arms can be crossed across the chest. Crossing the arms near the active muscles shortens the lever arm (moves the load closer to the fulcrum) making this variant useful for low fit individuals just beginning a training program.

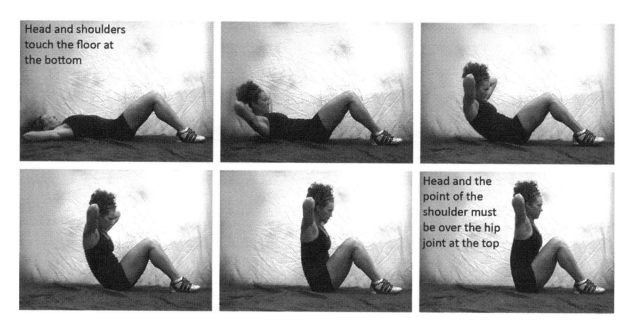

Figure 1. The Sit-up.

KETTLEBELL SWING

There are any number of specialized exercises that can be accomplished with kettlebells, the most valuable of which is the Kettlebell Swing. The primary purpose of this exercise is to develop the musculature around the hips, both in terms of improving repeated power output capacity and local muscular endurance. Execution of this weighted swing is fairly elementary but deceptively taxing. Beginners are urged to use a small kettlebell as technique is important for proper development, progress, and safety. Learn the movement pattern, get stronger, develop the necessary local muscular endurance, then progress to heavier implements.

There are a few preparatory steps to enter into a set of Kettlebell Swings. First is the selection of stance. It is recommended to assume the foot position for a Back Squat. At this width and toe angle, the arms will have adequate clearance when they swing through the legs. The next step is to simply pick up the kettlebell with both hands, stand up, hold it at arms length, and slightly bend the knees (figure 1A). To actually begin the swing phase, the hips are used to kick the kettlebell forward about 6-12 inches (figure 1B). This sets up the backward arc of the loading swing that takes the kettlebell backwards between the legs (figure 1C). In the loaded position the shins are near vertical, the shoulders are over the toes, the knees bent to about 110-120 degrees, the hips are well behind the heels, the back is in normal extension (no rounding), and the kettlebell has moved back under the butt - still held at arms length. This is a high velocity exercise so as soon as the kettlebell hits the apex of its backwards excursion, the hips violently open up, followed by fast knee extension. It is these movements, not any arm contribution, that propel the implement in its forward arc. The top position of the repetition is where the line of the shoulder-arm-kettlebell system rises to parallel to the floor or above (figure 1D).

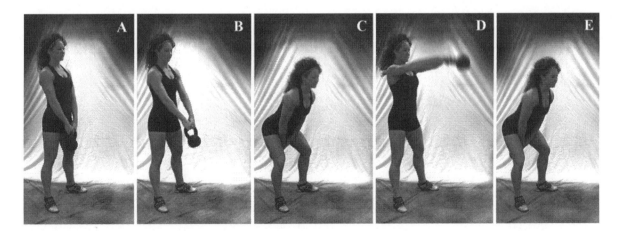

Figure 1. Key positions of the Kettlebell Swing.

This orientation establishes a nice objective criteria for determining completion of each repetition. As skill with the kettlebell and specific conditioning increases we can modify the criteria for the top position as swinging the kettlebell to a fully overhead position. This adds additional range of motion to the exercise and creates a requirement for higher power outputs to achieve the position, both valuable in furthering fitness. Or we can simply use a heavier kettlebell to drive fitness gain. After the top of the swing forward occurs, as expected there will be a backwards swing into the next repetition that will take you back to the loaded position (figure 1E) and the cycle of the swing repeats.

BURPEE

The Burpee or similar exercises - squat thrusts, mat drills, grass drills, and many more - have been used as a conditioning exercise since antiquity. The 1914 US Army Manual of Physical Training describes and depicts such an exercise and there are likely much older references to them in other military, physical culture, or sporting publications.

The Burpee, as currently *en vogue* and used by Mike "Yay Burpees!" Burgener, Olympic Weightlifting coach and CrossFit specialty certification instructor, uses the standard elements of all its predecessors but adds a little twist on the end, a jumping Jack. This little contribution adds to the physical demands, reduces the ability to do the exercise at a slow work rate, and provides an objective element in order to determine successful completion (getting the feet up off the ground and the hands overhead).

The execution speed of a Burpee has a learning curve. A beginner will do the exercise at a slower and more segmented pace than an experienced trainee. This is expected as coordination evolves with practice and physical capacity improves as well thus creating an ability for the more advanced trainee to work at a faster rate. The start position is a simple standing position, heels under hips (figure 1A). The first repetition begins with bending at the hips to a large degree and bending the knees to a lesser degree. The intent of this movement is to orient the torso more parallel to the ground and close enough to it for the palms to be placed in Push-up position (figure 1B). Once the hands are placed, the hips extend quickly to move the legs and feet back to Push-up position - this is akin to a Donkey kick (figure 1C). A very unfit or uncoordinated trainee may need to walk their legs back to a push up position here rather than kicking back. As the feet are extending to the rear, the elbows and shoulders are lowering the body to the bottom of the Push-up position (figure 1D). The body should not touch the floor at the bottom, if it does the advantage of the stretch reflex across the pectorals and deltoids is lost and the exercise becomes less powerful in execution. The stretch reflex helps drive the beginning of the return to start position. With a quick kick of the butt upwards (upside down V-up position) and a very quick and powerful push from the upper body the hands break contact with the ground. The knees are simultaneously drawn in under the chest and the feet planted firmly, preferably the whole foot (figure 1E). From this semi-squat position a jump of about 3-6 inches is performed (figure 1F). As fatigue sets in, the height will diminish but a requirement to break contact with the floor remains. You can actually use an overhead target, such as a Pull-up bar to establish a minimum height jump rather than using simple breaking contact with the floor. This makes quantification of work more accurate. During the jump, both hands must be lifted overhead. The method suggested here is to move them overhead as you would in diving into water, but the traditional Jumping Jack motion of getting the arms overhead is perfectly acceptable as well.

As ability improves in the Burpee, less time is spent in contact with the ground thus the speed in which each rep is completed is faster and it sometimes is a temptation not to use the complete range of motion. By using the performance criteria for the Push-up at the bottom of the exercise and the hands-over-head jump at the top, an objective criteria is set for proper performance and measurement at any repetition rate. Not everyone can start off doing a complete Burpee, with base strength generally the limitation. To include variant of a Burpee into training for beginners or the less than strong, the following progression may be useful:

Level 1 - Squat down, kick feet back to an "up" Push-up position, then reverse and stand up

Level 2 - Squat down, kick feet back, do a Push-up, bring feet back under, stand up

Level 3 - Squat down, kick feet back, do a Push-up, bring feet back under, jump up

Level 4 - Squat down, kick feet back, do a Push-up ballistically, push off the ground at the top of Push-up and tuck feet under body while in the air, jump up

Level 5 - Bend at waist and drop the entire body flat towards the floor, catch the bodyweight on the arms, do a ballistic Push-up, push off the ground at the top of Push-up and tuck feet under body while in the air, jump up

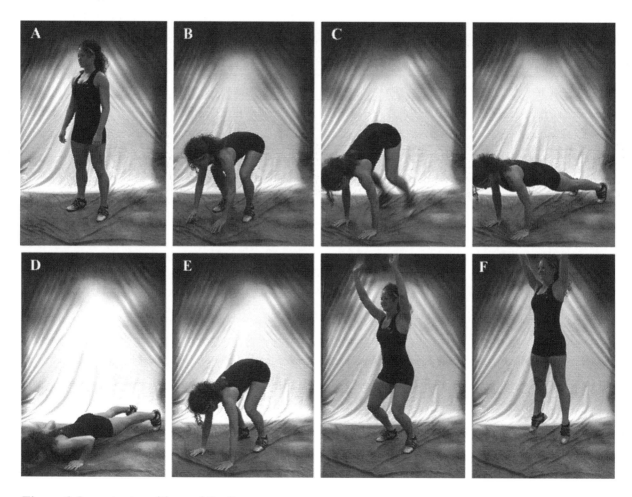

Figure 1. Important positions of the Burpee.

DUMBBELL HANG POWER SNATCH

The Dumbbell Hang Power Snatch is similar to the barbell version, yet it's done with one arm and adds a weighted jumping movement to the conditioning exercise repertoire that enhances mobility. The trainee begins with the dumbbell hanging in front of their hip and inner thigh, palm facing the body (figure 1A). The dumbbell will be in front of the hip on the same side as the hand holding it. The trainee will then flex the knees and hips as in the jump position for the Power Clean or Power Snatch (figure 1B). There is then a forceful extension of knees and hips together and a jump that carries the dumbbell upward (figure 1C). The jump occurs with straight elbows so that the full force of the jump travels through the trunk, shoulder, and arm to the dumbbell. The dumbbell will stay close to the body as the arm movement emulates that of the Power Snatch. The movement is finished when the weight is locked out overhead over the shoulder joint (figure 1D) and then moved to a standing position (figure 1E). The catch of the dumbbell overhead should occur simultaneously with feet as they land from the jump.

Most dumbbells will suffice for this movement, but dumbbells with a rotating handle are the best as they allow the arm to rotate freely under the weight. Since a solid (non-rotating handle) dumbbell will not rotate, there will be torque produced against the skin of the hand that may be uncomfortable, produce calluses, and make the movement slower. Dumbbell Hang Power Snatches aren't overly stressful on any muscle group (in contrast to Kettlebell Swings that are taxing on the hamstrings) and work really well for five to ten reps on each arm as part of a multi-element conditioning workout.

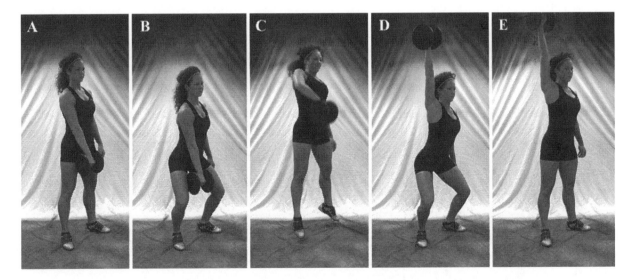

Figure 1. Important Dumbbell Snatch positions.

BODYWEIGHT SQUAT

There is another squat exercise that is also a valuable tool in the development of fitness, a simple bodyweight squat. Known by many other names over the course of exercise history, the bodyweight squat, the knee bend, the deep knee bend, the air squat, or simply the squat is a useful endurance development exercise. In very poorly fit individuals the Bodyweight Squat can be an initial strength stimulus, used until the trainee can progress to an unloaded bar. At that point they begin using Back Squats for strength development. The proper use of this exercise in all other populations is with higher repetitions in order to target the development of the metabolic machinery of local muscular endurance. Once you can do 20 Bodyweight Squats, the exercise cannot be a developer of strength as there is no means of advancing the intensity (weight) used in the exercise (refer back to chapters 2 and 4 for explanation).

To do a Bodyweight Squat we use the exact same lower body set up as in the Back Squat (figure 1A). The heels are directly under the shoulder joints and toes are pointed out slightly. The back is in normal extension and remains so throughout the exercise. It is recommended here to carry the arms extended to the front with the hands held at about waist level. They will serve as a counterbalance and steadying agent during the squat movement. To start the exercise simply drop the hips back and then bend the knees to lower the body to one of the two appropriate squat depths - hip crease below knee cap or full range of motion (figure 1B). As the body lowers into the bottom position, the hands stay at roughly the same position relative to the floor, this is accomplished by raising the arms at the same rate the body lowers. To finish the repetition, you simply stand up and reassume the start position.

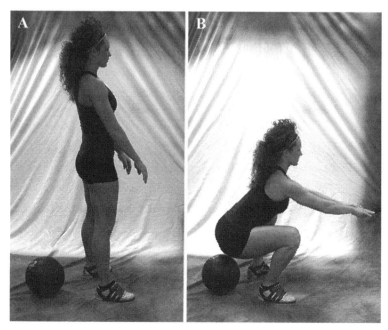

Figure 1. The top and bottom position of the Bodyweight Squat. The medicine ball is a target and does not have to be used.

As this exercise is done for many repetitions and fatigue will be a factor, providing a temptation to not completely resume extension in the start position, not hit proper depth, or both, it is useful to provide the body a depth target. Choose a medicine ball that, when touched by the butt at the bottom of the squat, places the body BELOW an approved depth. A medicine ball is used as it has very little bounce thus preventing an alternate means of cheating, bouncing off the depth target. A small Swiss ball would not be a good tool for this use as it rebounds significantly. A hard block of something (wood, stone, metal, etc) also would not make a good target as a miscalculation of depth and speed of approach to the bottom could prove a bit painful. A medicine ball has enough give to avoid this latter problem. Understand that the goal is to lightly touch the target, not HIT it.

THRUSTER

The Thruster is a compound lift that combines a Front Squat and a Press and can be done with a barbell or with dumbbells. The thruster uses the Front Squat ascent to initiate the bar's movement off of the shoulders in the same way that the Push Press utilizes the dip-and-drive to initiate momentum. Begin with the bar on the shoulders in the push press or jerk start position (grip outside the shoulders with slightly elevated elbows)(figure 1A). It is important that the bar does not move from the initial rack position, particularly at the bottom of the front squat. Too often trainees will attempt to hold the bar, with vertical forearms and wrists off of the shoulders. This puts the wrists in an awkward and consistent loading during the exercise. Such a posture will place stress on the wrists and can result in aching or injured wrists. This is also not mechanically optimal position since the force produced by the quick down and up movement inherent in a Thruster is dissipated by spring element of the bar-off-the-shoulder position.

When the bar is properly secured, the trainee will descend into a front squat (figure 1B). As with front and back squatting, it's important to keep the knees out so that the femurs are in line with the angle of the feet. After achieving proper depth, the trainee will forcefully drive up and out of the squat to generate momentum and transfer it into the press and final lock out at the top (figure 1C). Complete elbow extension is required for a repetition to count, full range of motion is important.

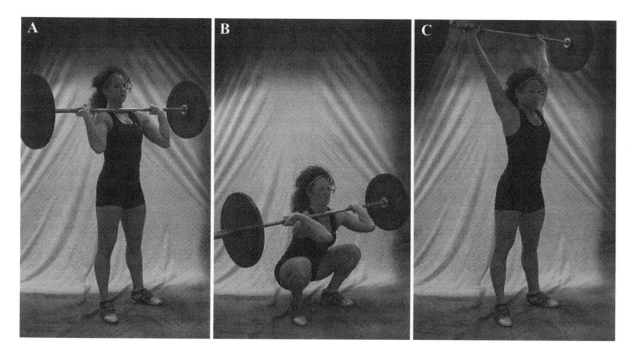

Figure 1. Key positions of the Thruster.

Although weights are used, Thrusters are primarily a conditioning exercise. Typically Thruster loads should not exceed 30% of a Front Squat max, 60% of a Press max, and/or 50% of a Push Press max. This loading is admittedly arbitrary, but such light loads ensure that enough repetitions can be completed to elicit a proper conditioning effect. Be warned, Thrusters done for higher repetitions require large amounts of energy to complete and are quite taxing even with light weights.

Dumbbell thrusters utilize the same concept, however the dumbbells should be turned so that the bells are facing anterior and posterior. If the trainee used the medial/lateral bell press position, they may have unpleasant contact between the bell and their head or ears. The forearm should maintain a vertical position throughout the front squat and press portions of the thruster. The use of dumbbells here provides an added and excellent mobility stimulus through a very large range of motion.

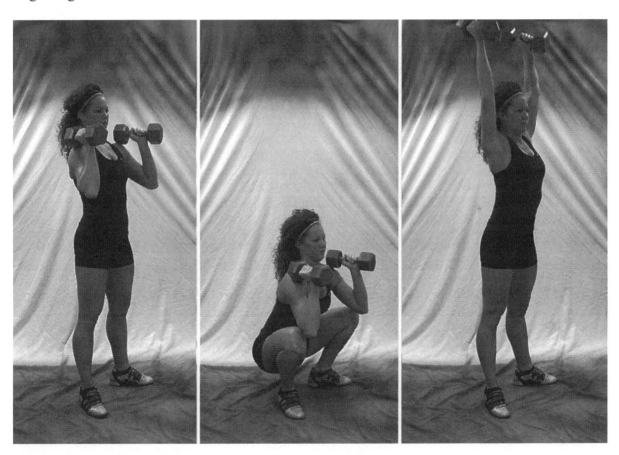

Figure 2. The Dumbbell Thruster.

MEDICINE BALL THROW

Medicine balls are quite old and excellent tools that have been used in physical conditioning for centuries. They can be tossed to the side, backward, or forward from different angles of release and trunk rotation. To keep it simple and build the most fitness (by demanding the most energy per repetition), the vertical Medicine Ball Throw to a target is presented here. This movement is similar to a Thruster in that it includes a Front Squat to ballistic Press, however it is finished by releasing the ball with enough force so that it travels vertically to a specified target height on a wall.

The trainee begins by facing the wall, a little more than arms length away, with the medicine ball in their hands. The "grip" should have the fingers pointing vertically on the side of the ball with the heel of the palm slightly underneath the curve of the ball - think 4 and 8 o'clock positions (figure 1A). This position allows the ball to sit in the palm as opposed to the trainee needing to provide pressure from the side to hold the ball in position. The elbows will maintain a vertical alignment during the subsequent front squat, press, and release (figure 1B,C,D,E). The Medicine Ball Throw aims to transfer the force from the legs during the front squat to the press at a high enough speed to push the ball into the air. As with all forms of squatting, care should be taken to track the knees along the long line of the foot (knees out) and to achieve full depth - even when tired.

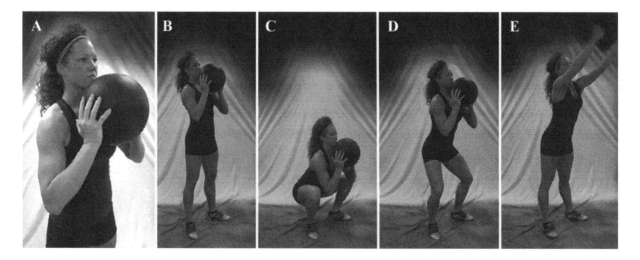

Figure 1. Basic Medicine Ball Throw positions.

Before actually doing the exercise a target needs to be selected to ensure a quantifiable and consistent amount of work is done with each repetition. Target heights on the wall are typically placed at a height between eight and twelve feet above the floor. Use a piece of tape, a dot of paint, or choose a specific brick in the wall to designate the target. In general medicine balls weighing between 15 to 30 pounds for men and 5 to 15 pounds for women are used. Lighter balls are used for lower fit individuals and progression is used to move the trainee to heavier balls and more difficult training over time. If heavier balls are not available the target height can be moved up to increase the work required per repetition. Exercises such as this can be deceivingly difficult; trainees must start with and adapt to lighter balls and lower target heights before advancing.

Also note that medicine balls, especially the new composite material balls more so than older style leather balls, can leave surface marks on walls. Further, these are weighted balls and can dent or break drywall or other lightly constructed walls. Find robust walls that will not be damaged and ensure that the property owner approves of you throwing things against the wall prior to actually doing it.

BOX JUMPS

Box jumps are a conditioning movement in which the trainee jumps with both feet from level ground to an elevated surface. The trainee starts by facing the box with a hip width stance (figure 1A). To initiate the jump, the body is lowered by flexing the hips, tilting the trunk slightly forward, the knees bend slightly, and the arms are swung to the rear quickly. In this bottom position the elbows are slightly bent and to the rear of the body and the hands are at or slightly behind the hips (figure 1B). Note that the jump position is not merely flexing the knees, both knee and hip extension are necessary for efficient jumping. This is a ballistic movement that uses the stretch reflex to produce rapid force generation. As in the Jerk, lowering into the jumping position is a quick movement and immediately subsequent extension of the hips and knees to propel the body vertically and slightly forward onto the box that is just a few inches in front of the toes (figure 1C). When landing on the box, it should be a soft touchdown where the knees and hips bend to cushion the impact (figure 1D). Trying to minimize the amount of noise made when landing on the box softens the landing and will prevent future soreness from repeated impacts. After landing the repetition is competed by standing up fully on the box. To return to the start position, the trainee steps back and off the box, one leg at a time, to the level ground (figure 1E).

If new to Box Jumping a trainee should ease into the exercise both by doing some practicing jumping for a two or three sets of no more than five to ten repetitions onto the lowest box available. This preview will allow selection of a starting box height and a starting repetition number for inclusion in future workouts. Failing to test the waters, so to speak, will generally lead to unnecessary soreness in the knees the day after jumping, a result of not starting at a low enough workload and easing the anatomical structures used into a new and jolting activity. The eyes should not stray from the box as it's easy to stumble or completely miss the box if the eyes are looking elsewhere (Can you hit a golf ball blindfolded?). Stumbles or misses can result in banging the shins on the edge of the box; a painful and potentially physically scarring experience. The necessity for task focus is doubly important when fatigued from a difficult conditioning workout - the type of workout in which this exercise is included. As technical skill and fitness advance, there is an option to hop backwards off the box. This reduces transition time back to the start position and increases the rate of jumps. More jumps equates to more work being completed and is a demonstration of improved fitness. The hop back off of the box should attempt to retake the exact same position where the exercise started, no one should randomly and wildly propel themselves backwards off a box. Recklessness is not mandatory for good fitness.

There are lots of examples of individuals leaping up on top of boxes well over 4 feet in height. While that is mildly impressive, remember that the intent for the Box Jump exercise here is in the development of endurance. You cannot jump near maximal heights for enough repetitions to produce an endurance stimulus (if you attempt this you will fail and risk injury). Start with small boxes, 12 inches or less in height, and then over time begin using higher boxes. In general you will not want to use a box more than six inches higher than your best standing vertical jump. If your best vertical jump is 24 inches you would begin by using the 12 inch box and then over a period of many months you would use progressively higher boxes until you reach a 30 inch box.

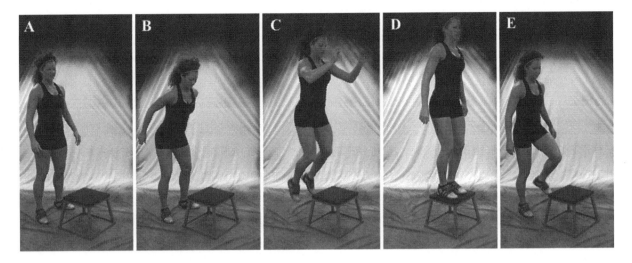

Figure 1. Basic Box Jump positions.

As you get older it is harder to have heroes, but it is sort of necessary.

Ernest Hemingway

MOBILITY EXERCISES

As laid out in chapter 5, mobility training can be done in a specialized training session but it can be accomplished as part of any normal workout - as long as attention is given to performing each exercise through the complete range of motion AND eliminating machine based exercises from the workout menu. The following exercises are intended to be used as developmental exercises that create mobility in individuals who have limited range of motion and movement skills. They are not intended to be part of every training session for everyone.

There are two general classifications of exercises included below; (1) Dynamic flexibility exercises that utilize active movement through the complete range of motion and (2) Static flexibility exercises that involve holding a stretched muscle and joint position for a brief period.

Dynamic Flexibility Exercises

Dynamic exercises are frequently used as preparative exercises prior to training or competition in order to ensure that the desired exercise positions can be attained. It is imperative that with each repetition of each exercise there is a defined attempt to increase the range of motion. While dynamic flexibility work is quite useful in trainees and athletes with poor to average mobility, it may possibly inhibit peak performance in individuals with already well developed flexibility and mobility or that require great deals of strength or power for success.

Static Flexibility Exercises

In the exercise arena there are very few new things. Static stretching has been part of exercise programs for likely as long as there have been humans. Representations of stretching appear in pre-Vedic Indian art of at least 5,000 years ago. It was formally presented as a contributing means to holistic health and enlightenment in the Rigveda about 3,500 years ago. Vestiges of these depictions and writings remain in practice to this day, some virtually unchanged, within the discipline of Yoga. Any time we stretch, we are doing something humans have been doing throughout recorded history. For something to have survived so long, it either has had to work towards achieving a goal or it has had to feel really good. Static stretching does both. When executed appropriately it will increase the range of motion around a joint AND it provides a pleasurable sensation if done delicately. Here we are most interested in improving range of motion and to accomplish this the stretch placed on a muscle or muscle group needs to push past the pleasurable to the edge of discomfort, but not pain. This is where the best gains are made.

Lower Body Dynamic Exercises

The following exercises target the hamstrings, hip flexors, and lower lumbar area of the back. As the hips and legs are likely the most important set of joints in the body relative to exercise, and because there is such a large mass of muscle associated with them dynamic flexibility exercises that target them provide an effective means of warming up the entire body. As such lower body exercises are included prior to upper body exercises in this application.

LATERAL SHUFFLE

Start with the feet hip to shoulder width apart. Drop the hips down to a jumping position by bending the knees to just about quarter squat depth. Keeping the back flat and the chest up, begin by stepping the lead foot out to the side then gathering the trail foot back in to about hip to shoulder width. Then by pushing off the trail foot, repeat the process for the given distance. Most importantly always stay low with the hips down and the back flat. Never let the feet come any closer together than six to eight inches. Always make the lead step lateral, never forward or backward.

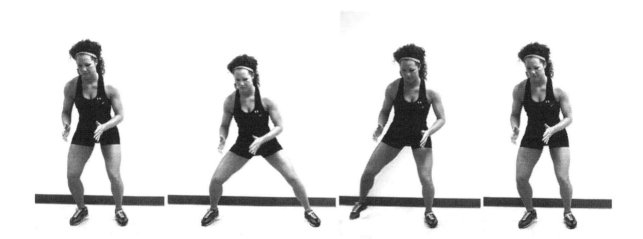

Figure 1. The Lateral Shuffle exercise.

WALKING TOE TOUCH

Begin with the toes on the line of the start point, standing tall with arms extended straight ahead with hands at eye level. Start with a step forward with the lead leg (figure 2 left) followed by a kicking motion with the trailing leg (figure 2 right). Keeping the leg as straight as possible (done by flexing the quadriceps during the kick) trying to touch the tip of the toe to the outstretched fingers. Take the second step with the opposite leg repeating the process trying to once again touch the toe to the finger of the opposite hand. This action will be repeated the length of the given distance or number of toe touches, usually around 10 yards or 10 touches.

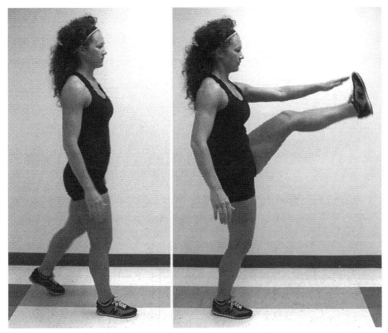

Figure 2. The Walking Toe Touch exercise.

Keep the legs as straight as possible during the kicking motion. Try to kick a little higher with each step to push the hamstring and low back through as much range of motion as possible. Depending on your level of flexibility and coordination, this exercise can be done by kicking the right toe to the left fingers and the left toe to the right fingers, or by kicking the same toe to the same hand.

HIGH KNEE TUCK

This is a walking exercise. As in the previous exercise, the trailing leg is pulled to a high stretched position as it moves to the lead position. The knee is pulled up then both hands are used to grasp the knee and pull it tightly into the chest and held for about a second. The hold is released and the next step is taken and the opposite knee is driven high to the front, grasped, and pulled tightly to the chest. Following the brief pause at the top, the cycle continues for 10 cycles or about 10 yards. It is important to pull the knee up and in, not just towards the chest. To add an additional mobility element to the exercise, rise up on the ball of foot and toes at the top of each repetition to add the need for balance.

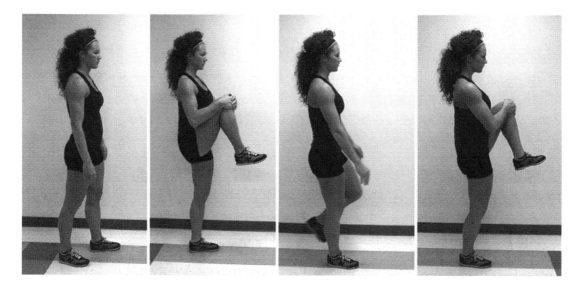

Figure 3. The High Knee Tuck exercise.

LEG SWINGS

Leg swings are a simple and basic hip mobility exercise that work medio-lateral range of motion. Stand with the bodyweight supported on one foot. Hold on to some structure to aid in balance. Start slowly and swing your unsupported leg across the body to the front (figure 4 left), when the end of the range of motion is reached, change the direction of the swing towards moving the leg laterally. When the end of the range of motion to the side is reached, change swing direction back towards the middle. Perform 10 escalating amplitude swings. Repetition 1 should be a small swing amplitude, swing 10 should be the largest amplitude of the set. Up to three sets of 10 repetitions can be done. The same number of repetitions should be done for both legs.

Front-to-back Leg Swings can also be done to work on anterio-posterior hip range of motion. The same principles apply, the only change being that the leg is swung back and forth.

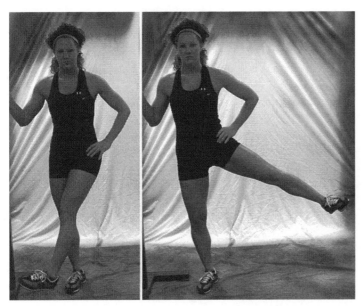

Figure 4. Leg Swings for hip mobility.

Upper Body Exercises

The following exercises target the joints and muscle of the shoulder joints. These joints are also important as they are involved with any interaction of the hands with any implement, weight, or other body during exercise and sport.

Y, T, W, & L

The Y & T portions of this exercise are done together and are derived from the Utkatasana pose in Yoga. First bend over at waist to about a 45 degree angle. This is important as this is where the resistance to movement comes from. Let the arms hang straight down directly below the should joints. The elbows should be straight. The Y is accomplished via a quick raise of the straight arms, thumbs pointed up, forward overhead to the position of a Y (torso is the stem, arms the uprights)(figure 5 left). Ten repetitions are done. Immediately after completion of the Y repetitions, the arms are moved from the hanging position to the side to form a T (torso is the stem, arms to crossbar). Ten repetitions are done before moving the W movement.

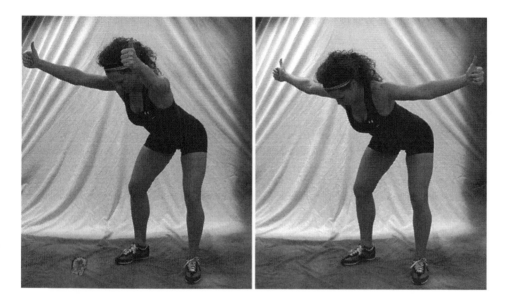

Figure 5. Top positions for the "Y" (left) and "T" (right) mobility exercises for the shoulder.

In the W component, you stand upright, bend elbows and pull them to the rear to a point that the hands are just in front of the body (figure 6 left). The elbows should be bent at about a 90 degree angle and will stay so throughout the exercise. Moving only at the shoulder joint move the arms up to where they are parallel to the floor (figure 6 right). During this motion the arms will be back as you squeeze the shoulder blades together. This movement looks much like a bird flapping its wings. Perform 10 repetitions before moving the L portion.

For the L section, stand upright with the arms raised to shoulder level and parallel to the floor. Bend the elbows to 90 degrees foward (figure 7 left). Keeping the orientation of the arm to floor and the elbow angle the same, rotate upper arm so the forearms point straight up towards toward the ceiling (figure 7 center). Still maintaining arm position, rotate at the shoulder and bring the forearms down pointing towards the floor (figure 7 right). Repeat this cycle for 10 repetitions.

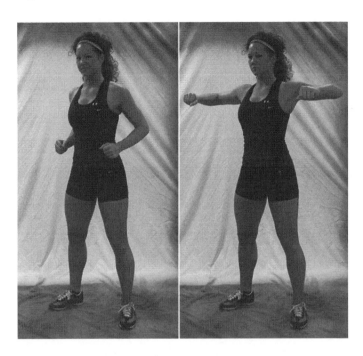

Figure 6. The "W" exercise for shoulder mobility.

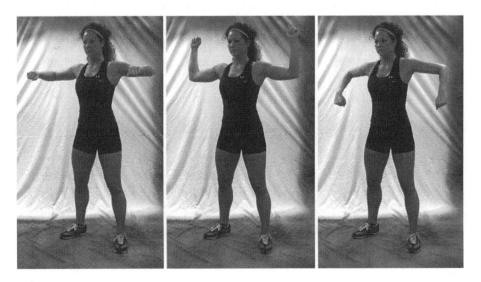

Figure 7. The "L" exercise for shoulder mobility.

WALL SLIDE

The Wall Slide is a simple shoulder exercise that works overhead range of motion and is similar to the free-standing Yoga pose Urdhva Hastasana. Place the heels, butt, shoulders, and arms against a wall (figure 8 left). At the start, the elbows will be at 90 degrees and the upper arm will be parallel to the floor. To complete the movement, the arms simply extend overhead until the elbows near complete extension and the hands touch (figure 8 right). It is important that all parts of the body, even the moving parts, maintain contact with the wall throughout the movement. Repeat for 10 repetitions.

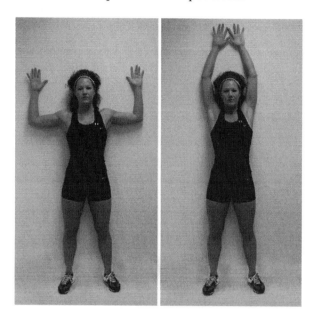

Figure 8. The Wall Slide exercise for shoulder mobility.

OVERHEAD SQUAT

The Overhead Squat is a loaded and moving variant of the Utkatasana posture in Yoga and combines a tremendous breadth of mobility elements into a single dynamic flexibility exercise. Virtually every joint system, upper and lower body, is involved in this movement that also requires coordinated effort and balance. To start each repetition, the bar should comfortably rest across the top of the shoulders at the base of the neck. The bar will be held with a Snatch grip (see Strength Exercises chapter). The feet are placed so the heels are slightly wider than the hips, toes are pointed out slightly. The bar is pressed overhead until the arms are fully extended the a simple squat follows. The bar should remain aligned over the back of the head (no farther forward than the ears. The elbows and shoulders should be involved in a hard press out during the entire movement and the chest should be up and back straight throughout. Ten repetitions are done with either an appropriate weight bar or a broomstick.

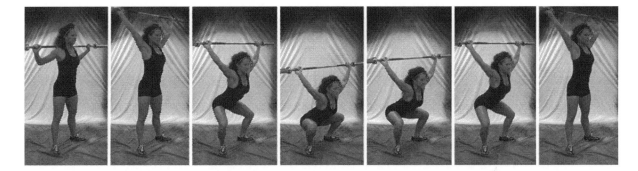

Figure 9. The Overhead Squat exercise.

Static Flexibility Exercises

At the end of a workout body temperature and muscle pliability is at its highest and this is when we most effectively use static stretching exercises to improve range of motion. Unlike in dynamic work, we begin static stretching with the upper body as it is a smaller muscle mass and will lose heat and its temperature-related elasticity more rapidly than the lower body. The stretches described here is a basic set of static stretches targeting the most important joints for general exercise ability.

PULL ACROSS – PULL OVER STRETCH

This combination stretch is derived from two Yoga positions, Garudasana (the Pull Across) and Gomukhasana (the Pull Over) and targets the Pectoralis major and minor, internal rotators of the upper arm, and Triceps brachii.

While standing upright, use your opposite arm, pull your arm in towards the chest and reach across the body as far as possible (figure 10). A beginner with limited range of motion will hold the stretch for 10 seconds. Progression in the duration of the hold out to about 30 seconds over the course of weeks and months will produce improved range of motion. At the end of the hold pull your arm up - upper arm as straight up as possible and forearm behind the head. Using the opposite arm, hold the elbow and pull the arm in behind the head and reach as far as possible towards the middle of the back with the hand of the stretched arm. Bend at the waist slightly away from the arm being stretched. Hold for 10 seconds. Progress as described. Once the stretch is completed with one arm, repeat with opposite arm.

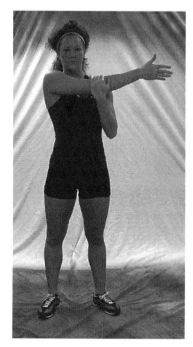

Figure 10. Pull Across exercise for shoulder mobility.

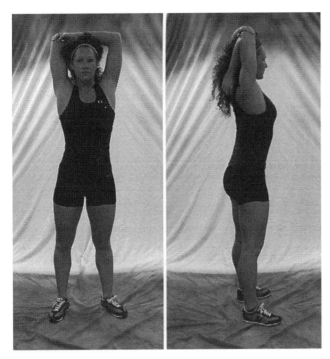

Figure 11. Pull Over exercise for shoulder mobility.

SIDE QUADRICEPS STRETCH

This stretch is a modification of the Yoga stretch, Ardha Supta Virasana, and targets the quadriceps, Iliacus, Psoas, and other hip flexors.

Lie on your side using the same side elbow as a prop for the upper body. Grasp the top of the foot and pull the heel back and up toward the butt and hold at the end of the range of motion for 10 seconds (figure 12). Be sure you are propped up on the elbow with knees, hips, and shoulders in line and that the pull is applied slowly and gradually. Turn over to the other side, assume the same position, and repeat the stretch with opposite leg.

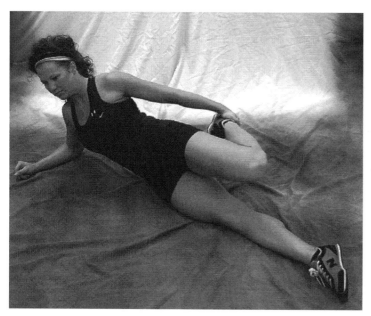

Figure 12. Side Quadriceps exercise for knee and hip mobility.

SUPINE KNEE FLEX

This stretch is essentially identical to the Yoga position, Ardha Pavana Muktasana, and targets the hip extensors, Gluteus maximus, Gluteus medius, Gluteus minimus, and the hamstrings.

Lie on your back with one leg straight and in contact with the floor. Wrap the hands around the opposite bent knee and pull it towards the chest slowly. At the end of the perceived range of motion, hold for 10 seconds. Make sure the hip of the straight leg is in line and flush with the floor as allowing it to elevate minimizes the stretch effects on the other leg. Release the stretch then repeat the process with the opposite leg.

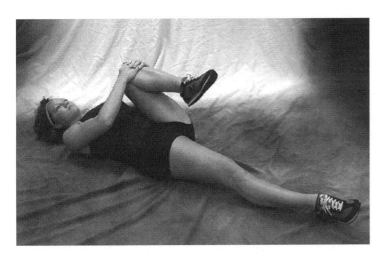

Figure 13. Supine Knee Flex exercise for posterior hip mobility.

SUMO SQUAT STRETCH

The Sumo Squat stretch described here is a variant of the Malasana position of Yoga. It targets the Gluteus maximus, Gluteus medius, Gluteus minimus, hamstrings, and adductors of the leg.

Place your feet slightly outside shoulder width - wider than your Back Squat stance - with heels flat and toes pointing slightly out. Lower your hips slowly to the bottom of a squat position, as low as possible. Ensure that the heels remain flat on the floor. Force your knees out, push your butt back, and keep the low back as flat as possible in the bottom position (figure 14). Push the knees out with your elbows to produce the best effect and hold the position for 10 seconds.

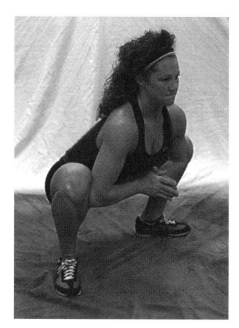

Figure 14. The Sumo Squat exercise for hip mobility.

HIP FLEXOR STRETCH

This stretch is a variant of the Yoga position, Anjaneyasana, and targets the hip flexors, Iliacus, Psoas, and the musculature of the groin region.

Place one leg forward with a bent knee, aligning your knee directly over the ankle (90 degrees at the knee, thigh to shin). The other leg should be directly behind with knee slightly off ground or resting very lightly on the ground as it is not to be a weight support. Slowly move your hips forward - without changing position of front foot or back knee - until the end of the range of motion (figure 15). Hold the position for 10 seconds, release, and then repeat with opposite leg.

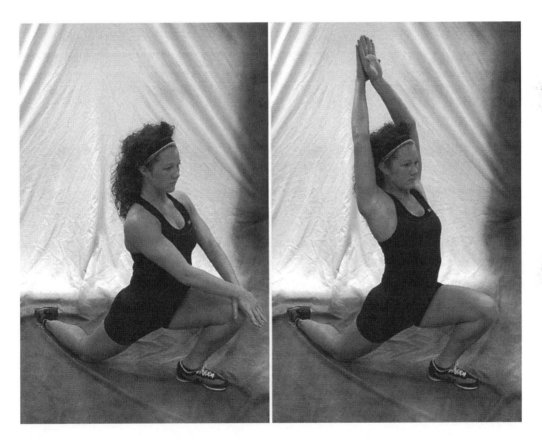

Figure 15. Two finishing positions for the Hip Flexor exercise for hip mobility; easy (left) and more difficult (right).

STANDING HAMSTRING STRETCH

This stretch is loosely based on the Uttanasana pose in Yoga and targets the hamstrings and low back.

From a standing position, with your feet under your hips (as in Jerk stance), slowly flex the hips (bend at the hips). As your shoulders lower to the front, your butt will be moving back. Keep the knees slightly bent (just barely), keep the palms on the upper thigh, and slide them downward in a slow controlled position until an easy stretch is felt in the back of the legs (figure 16). Most trainees will initially have difficulty getting their hands below the knee if the position is strictly maintained. At the end of the available range of motion, hold the position for 10 seconds.

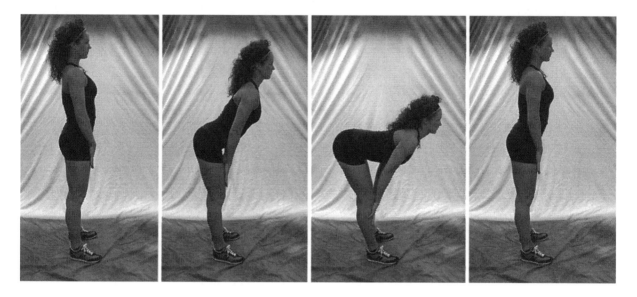

Figure 16. The Standing Hamstring exercise for hip mobility.

STRADDLE STRETCH

The Upavistha Konasana position in Yoga serves as a basis for many Yoga poses and is similarly modified here to produce a three position stretch that targets the Gastrocnemius, hamstrings, Erectors spinae, adductors of the leg, and the Sartorius.

From a sitting position with your upper body posture erect and vertical, spread the legs as far as possible laterally. The knees are straight or have only a minor bend in them throughout the stretch. Move your torso and reach with both hands slowly towards one foot as far as possible (figure 17). In someone with poor flexibility, they might only be able to get the hands past the knee cap. That is fine, it is the starting point from where progress begins. At the end of the range of motion hold the position (no bouncing) for 10 seconds. Release and return to the torso upright position and then reach for the opposite foot and hold for 10 seconds. Release and return to the upright position. Finally reach directly forward between the legs as far as possible and hold without bouncing for 10 seconds (figure 17 far right). Although rounding of the low back is quite permissible here, the straighter the back, the more profound the stretch.

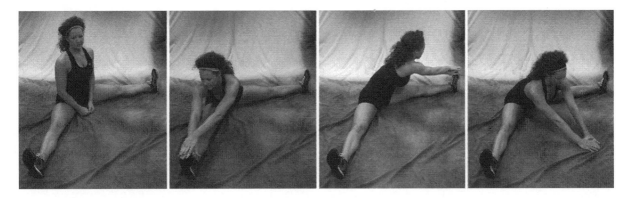

Figure 17. The Straddle exercise for hip mobility.

SPINAL TWIST STRETCH

Called the Hook and Look in many weight rooms, the Spinal Twist stretch is actually the Eka Pada Upavistha Parivrttasana position in Yoga. It's twisting nature targets the Erectors spinae, Internal obliques, External obliques, along with many other vertebral column related structures.

Sit erect with your left leg straight, place the right foot to the left side of the left knee. Place your left elbow on the right side of the bent right knee and elbow on the right side of the bent right knee and allow palm to support torso about 8-12 inches behind hips. Push your right knee with left elbow while turning the torso to the right and looking back as far as possible (figure 18). Make sure the cross over foot is flat and that the correct elbow is being used to push on the lateral portion of the knee. Hold for 10 seconds, release, then repeat to the opposite side.

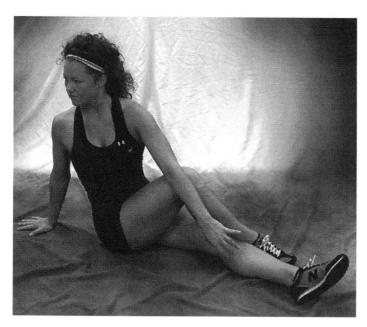

Figure 18. The Spinal Twist exercise for lumbar mobility.

BUTTERFLY STRETCH

This variant of the Baddha Konasana position in Yoga targets the adductors of the leg, the Sartorius, and other structures in the groin area.

Sit on the floor erect and pull the soles of your feet together. With your hands clasped around your ankles (either on the front of the ankle or just below on the mid-foot) pull yourself forward, low back flat, until you feel a stretch in the groin area. Use your elbows to push your knees down to produce the best stretch. As flexibility is advanced, the heels will need to be pulled closer to the body and knees pressed down more with the elbow to produce a stretch. Hold the stretch at the end of the range of motion for 10 seconds.

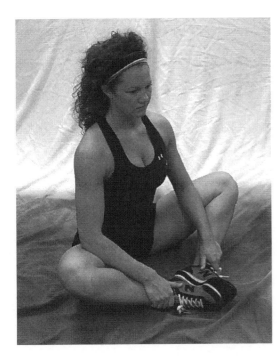

Figure 19. The Butterfly exercise for hip mobility.

CALF STRETCH

This is a small scale stretch that has no direct analogous pose in Yoga. However, there are any number of Yoga poses that create the exact same stretch as part of a more complex multi-body-part pose. The targets of this stretch are the two major calf muscles, the Gastrocnemius and the Soleus.

Place the toes or ball of the foot up on a vertical surface with the heel on the ground (figure 20). The angle of the foot - floor to wall - should be about 30 degrees for first time users of this stretch. As flexibility improves the foot angle can and should be increased to progress in range of motion. After the foot is placed, bend the knee slightly and slowing move the knee closer to the wall or vertical structure (figure 20A). With the knee bent, the soleus is provided an isolating stretch. Hold for 10 seconds. Release the stretch, straighten the knee, and again move the knee towards the wall or vertical structure (figure 20B). Performed with a straight knee the Gastrocnemius is now stretched. Hold for 10 seconds, release, and repeat the process on the opposite leg.

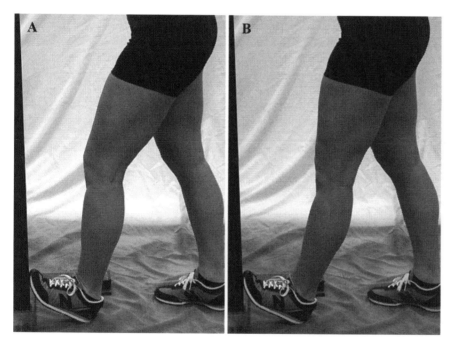

Figure 20. Calf stretch exercise for the soleus (A) and the gastrocnemius (B).

GETTING READY TO TRAIN

Out of clutter find simplicity.

Albert Einstein

Getting ready to exercise is a bit of an art ... sometimes a ritual ... always considered a necessity, as no one, in general, just gets up off the couch and goes full tilt into a workout. There are lots of examples of this in the animal kingdom, but not generally in humans. Humans think about and plan exercise for reasons other than survival.

Where

One of the first considerations of a workout is where it is to be conducted; in a gym, at home, on a trail, on a track, on the street, on playground monkey bars, or some other location. The workout you want to do has to be facilitated by your exercise environment. If you want to do squats (and who doesn't), you don't go to a spa where 5 pound dumbbells and a few hydraulic machines are the entire stock of resistance equipment. If you want to run 5 kilometers you don't jump in a pool. In a perfect world every training facility would have everything one would need to develop complete fitness, but alas they don't. You may have to shop around to find the best fit for you. There are a number of websites available that list clubs and gyms that have specific types of equipment or support certain modes of training. The startingstrength.com website has a good list of gyms that support basic barbell training, the CrossFit.com website has a list of some 2000 gyms that have a broad holding of basic multi-element training tools, national governing boards for specific Olympic sports (such as weightlifting, cycling, swimming, and track &field) have lists of coaches and facilities on their websites, and there are plentiful other similar listings around the world. There is no reason to do without proper equipment and resources, where there is a will there is a way to train correctly.

If you train outside, pay attention to the weather. Frostbite and heat illnesses are not appropriate training strategies.

Apparel

If you run, wear proper footwear to protect your feet. If you lift, wear shoes that make stable and repeatable technique the norm, not a chance occurrence. If you do multiple element training, wear shoes that facilitate correct running form and do not interfere with lifting stability, balance, and jumping force transfer.

Clothing is a bit of a mixed bag. The original Olympians trained and competed in the buff. The best cooling of the body is provided by direct exposure of the skin to the environment (not

287

considering sun-burn and such here). And less clothing provides the least restriction to movement. So there is somewhat of a basis for wearing limited clothing during training, as permitted by environmental conditions. Also, when people get fit, they like to wear less to show off their hard-won fitness gains. It's good to be proud of your gains BUT certain activities require certain apparel considerations. In a weight room or in room with exercise machines used by multiple people, a barrier between the skin and contact surfaces on the machines are needed to diminish the risk of bacterial infection spread among users (reviewed in 1). Staph from one person's skin-to-pad contact can infect many other people who put their skin on the same equipment. Repetitive cleaning of equipment throughout the day can limit transmission but it's easier for all involved to just wear clothes that stop skin-to-pad contact - simply wearing a shirt attenuates the spread of disease.

Barbells present somewhat of a similar issue. Some people will occasionally scrape the skin on their shins with the knurling on the bar leaving a little blood from the scratch on the bar (some people train their entire lives without doing this, some people are constantly doing this). Wearing knee socks or sweat pants during exercises that work off the floor prevents potential blood borne pathogen transmission. Also with barbell exercises that have the bar supported on the shoulders (front or back), a shirt is recommended as sweat makes the skin slippery and the bar has a chance of sliding out of position. A sliding and misplaced bar reduces exercise efficiency and may increase the risk of accident.

Other than those issues relative to shoes (covered in previous chapters) and clothes, everything else about training apparel is wide open. Slave to fashion or minimalist couture is unimportant, its the training that is important. Cheryl Tiegs once proclaimed that "It's very important to have the right clothing to exercise in. If you throw on an old T-shirt or sweats, it's not inspiring for your workout." We'd like to think that the results of training are what is inspiring, but if cool gear gets you to the gym, that works too.

The Warm-up

This is another mythology laced part of a workout. The simple purpose of a warm-up is to prepare the body to effectively produce force for the duration of the workout. It is not intended to enhance performance, it is not intended to reduce injury, it is not intending to improve flexibility, just prepare the body to train at its present fitness status.

This previous statement is quite contrary to the position espoused by many exercise, sport, and clinical professionals. They propose that warm-ups are required in order to prevent injury and to enhance performance. This has been a mindset for decades, one with very little factual support. In fact, if a warm-up includes stretching, as is generally the case, the ability to generate force goes down (2,3) and running performance goes down (4). Injury rate following warm-up stretching is no different than if no stretching is done (5,6). So it appears as though one traditional element of pre-exercise warm-ups, stretching, is wasted time in injury prevention and empty effort linked to inhibition of quality exercise performance. Now realize that there is a purpose for stretching, improved range of motion, however the time to do that is not during a pre-exercise warm-up, it is much more effectively carried out at the end of a training session, when the muscles have become much more compliant and fatigued (see the Mobility chapter). Under these conditions stretching is productive at increasing joint flexibility. However, if there is already satisfactory flexibility - meaning that the complete range of motion required of an exercise skill or set of skills is present - no additional stretching work is needed.

So how should warm-ups be constructed? Let's begin with how they should not be constructed. An endurance trainee whose target distance is 5-10K (3-6 miles) should not be jogging for a couple miles before a training run. Why would we want to include long-slow-distance training in every workout? We already know that it cannot help us improve running speed. And continuous endurance training will interfere with the rate of progression of other fitness elements if included in workouts intended to develop those other fitness elements. Also the repetitive impact nature of distance running and the prevalence of over-use injury associated with high mileage would suggest that elimination of any miles not directly contributing to fitness development would payoff with more efficient use of training time and a reduction in injury risk.

To elevate body temperature to a point that muscle contraction and the metabolic machinery operate optimally during a running workout, one simply needs to do an ascending intensity exercise ramp. Start at walking pace for a minute, walk faster for a minute, jog for a minute, run at near training pace for a minute, ease back to a walk for a minute, then start your training session. A similar pattern of loading would be followed in preparation for rowing or any other continuous endurance exercise session. Five minutes of simple exercise provides everything needed to facilitate entry into an endurance workout. Anything beyond this is misuse of time and adds unnecessary joint impacts. Note that these are recommendations for fitness trainees, not for specific event and distance endurance athletes, although similar concepts are in operation with those populations as well.

For strength training sessions, a brief rowing (preferable), cycling, treadmill, or other exercise bout is needed to increase body temperature for the same reasons as with running. No more than 3-5 minutes of escalating intensity exercise is needed to produce the desired general body temperature increase. Unlike the running workout, where the warm-up activity is both general and specific to the training activity, a strength warm-up must include an exercise specific component. In this context, specific means an increasing weight ramp while performing the first exercise of the training session. The ramp starts with the bar and ends with a weight about 5-10% lighter than the intended training weight. No more than 20 warm-up repetitions should be used and they should be grouped in sets with descending repetitions (as the warm-up weights get heavier, fewer repetitions are done in each warm-up set). This is a warm-up, not a training stimulus. Also unlike running or other continuous endurance activities, the nature of the movement trained changes with each weight exercise included in a workout. This results in smaller scale specific warm-ups being inserted between exercises. There is no rowing, cycling, or running in between exercises, just 8 to 12 repetitions of the new exercise grouped and loaded in the same pattern as the first exercise. The body is already warm and ready to train from the first warm-up and exercise, we are now simply warming up the specific motor patterns involved in the new exercise, along with any musculature not involved in the first exercise.

It is not unheard of for Olympic lifters and powerlifters to forgo any type of general warm-up and proceed directly to an exercise specific warm-up. While not a fast and effective means of elevating body temperature, a warm-up is still accomplished, generally using more repetitions with the lighter end of the weight ramp before progressing to lower and heavier repetitions. This does increase body temperature to a lesser extent, but it retains a degree of muscle rigidity and force transfer, a benefit in lifting performance. Too much endurance activity and/or stretching prior to a lifting session reduces muscle force and power output capacity. There is a narrow margin of too much and not enough warm-up here. Only individual coaching or training experience can discern the line between the two.

For multi-element training sessions the warm-ups can be a bit more involved as there may be many exercises included in the training session and no break between them to allow for separate specific warm-ups, as done in lifting workouts. The structure of such a warm-up is dependent on the exercises included in the actual workout, but an example might be to do 3 to 5 minutes on the Concept 2 with an escalating frequency stroke rate (20-25-30-35) followed by three repeats of a circuit composed of bodyweight squats (10-10-10), push-ups (5-5-5), and pull-ups (ability specific and lower repetitions - not to failure). About one or two minutes after completion of the last circuit, the training session would begin.

The idea behind all of these warm-ups is to prepare for the workout, not to do so much work as to disrupt homeostasis and induce adaptation. If we do, we are programming incorrectly, giving away valuable future progress, developing unintended fitness elements, and are running the risk of overtraining.

After its over

We've all been told that when we get done with a training session that we need to continue low intensity exercise until the heart rate drops to an arbitrary number, usually 100 beats per minute. We are also told not to sit down and never to lie down immediately after exercising for fear of "blood pooling" or having a cardiac event.

The basis for the concept of cool down is derived from a misapplication of the science around cardiac arrhythmias (irregular heart beats). In the past, after a maximal treadmill exercise test of a patient suspected of previously having an arrhythmia, the patient would be immediately laid on an exam table after exhaustive running. Due to the change in the nature of the pressures exerted on the heart from moving from standing to lying (orthostatic challenge), the patient had a high percentage chance of experiencing the arrhythmia in the presence of the physician. So in cardiac diseased populations, lying down immediately after hard exercise may potentially provoke an arrhythmia. This has never been seen in healthy populations and the logic for using this concept in healthy and athletic populations is absent. Not a single healthy, disease free, individual has ever been reported to die or be injured after abruptly ceasing exercise and remaining standing, immediately sitting down, or immediately lying down. So the bottom line is that when you are done with your workout, you are done. There is no advantage in maintaining low level movement over sitting down or lying down after finishing a workout. Even if you want to get the heart rate down to some arbitrary level (there is no real data to support this practice either), which is more effective at getting it down, more exercise or stopping exercise?

There is also a proposition that continued movement keeps the blood circulating after training and aids in clearance of circulating metabolites such as lactic acid. This concept is contradictory to the desire to reduce heart rate to 100 beats per minute. Besides, if lactate clearance is a problem, that needs to be addressed through intelligent long-term exercise programming, not as an add-on at the end of a workout. Probably the best reason for doing additional activity after finishing a bout of exercise is for performing a victory lap, a very unique and specific application.

Recovery rates are different between types of training. After a hard strength session you should be able to go directly from your last set to the shower ... after a minute or so of recovery (and of course only after re-racking your plates). After a hard continuous endurance session you should be able to hit the shower after a short few minutes of recovery. After a hard mixed-element training session you will likely be immobile for several minutes before you even feel like heading to the shower.

Exercise Can Kill You

When you decide to begin a program of exercise to improve fitness, you are acknowledging that you have less than optimal levels of one or all components of fitness. This means that you will be unaccustomed to doing the activities included in your program either in exercise type, volume of training, or intensity of training, or all of the above. Most people just charge on in and begin exercising without a thought of what the possible outcomes of their participation might be, other than the intended outcome of becoming more fit.

The fact that most people begin training on a whim and do not ever consult a physician regarding exercise is not really problematic. The American College of Sports Medicine does not recommend that all people beginning an exercise program have a physician's consultation prior to the start of training. Children, teens, men younger than 45, and women younger than 55 who do not have any symptoms, history, and have two or less risk factors of cardiovascular disease can begin exercising without a physician's examination.

But if we refer back to Selye's perspective, exercise could be lethal. And this is still true. People die each year during and after exercise. In most instances there was an underlying pathology that was exacerbated by exercise and resulted in the untimely demise. This is the primary benefit of having a physical prior to beginning a program of training, to identify active disease processes in order to modify training. A pre-participation physical does not tell us anything about an individuals exercise tolerance or whether they are able to exercise (everyone can exercise in some form), it simply identifies disease states that have the potential to negatively interact with exercise. Note here that your garden variety turn-your-head-and-cough exam will not identify any pathology other than the most obvious. Much more aggressive means are needed, and unfortunately those means are intrusive, expensive, and not covered by most medical insurance plans.

There are other deaths that do occur not from an unknown pathology being provoked by exercise, but from exercise itself. People fall, people drop things on themselves, people try to do more work than their body can tolerate. The first two items deal with safety and awareness of the exercise environment. Paying attention to where you are at and to the equipment you are using will pay dividends by preventing accidental injury or death (all accidents cannot be prevented however). The last item is an issue of judgement. Someone, the trainee, the coach, the trainer, has decided to push the volume or intensity (or both) of training to the point where systemic failure occurs. The easiest example of this is with exercise in the heat, where death can occur in just a matter of hours if body temperature is allowed to rise unrestricted. In the heat, there must be a lower volume and intensity of work in order to allow the body to regulate temperature.

When all is said and done however, exercise participation is governed by personal choice. In adult populations, the trainee is the ultimate deciding authority. Just as an adult can choose to be sedentary or to exercise, an adult trainee can choose to not seek, or ignore, medical and exercise advice.

REFERENCES

Cohen, P.R. The skin in the gym: a comprehensive review of the cutaneous manifestations of community-acquired methicillin-resistant Staphylococcus aureus infection in athletes. Clinical Dermatology 26(1):16-26, 2008.

Fowles, J.R., D.G. Sale, and J.D. MacDougall. Reduced strength after passive stretch of the human plantar flexors. Journal of Applied Physiology 89:1179–1188, 2000.

Kokkonen, J., A.G. Nelson, and A. Cornwell. Acute muscle stretching inhibits maximal strength performance. Research Quarterly in Exercise and Sport 69:411–415, 1998.

Young, W.B., and D.G. Behm. Effects of running, static stretching and practice jumps on explosive force production and jumping performance. Journal of Sports Medicine and Physical Fitness 43(1):21–7, 2003.

Pope RP, Herbert RD, Kirwan JD, Graham BJ. A randomized trial of preexercise stretching for prevention of lower-limb injury. Medicine and Science in Sports and Exercise 32(2):271-7, 2000.

Shrier, I. Stretching before exercise does not reduce the risk of local muscle injury: a critical review of the clinical and basic science literature. Clinical Journal of Sports Medicine 9:221-227, 1999.

There is nothing like a challenge to bring out the best in man.

Sean Connery

PHYSICS, PHYSIOLOGY, AND FOOD

"To some people, diet is like a religion."

– Tony Budding

When people think about "diet," they almost always think of losing weight. Pritikin, Atkins, Weight Watchers, Jenny Craig, South Beach, SlimFast, Nutrisystem, Learn, Paleolithic, Zone—diets galore and hype galore. All are touted to provide you the means to a "healthy" weight. What do all these diets have in common . . . besides costing you money if you buy the books, supplements, or the prepackaged special foods that go with them? They all do three basic things: (1) they modify the composition of your diet (limit your food selection), (2) either directly or indirectly limit your caloric intake, and (3) expect you to exercise as part of your diet. So they all are all basically variations on the same theme, but there is a tremendous amount of controversy about which diet is superior.

Currently, the biggest debate, and debacle, is low-fat versus low-carbohydrate. Who would have ever guessed that a simple manipulation of a couple macronutrients would be such of point of contention with fitness professionals, physicians, the media, and the public in general? Who would have thought that the tremendous amount of federal and private funds expended on nutrition and obesity research would create such a wealth of wrong thinking?

Wrong thinking? How could someone suggest that some of the best minds in obesity research aren't producing useful information? They are forgetting basic physics, and they are also forgetting to consider the basic reasons why we eat.

What everyone – clinicians, scientists, trainers, and trainees - also seem to forget or refuse to believe is that diet does not make you fit. In the hierarchy of fitness gain, getting your training program in order is more important than your diet. Sacrilege I know, but the truth is sometimes painful. *Diet supports fitness gain, it does not drive it.*

PHYSICS OF BODYWEIGHT

One of the largest motivations for people to start dieting or exercising is weight loss. Whether it is to get into the pair of jeans you wore two years ago, make a weight class, or to expose your hidden six pack, weight loss is a strong motivator and an easy target for market exploitation because most people do not think about it simply and logically. So let's look at weight loss objectively.

Let's first consider the current debate about dietary composition in the light of some simple laws of physics. The various kinds of diets prescribed, marketed, and researched are distinguished by their composition—by the kinds of foods and/or by the ratios of macronutrients (protein, carbohydrate, and fat) that they stipulate. Variations in composition make these diets easy to differentiate and easy to describe, but does the composition of your diet really matter?

The Law	Energy can be neither created nor destroyed, only conserved
The Formula	$\Delta Energy_{Universe} = \Delta Energy_{System} + \Delta Energy_{Surrounding} = 0$
The Concept	Energy going into a system must equal that retained and lost
The Application	Energy In = Energy Expended + Energy Stored
The Example	Calories In = Metabolic Cost of Life + Metabolic Storage
What it Means	Food In = Energy Expended + Macronutrient Storage
Real World Condition A	Food In = Energy Expended = No Weight Gain
Real World Condition B	Food In > Energy Expended = Weight Gain
Real World Condition C	Food In < Energy Expended = Weight Loss

Figure 1. First law of thermodynamics and its application to diet and exercise.

Whether anyone likes to admit it or not, for sheer weight loss, it probably doesn't. It is the total amount of energy consumed (calories) that matters. And this is not an arguable point. There is this pesky little physical law of the universe that forms the basis of all weight loss and weight gain. The second law of thermodynamics states that energy cannot be created or destroyed but is always conserved. In other words, energy that enters a system will necessarily equal the energy that remains in the system or leaves the system. Food, as far as the body is concerned, is merely a form of energy, and the amount of calories you take in (eat and drink) must equal the amount of calories stored in the body or expended through metabolism. Nowhere in this inalterable equation is the quality of the diet or composition of the diet a consideration, only the math of caloric deficit or surplus. It's old, but the phrase "calories count" is still as viable today as it was when the first diet hucksters tried to cash in on the vain American obsession with skinniness. So, according to the law of energy conservation, you eat according to the food pyramid and keep the numbers of calories you eat to less than you expend, you can lose weight. If you go low-fat and low-calorie, you can eat and drink nothing but Choco Cap'n Crunch and Coke in appropriate quantities and you can lose weight. If you go low-carbohydrate, you can eat and drink nothing but bacon and diet Coke in appropriate quantities and you can lose weight. If you go low-protein, you probably can't think clearly enough to comprehend this, but the same energetic relationships apply.

While we don't recommend any of these examples for trainees, it is prudent for trainers and trainees to understand simple dietary concepts and how they relate to the diets that are receiving the lion's share of media and clinical attention. There is some very simple calorie-based logic underlying both the low-fat and low-carbohydrate diets. The low-fat diet presumes, quite correctly, that since fat is a very energy-dense macronutrient at 9 calories (kilocalories, to be precise, but we'll just call them calories, per popular use) per gram, reducing how much fat you eat will reduce your caloric intake significantly. The average American gets somewhere around 34 percent of total dietary calories from fats in food. Reducing this intake to 20 percent would be enough of a caloric reduction for someone to lose about a pound a week—if the calories were not replaced with carbohydrate or protein. (However, even replacing them on a gram-for-gram basis would likely net a weight loss of about a pound every ten days or so, since both carbohydrate and protein contain 4 calories per gram.) If you can hang with the food choices of the low-fat diet, you can effectively lose weight.

But high-carbohydrate diets have an innate problem that makes compliance with them difficult over the long term. Carbohydrate consumption stimulates insulin secretion (and this happens whether it is a "good" carbohydrate or a "bad" carbohydrate). Insulin stimulates the transport of that newly digested carbohydrate, now in the form of blood sugar, to be moved out of the blood into the various tissues of the body. The inevitable result of insulin action, a reduction in blood sugar, stimulates hunger, which is a response to depressions in blood sugar. You get hungry more frequently on a low-fat diet. That tiny little problem usually dooms low-fat diets to failure and abandonment in a matter of weeks. For a chance at success with a low-fat diet, not only do you need to change the foods you eat, you also need to change how you eat. Instead of three squares a day, it is much more effective to eat four or five smaller meals with little snacks between. Spreading the food relatively uniformly across the waking day helps minimize the time between insulin concentration troughs, thereby helping limit between-meal hunger pangs. It is interesting to note that, in the last decade, the government-sponsored campaign against dietary fat has resulted in a decrease in the percent of fat in the American diet (it peaked out at over 42 percent a number of years ago). But, over the same time, the average body weight and body fat of the average citizen has increased despite the decrease in dietary fat. Oops. Looks like there was a misfire with this magic bullet for health. A blanket promotion of a low-fat lifestyle as a means toward national health does no good if we fail to consider the basic physics of eating and the fact that, for weight loss, it is calories - not food selection that really count. We may be eating less fat but we are negating that reduction by adding a caloric excess of low-fat foods in their stead.

The highly touted low-carbohydrate diet has some quite clever elements that are biologically effective and promotionally effective. "Eat as much protein and fat as you like" is one element that almost every one of its practitioners loves. "Wait, I'm on a diet and I can eat as much as I want? Sign me up!" Despite its outward appearance, though, a low-carbohydrate diet is not a high-calorie diet. Two interesting things will initially prevent over-consumption of calories. First, fat is a very satisfying macronutrient. A protein- and fat-rich meal will satisfy hunger more effectively than a high-carbohydrate meal. Second, severely limiting carbohydrate consumption limits insulin secretion, and the dieter will not experience the swings in blood glucose seen in the low-fat diet. With a more consistent level of blood sugar throughout the day, the low-carbohydrate dieter will experience fewer hunger pangs (and mood and energy swings). Less perceived hunger results in a self-selected reduction in calories consumed. So eating "as much as you want" actually turns out to be less than you normally would eat with a typical American pattern of eating lots of carbohydrates along with your fats and proteins. There is a misconception out there that low-carbohydrate diets drop your body fat faster and to a greater magnitude than low-fat diets. You do lose "weight" very quickly in the early stages of the low-carbohydrate diet. This is because the body mobilizes and uses its existing carbohydrate stores (i.e., glycogen and glucose) when you stop consuming them in your meals. That elimination of stored carbohydrate carries with it an elimination of water weight as well. Any time carbohydrate is stored in a cell, it is stored in conjunction with water. Get rid of the carbohydrate and you will also get rid of the water. The end result is a rapid loss of body weight that is composed mostly of stored sugars and water and minimally of fat. But that loss of carbohydrate and water is fast enough and large enough for most dieters to perceive a difference in the mirror and on the scales. Success makes you feel good and contributes to staying on the diet longer. Once the initial carbohydrate losses have petered out, the body will then begin to tap into stored fat and the rate of fat loss will increase and be similar in rate and magnitude to that seen in a successful long-term low-fat diet.

Despite all the hype and hyperbole, there is enough research produced to date to demonstrate that any of the aforementioned diets will result in about a pound of weight loss per month. Hey! That's not what the commercials say. Well, hit pause on your DVR when the diet ads are on and read the disclaimers about the big weight losses shown; "Results not typical" is always be in the small print that flashes across the bottom of the screen for a microsecond. If we really evaluate all the research out there on all the diets, it is apparent that small to moderate weight loss is all we can expect to happen with any diet. And we can only expect it *if* the dieter persists with the regimen over the long haul. This typically doesn't happen. The average "diet" lasts only a matter of weeks, and even the longer-term success stories generally relapse to gaining weight eventually. And this is not just an observation of the general public, it happens to the Hollywood elite who endorse so many diets and diet products, just check the tabloids to watch the paparazzi document weight gains and losses of event the most svelte and enticing figures. So dieting for weight loss seems to be at best a transient and very short-term fix for what is considered to be a national health epidemic.

This isn't new information. The medical and health professions have failed to get the nation to make progress toward "healthy" body weights with thirty years of beating the dead horse of dietary modification. We failed to meet the National Institutes of Health and Surgeons General Healthy People 2000 and 2010 goals in this area. In fact, there was no progress in weight or exercise habits over the 20 year span (Don't believe it? Visit healthypeople.gov and check the data for yourself). And without retooling or reconsidering, the same basic goals are set for Healthy People 2020. Why do we continue in the futile effort to find just the right dietary intervention for the entirety of the American population? Job security for clinical researchers in obesity? Catering to the endless need for promotional fodder of the political machine in its quest to appear as though it is saving us from certain death? Whatever the motive, it may even be well intended, but the results have consistently fallen short.

Dietary intervention is not the only way to fight obesity. Everyone seems to loudly promote the energy-consumed component of the first law of thermodynamics—the "eat less" part—and forgets about the other component, the effective and easily manipulated one, the energy-expended component—"exercise more." In actuality, the diet industry and at least one government regulatory agency have not forgotten exercise. They do pay a very small, lawsuit-minimizing, amount of attention to it. That small disclaimer on every diet ad that says "results not typical" also says "part of a comprehensive program of diet and exercise." So let's think about exercise for a moment. The medical community, the exercise industry, and even Hollywood have framed everything, eating and exercising, as a means to being skinny, beautiful, and therefore healthy. But skinny is not the primary concern we should have when we eat. How much we weigh is not the important issue here.

We need to consider function when we consider health. We need to consider our ability to survive and our ability to manage the challenges of our daily lives and recreational pursuits. With exercise we consume food to fuel our efforts at gaining fitness and to create a better quality of life. When we target physical fitness, everything else tends to fall in line over time, including body fat.

WHAT DO WE REALLY NEED?

We should never blindly follow conventional wisdom. This includes even authoritative dietary advice. Even the hallowed RDAs (now called DGs) are suspect in that they have been found to flawed, with "several critical weaknesses, including use of an incomplete body of relevant science; inaccurately representing, interpreting, or summarizing the literature; and drawing conclusions and/or making recommendations that do not reflect the limitations or controversies in the science" (1). And although we are socially conditioned to reduce the amount of food we eat, we need to be cautious of when we do so. Most people will acknowledge that performance will be less than maximal if pre-event meals are lacking but often fail to consider the effects of reducing intake before training sessions. A profoundly problematic oversight. All elements of fitness can be diminished in short term function by inadequate caloric availability. Something as simple as 12 hours of not eating can reduce something as elementary as balance (2). This affects a trainee's ability to utilize correct, consistent, effective, and safe exercise technique and thereby reduces the quality of a workout.

It remains that we need to understand what we need to eat and why. We need to understand how training affects both the number of calories we need to consume and how it dictates the composition of our dietary needs. We can do this simply by working backward from conventional dietary prescription methods that start with appearance and begin here with how training drives the body's metabolic and dietary needs.

In general, effective exercise programming stresses glycolytic and phosphagenic metabolism. Aerobic adaptations piggyback on top of adaptations to those systems. Glycolytic adaptations require carbohydrate to be present, phosphagenic adaptations rely, in part, on high-phosphagen foods (meats), and aerobic adaptations involve the oxidation of carbohydrate and fat. So right off the bat, it appears that extremely low-fat and extremely low-carbohydrate diets won't meet the nutritional needs of most trainees. Let's be a little more specific and evaluate the metabolic needs of the three common exercise modes used in training: mobility exercises, endurance exercises, and strength exercises.

Exercises with mobility aspects within them are usually done with bodyweight and although an individual move is completed in a matter of seconds (a Pull-up, a Muscle-up, etc.), they are typically done for many repetitions and for many many seconds. These exercises expend stored high-energy phosphates and tap into stored carbohydrate. Endurance exercises are done for a few up to many minutes and are driven primarily by stored carbohydrate (with a little fat if the intensity is low enough). Strength exercises in the low end of the repetition continuum are dependent on stored high-energy phosphates but as the repetitions get out into the double digits, anaerobic glycolysis is active and some carbohydrate gets used to power sets. If we are doing mixed-modal training, we are doing all these types of work, often blended indistinguishably. So it is easy to see that we can't eliminate any of the macronutrients from a training diet and that low-carbohydrate diets might not be a wise choice to support training. In fact, it is well known that low-carbohydrate diets reduce the amount of stored carbohydrate and it is similarly well known that lowering carbohydrate stores in the muscle and liver predisposes trainees to early fatigue. Interval training can tire your butt out all on its own; you don't need to have your diet helping to induce fatigue and slow recovery.

It is not as easy to see that low-fat diets are not so relevant to fitness, and then there's the hurdle of getting over the popular belief that they automatically help prevent heart disease. First off, let's consider fat as a good thing, in the diet and in the body. Just sitting there reading this chapter you are deriving about 66 percent or more of the energy you are using from fat stored in your body. If we extend that ratio to the average non-exercising American who might be expending 2500 calories per day, 1650 calories are coming from fat metabolism. If we use the average daily protein requirement numbers proposed by the American Dietetic Association (0.8 grams per kilogram of body weight per day), a 165-pound trainee would need to consume 240 calories of dietary protein per day. Simple subtraction provides us the number of carbohydrate calories Joe Couch would then need to consume per day, 610 calories. These numbers hardly paint the picture of the need for a low-fat diet; rather, they suggest fat is an essential element of the diet (it has been since the emergence of mankind).

And as for the heart-disease-prevention angle used to promote low-fat diets, most recent comparative research has shown that cardiovascular disease risk decreases similarly with low-fat and low-carbohydrate diets - neither is heart-healthier than the other. Now let's add exercise into the picture, since surely exercise increases the need for carbohydrate? Yes, in fact, it does, but how much? A broad assessment of all exercise modalities might indicate that if 400 calories worth of exercise is added to Joe Couch's daily habits, about 300, or 75 percent, of the calories used to power exercise would come from carbohydrate, with the other 25 percent coming from fat. If we add those 300 calories to the 610 calories derived from carbohydrate needed for sedentary existence, that brings us to about 30-35 percent of our total caloric need from carbohydrate. That's not "low-carb," but it is pretty low compared to the 55 percent or more carbohydrate content pushed by the clinical and aerobic fitness communities.

The final micronutrient for consideration is protein, the building blocks of all structural and metabolic enzyme proteins. When we recover from exercise we don't just replete the expended energy substrates (fat and carbohydrate); we also have to replace any broken down structural proteins and enzymes that resulted from the exercise bout. That means we have to match protein intake to protein broken down just to maintain the status quo of fitness. With regular aerobic exercise (of the long-slow-distance ilk) it has been shown that up to 1.8 grams of dietary protein per kilogram of body weight are required to maintain a positive nitrogen balance (3). A positive nitrogen balance means that you have enough protein building blocks to support fitness gain. With intense weight training, up to 2.4 grams of protein consumption per kilogram body weight are needed to maintain a positive nitrogen balance (4). With a compromise of 2.2 grams of dietary protein per kilogram of body weight per day intake (in between 1.8 and 2.5 g/kg/day) more than 24 percent of the diet would need to be protein to support the fitness gains possible with training.

So where does this leave us? If we want to choose a named diet that best supports the demands of training, we would not choose low-fat, and we would not choose low-carbohydrate. We need to have a diet that delivers a moderate quantity of every macronutrient—fat, carbohydrate, and protein—according to the demands of the basic physics and physiology of exercise adaptation (figure 2).

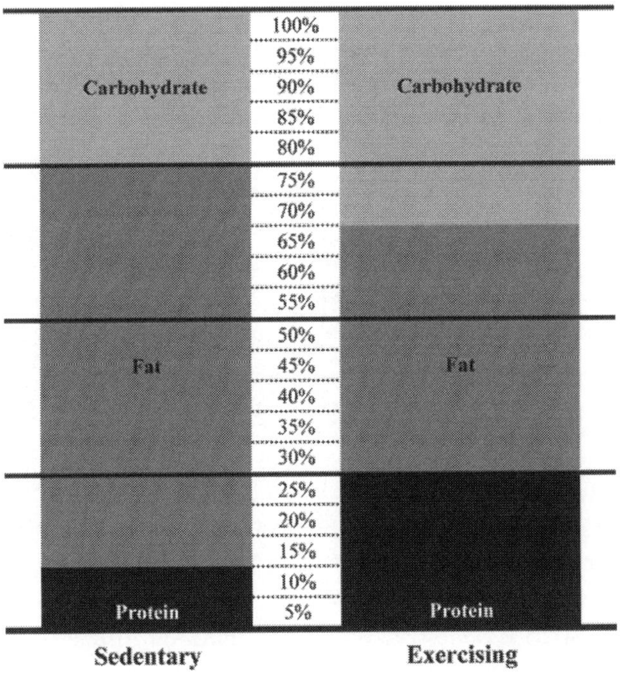

Figure 2. Comparison of relative requirements for macronutrients at rest and in support of mixed modal exercise.

We need less carbohydrate than conventionally thought but more than the truly low-carbohydrate diets. We need somewhere between the American Dietetic Association recommendation for fat content, 30 percent, and 40 percent — not the exorbitantly low quantities suggested by lots of low-fat diets. And we need more protein than most clinicians generally prescribe. Of all the diets listed in the first paragraph, the Zone is a decent fit. Although not an exact match or even a recommendation, the metabolic and structural stress placed on the body by exercise training will be accommodated by the 40 percent carbohydrate, 30 percent fat, and 30 percent protein recommendations of the Zone (compared to other marketed diet plans). But really you don't need to buy a diet, you just need to eat intelligently. If you love bacon and apple pie, you can have it with no worries and no guilt, as long they don't form the sole nutritional basis of your diet ... and you exercise.

PACKING ON THE POUNDS

Weight gain. A dirty word(s) to some, the pinnacle of training success to others. What is really the discriminating issue here is the composition of the weight gain; fat, protein, or carbohydrate. To be fit, we generally need to add protein (muscle) without adding substantial fat.

Weight gain is subject to the first law of thermodynamics, just like weight loss (see figure 1). If we consume excess calories without exercising, the majority of the excess will be stored as fat. And it doesn't matter if the source of the excess was carbohydrates, fat, or protein. Fat is the body's preferred, and most efficient, form of energy storage so any excess macronutrient gets digested, broken down, and then re-assembled as stored fat. Over time, human physiology has developed, just like in animals, the ability to store energy (fat) in order survive austere times with low food availability. We do it quite well. But we don't want to add fat mass when we gain weight as a result of training intended to induce weight gain, we want lean body mass added.

This is an aspect of the art of applied nutrition; how to gain muscle mass without adding fat mass. There is much debate on this particular nuance of diet and exercise with many opinions on the table. In general they are pretty similar in concept, eat enough protein to support creation of new muscular architecture and enough calories to support exercise and the metabolic cost of building new muscle and connective tissue (along with the other peripheral structural adaptations that occur in the skeletal and cardiovascular systems). Where they differ is in the degree of caloric excess required to support the muscle building process. Lots of people have success with varying degrees of success with varying amounts of caloric excess. A beginner can make huge advances in strength by consuming an excess of 1000 calories or more per day. But this degree of excess can lead to a moderate increase in stored body fat. For some, this fat gain may not be problematic, a high school football player or shot putter for example. But for others the increased fat mass may be quite undesirable for performance reasons (power-to-weight ratio in cyclists for example) or for aesthetic reasons (the quest for the perfect set of abs). To minimize the amount of fat gain while still supporting muscular strength, size, and fitness gain is tricky, with lots of individual variation making one-size-fits-all recommendations difficult. But with that said, consuming less than 500 excess calories per day will likely prove to be inadequate to support the anabolic processes leading to strength gain as well as a more calorically dense diet. The smaller caloric excess can simply support a smaller degree of fitness gain, so it will take longer to produce the desired adaptation ... but they will still come at some point.

A frequently overlooked weight gain consideration is in those individuals desiring improved endurance. The power-to-weight ratio is often cited as a reason that endurance trainees should not gain weight. This is correct if the gain is fat mass. But if the weight gain is muscle mass and performance relevant proteins and energy stores, it is a performance enhancing gain. If we want to increase our ability to do long duration running, we need to maximize carbohydrate storage. If we add carbohydrate storage, won't that increase body weight? Yes. And it also delays the onset of fatigue - we can run longer. If we add muscle mass that is aerobically enhanced will that cause weight gain? Yes. And it will improve running velocity - we run faster. So even endurance trainees need to consume a caloric excess in order to support fitness gain. Basic physics and the physiology of adaptation demand it.

WHAT IT ALL MEANS

Understanding nutrition is not that hard when we get rid of the hype and misinterpretations promulgated by clinicians, supplement manufacturers, and our fellow exercise professionals. Exercise is about adaptation. Nutrition is about the support of that adaptation. When we think of it this way, there is a hierarchy of adaptive support that diet must provide:

1 – Get your training program in order. Fitness comes from training not engineered eating.

2 – Ensure that the gross caloric content of the diet meets caloric expenditure in order to maintain fitness or mildly (moderately?) exceeds caloric expenditure for adaptations to occur.

3 – Include a selection of foods that provides a balance of macronutrients that meets the demands of training and recovery - consumption must reflect actual biological need in order for adaptations to occur optimally (in rate and magnitude).

4 – Cover your nutritional bases and make sure micronutrient intake is adequate to support macronutrient utilization. This means eating a variety of foods.

5 – Only after 1 through 4 are attended to do we deal with peripheral issues such as food quality, timing, ergogenic aids, and such. These are only minor tweaks of the overall adaptive system providing very limited benefits, benefits that will be unrealized if 1 through 4 are not in place.

Most articles, books, and fitness personalities jump the gun on this hierarchy and consider the peripheral issues before taking care of the basics. Hopefully here we have established:

A basic appreciation of the physics of eating

The concept that "diet" and "dieting" are two distinct entities

That survival and training – not socially driven concepts of health and beauty - drive dietary composition.

Every coach and trainer should be cognizant of these basic concepts and be able to explain them to their clients as training success hinges on our ability to get trainees to buy in to better nutrition to support better training. Every trainee should understand these ideas and application as they will become fitter more quickly if they adhere to them.

We have specifically chosen not to address the issues related to food quality, timing, and ergogenic aids here, as this book is about the basics of getting fit and the basics are simple - items 1 though 4 in the nutritional hierarchy above. If you make it to the advanced level of training progression, consideration of the items listed in item 5 are merited in a more detail treatment than can be delivered here.

REFERENCES

(1) Hite, A.H., et al. In the face of contradictory evidence: Report of the Dietary Guidelines for Americans Committee. Nutrition 26:915-924, 2010.

(2) Johnson, S. and K. Leck. The effects of dietary fasting on physical balance among healthy young women. Nutrition Journal 2:18, 2010.

(3) Friedman, J.E. and P.W. Lemon. Effect of chronic endurance exercise on retention of dietary protein. International Journal of Sports Medicine 10(2):118-123, 1989.

(4) Tarnopolsky, M.A., et al. Evaluation of protein requirements for trained strength athletes. Journal of Applied Physiology 73(5):1986-1995, 1992.

"The scientific truth may be put quite briefly; eat moderately,
have an ordinary mixed diet, and don't worry."

- Robert Hutchison
in the Newcastle Medical Journal, Vol 12, 1932.

EXERCISE PERFORMANCE STANDARDS

Performance standards are by nature a crude estimate of what we think someone should be capable of in a certain task under certain conditions. The lifting standards presented here are adult standards (>18 years old) based on competitive weightlifting and powerlifting (un-aided) classification systems in use from the 1960's to the present. Adjustments for the inevitability of aging are included. Standards are based on lifts completed with no supportive gear (a belt is acceptable) and using complete range of motion exercises as described in each lift's official international competitive rules and/or as described and pictured within this text. It is assumed that the lifts are chemically unassisted. Also included here are selected calisthenic based and endurance exercise standards. Failure to use complete range of motion or proper technique on any exercise voids the measurement. Definitions of the Novice through Elite stratifications included in the following tables are those found in Practical Programming for Strength Training and refer specifically to the adaptive status of the trainee (Rippetoe & Kilgore, 2006). Standards listed for weighted exercises are for a single maximal repetition (1RM, Max, PR, PB, etc). The elite column does not represent the highest level of performance possible rather it is the lowest end of the elite standard.

Standards Presented

Bench Press
Power Clean
Deadlift
Press
Power Snatch
Back Squat
Push-up
Pull-up
Sit-up
One Mile Run
1000 Meter Row

BENCH PRESS STANDARDS - POUNDS

Men

Body Weight	Untrained	Novice	Intermediate	Advanced	Elite
114	85	110	130	180	220
123	90	115	140	195	240
132	100	125	155	210	260
148	110	140	170	235	290
165	120	150	185	255	320
181	130	165	200	275	345
198	135	175	215	290	360
220	140	185	225	305	380
242	145	190	230	315	395
275	150	195	240	325	405
319	155	200	245	335	415
320+	160	205	250	340	425
Over 40 years old					
114	75	95	110	155	190
123	80	100	120	170	205
132	85	110	135	180	225
148	95	120	145	200	250
165	105	130	160	220	275
181	110	140	170	235	295
198	115	150	185	250	310
220	120	160	195	260	325
242	125	165	200	270	340
275	130	170	205	280	350
319	135	175	210	290	355
320+	140	180	215	295	365
Over 50 years old					
114	65	85	100	135	165
123	70	90	105	150	180
132	75	95	120	160	200
148	85	105	130	180	220
165	90	115	140	195	245
181	100	125	150	210	260
198	105	135	160	225	275
220	110	140	170	235	290
242	115	145	175	240	300
275	120	150	180	250	310
319	125	155	185	255	315
320+	130	160	190	260	325
Over 60 years old					
114	50	60	75	105	130
123	55	70	80	115	140
132	60	75	90	125	150
148	65	80	100	135	170
165	70	85	105	150	185
181	75	90	115	160	200
198	80	95	125	170	210
220	85	100	130	175	220
242	90	105	135	180	230
275	95	110	140	190	235
319	100	115	145	195	240
320+	105	120	150	200	250

Women

Body Weight	Untrained	Novice	Intermediate	Advanced	Elite
97	50	65	75	95	115
105	55	70	80	100	125
114	60	75	85	110	135
123	65	80	90	115	140
132	70	85	95	125	150
148	75	90	105	135	165
165	80	95	115	145	185
181	85	110	120	160	195
198	90	115	130	165	205
199+	95	120	140	175	220
Over 40 years old					
97	45	55	65	80	100
105	50	60	70	85	110
114	55	65	75	95	115
123	60	70	80	100	120
132	65	75	85	110	130
148	70	80	90	115	140
165	75	85	100	125	160
181	80	95	105	140	170
198	85	100	115	145	180
199+	90	105	120	150	190
Over 50 years old					
97	40	50	60	70	90
105	45	55	65	75	95
114	50	60	70	85	100
123	55	65	75	90	105
132	60	70	80	95	115
148	65	75	85	105	125
165	70	80	90	110	140
181	75	85	95	125	150
198	80	90	100	130	155
199+	85	95	105	135	160
Over 60 years old					
97	30	35	40	55	70
105	35	40	45	60	75
114	40	45	50	65	80
123	45	50	55	70	85
132	50	55	60	75	90
148	50	55	60	80	95
165	55	60	65	85	105
181	55	65	70	95	115
198	60	70	75	100	120
199+	60	75	80	105	130

BENCH PRESS STANDARDS - KILOGRAMS

Men

Body Weight	Untrained	Novice	Intermediate	Advanced	Elite
52	37.5	50.0	60.0	82.5	100.0
56	40.0	52.5	62.5	90.0	110.0
60	45.0	57.5	70.0	95.0	117.5
67	50.0	65.0	77.5	107.5	132.5
75	55.0	70.0	85.0	115.0	145.0
82	60.0	75.0	90.0	125.0	157.5
90	62.5	80.0	97.5	132.5	162.5
100	62.5	82.5	102.5	137.5	172.5
110	65.0	85.0	105.0	142.5	180.0
125	67.5	87.5	107.5	147.5	185.0
145	70.0	90.0	112.5	152.5	190.0
145+	72.5	92.5	115.0	155.0	192.5
Over 40 years old					
52	35.0	42.5	50.0	70.0	87.5
56	37.5	45.0	55.0	77.5	92.5
60	40.0	50.0	62.5	82.5	102.5
67	42.5	55.0	65.0	90.0	115.0
75	47.5	60.0	72.5	100.0	125.0
82	50.0	65.0	77.5	107.5	135.0
90	52.5	67.5	85.0	115.0	140.0
100	55.0	72.5	87.5	117.5	147.5
110	57.5	75.0	90.0	122.5	155.0
125	60.0	77.5	92.5	127.5	157.5
145	62.5	80.0	95.0	132.5	162.5
145+	65.0	82.5	97.5	135.0	165.0
Over 50 years old					
52	30.0	37.5	45.0	62.5	75.0
56	32.5	40.0	47.5	67.5	82.5
60	35.0	42.5	55.0	72.5	90.0
67	37.5	47.5	60.0	82.5	100.0
75	40.0	52.5	65.0	87.5	112.5
82	45.0	57.5	67.5	95.0	117.5
90	47.5	60.0	72.5	102.5	125.0
100	50.0	62.5	77.5	107.5	132.5
110	52.5	65.0	80.0	110.0	135.0
125	55.0	67.5	82.5	112.5	140.0
145	57.5	70.0	85.0	115.0	142.5
145+	60.0	72.5	87.5	117.5	147.5
Over 60 years old					
52	22.5	27.5	35.0	47.5	60.0
56	25.0	32.5	37.5	52.5	62.5
60	27.5	35.0	40.0	57.5	67.5
67	30.0	35.0	45.0	60.0	77.5
75	32.5	37.5	47.5	67.5	85.0
82	35.0	40.0	52.5	72.5	90.0
90	37.5	42.5	55.0	77.5	95.0
100	37.5	45.0	57.5	80.0	100.0
110	40.0	47.5	60.0	82.5	105.0
125	42.5	50.0	62.5	85.0	107.5
145	45.0	52.5	65.0	87.5	110.0
145+	47.5	55.0	67.5	90.0	112.5

Women

Body Weight	Untrained	Novice	Intermediate	Advanced	Elite
44	22.5	30.0	35.0	42.5	52.5
48	25.0	32.5	37.5	45.0	57.5
52	27.5	35.0	37.5	50.0	62.5
56	30.0	37.5	40.0	52.5	65.0
60	32.5	40.0	42.5	57.5	67.5
67	35.0	40.0	47.5	62.5	75.0
75	37.5	42.5	52.5	65.0	85.0
82	37.5	50.0	55.0	72.5	90.0
90	40.0	52.5	60.0	75.0	95.0
90+	42.5	55.0	62.5	80.0	100.0
Over 40 years old					
44	20.0	25.0	30.0	37.5	45.0
48	22.5	27.5	32.5	40.0	50.0
52	25.0	30.0	35.0	42.5	52.5
56	27.5	32.5	37.5	45.0	55.0
60	30.0	35.0	37.5	50.0	60.0
67	32.5	37.5	40.0	52.5	62.5
75	35.0	40.0	45.0	57.5	72.5
82	35.0	42.5	47.5	62.5	77.5
90	37.5	45.0	52.5	65.0	82.5
90+	40.0	47.5	55.0	67.5	87.5
Over 50 years old					
44	17.5	22.5	27.5	32.5	40.0
48	20.0	25.0	30.0	35.0	42.5
52	22.5	27.5	32.5	37.5	45.0
56	25.0	30.0	35.0	40.0	47.5
60	27.5	32.5	35.0	42.5	52.5
67	30.0	35.0	37.5	47.5	57.5
75	32.5	37.5	40.0	50.0	62.5
82	35.0	40.0	42.5	57.5	67.5
90	35.0	40.0	45.0	60.0	70.0
90+	37.5	42.5	47.5	62.5	72.5
Over 60 years old					
44	12.5	15.0	17.5	25.0	30.0
48	15.0	17.5	20.0	27.5	32.5
52	17.5	20.0	22.5	30.0	35.0
56	20.0	22.5	25.0	32.5	37.5
60	22.5	25.0	27.5	35.0	40.0
67	22.5	25.0	27.5	37.5	42.5
75	25.0	27.5	30.0	40.0	47.5
82	25.0	30.0	32.5	42.5	52.5
90	27.5	32.5	35.0	45.0	55.0
90+	27.5	35.0	37.5	47.5	60.0

POWER CLEAN STANDARDS - POUNDS

Men

Body Weight	Untrained	Novice	Intermediate	Advanced	Elite
114	55	105	125	175	205
123	60	110	135	185	225
132	65	120	150	200	240
148	75	135	165	225	265
165	80	145	180	245	290
181	85	160	195	265	310
198	90	165	205	280	325
220	95	175	215	295	345
242	100	165	225	305	355
275	105	190	230	315	365
319	110	195	235	320	375
320+	115	200	240	330	385
Over 40 years old					
114	45	90	110	150	175
123	50	95	115	160	195
132	55	105	130	175	205
148	65	115	140	195	230
165	70	125	155	210	250
181	75	140	170	230	270
198	80	145	175	240	280
220	85	150	185	255	295
242	90	155	195	260	305
275	90	165	200	270	315
319	95	170	205	275	325
320+	100	175	210	285	335
Over 50 years old					
114	40	80	95	135	155
123	45	85	105	140	170
132	50	90	115	150	185
148	60	105	125	170	200
165	65	110	135	185	220
181	70	120	150	200	235
198	75	125	155	215	245
220	80	135	165	225	260
242	85	140	170	230	270
275	85	145	175	240	280
319	90	150	180	245	285
320+	95	155	185	250	295
Over 60 years old					
114	30	60	75	105	120
123	35	65	80	110	130
132	40	70	90	115	140
148	45	80	95	130	155
165	50	85	105	140	170
181	55	90	115	155	180
198	55	95	120	160	190
220	60	100	125	170	200
242	60	105	130	180	205
275	65	110	135	185	215
319	65	115	140	190	220
320+	70	120	145	195	225

Women

Body Weight	Untrained	Novice	Intermediate	Advanced	Elite
97	30	60	70	95	115
105	35	65	75	100	125
114	40	70	80	110	135
123	40	75	85	115	145
132	45	80	90	120	150
148	50	90	100	135	165
165	50	95	110	145	185
181	55	100	120	155	195
198	60	110	125	165	205
199+	65	115	135	175	220
Over 40 years old					
97	25	50	60	80	100
105	30	55	65	85	110
114	35	60	69	95	115
123	35	65	70	100	125
132	40	70	80	105	130
148	45	75	85	115	145
165	45	85	95	125	160
181	50	90	105	135	170
198	55	95	110	145	180
199+	60	100	115	150	190
Over 50 years old					
97	20	45	55	75	90
105	25	50	60	80	95
114	30	55	65	85	100
123	30	60	70	90	110
132	35	65	75	95	115
148	40	70	80	105	125
165	40	75	85	110	140
181	45	80	90	120	150
198	45	85	95	125	160
199+	50	90	105	135	170
Over 60 years old					
97	15	35	40	55	70
105	20	40	45	60	75
114	25	40	45	65	80
123	25	45	50	70	85
132	25	45	55	75	90
148	30	50	60	80	100
165	30	55	65	85	110
181	35	60	70	90	115
198	35	65	75	95	120
199+	40	70	80	105	130

POWER CLEAN STANDARDS - KILOGRAMS

Men

Body Weight	Untrained	Novice	Intermediate	Advanced	Elite
52	25.0	47.5	57.5	80.0	92.5
56	27.5	50.0	62.5	85.0	102.5
60	30.0	55.0	67.5	90.0	110.0
67	35.0	60.0	75.0	102.5	120.0
75	37.5	65.0	82.5	112.5	132.5
82	37.5	72.5	87.5	120.0	140.0
90	40.0	75.0	92.5	127.5	147.5
100	42.5	80.0	97.5	135.0	155.0
110	45.0	82.5	102.5	140.0	160.0
125	47.5	85.0	105.0	142.5	165.0
145	50.0	87.5	107.5	145.0	170.0
145+	52.5	90.0	110.0	150.0	175.0
Over 40 years old					
52	20.0	40.0	50.0	67.5	80.0
56	22.5	42.5	52.5	72.5	87.5
60	25.0	47.5	60.0	80.0	92.5
67	30.0	52.5	62.5	87.5	105.0
75	32.5	57.5	70.0	95.0	112.5
82	35.0	62.5	77.5	105.0	122.5
90	35.0	65.0	80.0	110.0	127.5
100	37.5	67.5	82.5	115.0	135.0
110	40.0	70.0	87.5	117.5	140.0
125	40.0	75.0	90.0	122.5	142.5
145	42.5	77.5	92.5	125.0	147.5
145+	45.0	80.0	95.0	130.0	152.5
Over 50 years old					
52	17.5	35.0	42.5	62.5	70.0
56	20.0	37.5	47.5	65.0	77.5
60	22.5	40.0	52.5	67.5	85.0
67	27.5	47.5	57.5	77.5	90.0
75	30.0	50.0	62.5	85.0	100.0
82	32.5	55.0	67.5	90.0	107.5
90	35.0	57.5	70.0	97.5	112.5
100	37.5	60.0	75.0	102.5	117.5
110	37.5	62.5	77.5	105.0	122.5
125	40.0	65.0	80.0	107.5	127.5
145	40.0	67.5	82.5	110.0	130.0
145+	42.5	70.0	85.0	112.5	135.0
Over 60 years old					
52	12.5	27.5	35.0	47.5	55.0
56	15.0	30.0	37.5	50.0	60.0
60	17.5	32.5	40.0	52.5	65.0
67	20.0	35.0	42.5	60.0	70.0
75	22.5	37.5	47.5	62.5	77.5
82	25.0	40.0	52.5	70.0	82.5
90	25.0	42.5	55.0	72.5	85.0
100	27.5	45.0	57.5	77.5	90.0
110	27.5	47.5	60.0	82.5	92.5
125	30.0	50.0	60.0	85.0	97.5
145	30.0	52.5	62.5	87.5	100.0
145+	32.5	55.0	65.0	90.0	102.5

Women

Body Weight	Untrained	Novice	Intermediate	Advanced	Elite
44	12.5	27.5	32.5	42.5	52.5
48	15.0	30.0	35.0	45.0	57.5
52	17.5	32.5	35.0	50.0	60.0
56	17.5	35.0	37.5	52.5	65.0
60	20.0	37.5	40.0	55.0	67.5
67	22.5	40.0	45.0	60.0	75.0
75	22.5	42.5	50.0	65.0	85.0
82	25.0	45.0	55.0	70.0	90.0
90	27.5	50.0	57.5	75.0	95.0
90+	30.0	52.5	62.5	80.0	100.0
Over 40 years old					
44	10.0	22.5	27.5	37.5	45.0
48	12.5	25.0	30.0	40.0	50.0
52	15.0	27.5	32.5	42.5	52.5
56	15.0	30.0	35.0	45.0	57.5
60	17.5	32.5	37.5	47.5	60.0
67	20.0	35.0	40.0	52.5	65.0
75	20.0	37.5	42.5	57.5	72.5
82	22.5	40.0	47.5	60.0	77.5
90	25.0	42.5	50.0	65.0	82.5
90+	27.5	45.0	52.5	67.5	87.5
Over 50 years old					
44	10.0	20.0	25.0	35.0	40.0
48	10.0	22.5	27.5	37.5	42.5
52	12.5	25.0	30.0	40.0	45.0
56	12.5	27.5	32.5	40.0	50.0
60	15.0	30.0	35.0	42.5	52.5
67	17.5	32.5	37.5	47.5	57.5
75	17.5	35.0	40.0	50.0	62.5
82	20.0	37.5	42.5	55.0	67.5
90	20.0	37.5	45.0	57.5	72.5
90+	22.5	40.0	47.5	62.5	77.5
Over 60 years old					
44	7.5	15.0	17.5	25.0	32.5
48	7.5	17.5	20.0	27.5	35.0
52	10.0	17.5	20.0	30.0	37.5
56	10.0	20.0	22.5	32.5	40.0
60	10.0	20.0	25.0	35.0	42.5
67	12.5	22.5	27.5	37.5	45.0
75	12.5	25.0	30.0	37.5	50.0
82	15.0	27.5	32.5	40.0	52.5
90	15.0	30.0	35.0	42.5	55.0
90+	17.5	32.5	27.5	47.5	60.0

DEADLIFT STANDARDS - POUNDS

Men

Body Weight	Untrained	Novice	Intermediate	Advanced	Elite
114	95	180	205	300	385
123	105	195	220	320	415
132	105	210	240	340	440
148	125	235	270	380	480
165	135	255	295	410	520
181	150	275	315	440	550
198	155	290	335	460	565
220	165	305	350	480	585
242	170	320	365	490	595
275	175	325	375	500	600
319	181	335	380	505	610
320+	185	340	390	510	615
Over 40 years old					
114	85	155	175	260	330
123	90	170	190	275	355
132	100	180	205	290	380
148	110	200	230	325	415
165	120	220	255	355	445
181	130	240	270	375	475
198	135	250	290	395	485
220	140	260	300	415	505
242	145	275	315	420	510
275	150	280	325	430	515
319	155	290	330	435	525
320+	160	295	335	440	530
Over 50 years old					
114	75	135	155	230	295
123	81	150	165	245	315
132	85	160	185	260	335
148	95	180	205	290	365
165	105	195	225	310	395
181	115	210	240	335	420
198	120	220	255	350	430
220	124	230	265	365	445
242	130	245	275	370	450
275	135	247	285	380	455
319	140	255	290	385	465
320+	145	260	295	390	470
Over 60 years old					
114	55	105	115	170	220
123	60	110	125	180	235
132	65	120	135	195	250
148	70	135	155	215	275
165	75	145	170	235	295
181	85	155	180	250	315
198	90	165	190	260	325
220	95	175	200	275	335
242	100	180	210	280	340
275	100	185	215	285	345
319	105	190	220	290	350
320+	105	195	225	295	355

Women

Body Weight	Untrained	Novice	Intermediate	Advanced	Elite
97	55	105	110	175	230
105	60	115	130	190	240
114	65	120	140	200	255
123	70	130	150	210	265
132	75	135	160	220	275
148	80	150	175	240	295
165	90	160	190	260	320
181	95	175	205	275	330
198	100	195	215	285	350
199+	110	195	230	300	365
Over 40 years old					
97	50	90	95	150	200
105	55	100	110	165	210
114	55	105	120	170	220
123	59	110	130	180	230
132	65	115	140	190	240
148	70	130	150	205	255
165	75	140	165	225	275
181	80	150	175	235	285
198	90	170	185	245	300
199+	95	175	200	260	315
Over 50 years old					
97	40	80	85	135	175
105	45	85	100	145	185
114	50	90	105	150	195
123	55	100	115	160	200
132	57	105	120	170	210
148	65	115	135	180	225
165	70	125	145	200	245
181	75	135	155	210	250
198	80	145	165	220	265
199+	85	150	175	230	275
Over 60 years old					
97	30	60	65	100	130
105	35	65	75	110	140
114	40	70	80	115	145
123	40	75	85	120	150
132	45	80	90	125	155
148	45	85	100	135	170
165	50	90	110	150	180
181	55	100	120	155	190
198	60	105	125	160	200
199+	65	110	130	170	210

DEADLIFT STANDARDS - KILOGRAMS

Men

Body Weight	Untrained	Novice	Intermediate	Advanced	Elite
52	42.5	82.5	92.5	135.0	175.0
56	47.5	87.5	100.0	145.0	187.5
60	50.0	95.0	110.0	155.0	200.0
67	57.5	107.5	122.5	172.5	217.5
75	62.5	115.0	135.0	185.0	235.0
82	67.5	125.0	142.5	200.0	250.0
90	70.0	132.5	152.5	207.5	257.5
100	75.0	137.5	160.0	217.5	265.0
110	77.5	145.0	165.0	222.5	270.0
125	80.0	147.5	170.0	227.5	272.5
145	82.5	152.5	172.5	230.0	277.5
145+	85.0	155.0	177.5	232.5	280.0
Over 40 years old					
52	37.5	67.5	80.0	117.5	150.0
56	40.0	77.5	87.5	125.0	160.0
60	45.0	82.5	92.5	132.5	172.5
67	50.0	90.0	105.0	147.5	187.5
75	55.0	100.0	115.0	160.0	202.5
82	60.0	110.0	122.5	170.0	215.0
90	60.0	112.5	132.5	180.0	220.0
100	62.5	117.5	137.5	187.5	230.0
110	65.0	122.5	142.5	190.0	232.5
125	67.5	127.5	147.5	195.0	235.0
145	70.0	132.5	150.0	197.5	237.5
145+	72.5	135.0	152.5	200.0	240.0
Over 50 years old					
52	35.0	62.5	70.0	105.0	135.0
56	37.5	67.5	75.0	110.0	142.5
60	40.0	72.5	85.0	117.5	152.5
67	42.5	82.5	92.5	132.5	165.0
75	47.5	90.0	102.5	140.0	180.0
82	52.5	95.0	110.0	152.5	190.0
90	55.0	100.0	115.0	160.0	195.0
100	57.5	105.0	120.0	135.0	202.5
110	60.0	110.0	125.0	167.5	205.0
125	62.5	112.5	130.0	172.5	207.5
145	65.0	115.0	132.5	175.0	210.0
145+	67.5	117.5	135.0	177.5	212.5
Over 60 years old					
52	25.0	47.5	52.5	77.5	100.0
56	27.5	50.0	57.5	82.5	107.5
60	30.0	55.0	62.5	90.0	112.5
67	32.5	62.5	70.0	97.5	125.0
75	35.0	65.0	77.5	107.5	135.0
82	37.5	70.0	82.5	112.5	142.5
90	40.0	75.0	87.5	117.5	147.5
100	42.5	80.0	90.0	125.0	152.5
110	45.0	82.5	95.0	127.5	155.0
125	45.0	85.0	97.5	130.0	157.5
145	47.5	87.5	100.0	132.5	160.0
145+	47.5	90.0	102.5	135.0	162.5

Women

Body Weight	Untrained	Novice	Intermediate	Advanced	Elite
44	25.0	47.5	50.0	80.0	105.0
48	27.5	52.5	60.0	85.0	110.0
52	30.0	55.0	62.5	90.0	115.0
56	32.5	60.0	67.5	95.0	120.0
60	35.0	62.5	72.5	100.0	125.0
67	37.5	67.5	80.0	110.0	135.0
75	40.0	72.5	85.0	117.5	145.0
82	42.5	80.0	92.5	125.0	150.0
90	45.0	87.5	97.5	130.0	160.0
90+	50.0	90.0	105.0	137.5	165.0
Over 40 years old					
44	22.5	40.0	42.5	67.5	90.0
48	25.0	45.0	50.0	75.0	95.0
52	25.0	47.5	55.0	77.5	100.0
56	27.5	50.0	60.0	82.5	105.0
60	60.0	52.5	62.5	87.5	110.0
67	32.5	60.0	67.5	92.5	115.0
75	35.0	62.5	75.0	102.5	125.0
82	37.5	67.5	80.0	107.5	130.0
90	40.0	77.5	82.5	112.5	137.5
90+	42.5	80.0	90.0	117.5	142.5
Over 50 years old					
44	17.5	35.0	40.0	62.5	80.0
48	20.0	37.5	45.0	65.0	85.0
52	22.5	40.0	47.5	70.0	87.5
56	25.0	45.0	52.5	72.5	90.0
60	25.0	47.5	55.0	77.5	95.0
67	30.0	52.5	62.5	82.5	102.5
75	32.5	57.5	65.0	90.0	112.5
82	35.0	62.5	70.0	95.0	115.0
90	37.5	65.0	75.0	100.0	120.0
90+	40.0	67.5	80.0	105.0	125.0
Over 60 years old					
44	12.5	27.5	30.0	45.0	60.0
48	15.0	30.0	35.0	50.0	62.5
52	17.5	32.5	37.5	52.5	65.0
56	17.5	35.0	40.0	55.0	67.5
60	20.0	37.5	40.0	57.5	70.0
67	20.0	37.5	45.0	62.5	77.5
75	22.5	40.0	50.0	67.5	82.5
82	25.0	45.0	55.0	70.0	87.5
90	27.5	47.5	57.5	72.5	90.0
90+	30.0	50.0	60.0	77.5	95.0

PRESS STANDARDS - POUNDS

Men

Body Weight	Untrained	Novice	Intermediate	Advanced	Elite
114	55	75	90	110	130
123	60	80	100	115	140
132	65	85	105	125	150
148	70	95	120	140	170
165	75	100	130	155	190
181	80	110	140	165	220
198	85	115	145	175	235
220	90	120	155	185	255
242	95	125	160	190	265
275	95	130	165	195	275
319	100	135	170	200	280
320+	100	140	175	205	285
Over 40 years old					
114	45	65	80	95	115
123	50	70	85	100	125
132	55	75	90	110	130
148	60	85	105	125	150
165	65	90	115	135	165
181	70	95	120	145	190
198	75	100	125	150	205
220	80	105	135	160	220
242	85	110	140	165	230
275	85	115	145	170	240
319	90	120	150	175	245
320+	90	125	155	180	250
Over 50 years old					
114	40	55	70	85	100
123	45	60	75	90	105
132	50	65	80	95	115
148	55	70	90	105	130
165	60	75	100	120	145
181	60	80	105	125	170
198	65	85	110	135	160
220	70	90	115	140	195
242	70	95	120	145	200
275	70	100	125	150	210
319	75	105	130	155	215
320+	75	110	135	160	220
Over 60 years old					
114	30	45	50	65	75
123	35	45	55	65	80
132	35	50	60	70	85
148	40	55	70	80	100
165	45	55	75	90	110
181	45	65	80	94	125
198	50	65	85	100	135
220	50	70	90	105	145
242	55	70	90	110	150
275	55	75	95	110	155
319	60	80	95	115	160
320+	60	80	100	120	165

Women

Body Weight	Untrained	Novice	Intermediate	Advanced	Elite
97	30	40	50	65	85
105	35	45	55	70	90
114	35	50	60	75	100
123	40	50	60	80	105
132	40	55	65	85	110
148	45	60	70	95	120
165	50	65	75	105	135
181	50	70	80	110	140
198	55	75	85	115	150
199+	60	80	95	125	160
Over 40 years old					
97	25	35	45	55	75
105	30	40	50	60	80
114	30	45	55	65	85
123	35	45	55	70	90
132	35	50	60	75	95
148	40	55	60	85	105
165	45	55	65	90	120
181	45	60	70	95	125
198	50	65	75	100	130
199+	55	70	85	110	140
Over 50 years old					
97	20	30	40	50	65
105	25	35	40	55	70
114	25	40	45	55	75
123	30	40	45	60	80
132	30	45	50	65	85
148	35	45	55	75	90
165	40	50	60	80	105
181	40	55	60	85	110
198	45	60	65	90	115
199+	45	65	75	95	125
Over 60 years old					
97	15	25	30	35	50
105	20	25	30	40	55
114	20	30	35	45	60
123	25	30	35	45	60
132	25	30	35	50	65
148	25	35	40	55	70
165	30	35	45	60	85
181	30	40	45	65	80
198	30	45	50	65	85
199+	35	45	55	70	90

PRESS STANDARDS - KILOGRAMS

Men

Body Weight	Untrained	Novice	Intermediate	Advanced	Elite
52	22.5	32.5	40	50	60
56	25	35	45	52.5	65
60	27.5	37.5	47.5	57.5	70
67	30	42.5	55	62.5	77.5
75	32.5	45	57.5	70	85
82	35	50	62.5	75	100
90	37.5	52.5	65	77.5	105
100	40	55	70	82.5	115
110	42.5	57.5	72.5	85	120
125	42.5	60	75	87.5	122.5
145	45	60	75	90	125
145+	45	62.5	77.5	92.5	130
Over 40 years old					
52	20	30	37.5	42.5	52.2
56	22.5	32.5	40	45	57.5
60	25	35	42.5	50	60
67	27.0	40	47.5	57.5	67.5
75	28	40	52.5	60	75
82	32.5	42.5	55	65	85
90	35	45	57.5	67.5	92.5
100	37.5	47.5	60	72.5	100
110	40	50	62.5	75	105
125	40	52.5	65	77.5	107.5
145	42.5	55	67.5	80	110
145+	42.5	57.5	70	82.5	112.5
Over 50 years old					
52	17.5	25	32.5	37.5	45
56	20	27.5	35	40	47.5
60	22.5	30	37.5	42.5	52.5
67	25	32.5	40	47.5	60
75	27.5	35	45	55	65
82	27.5	37.5	47.5	57.5	77.5
90	30	40	50	60	82.5
100	32.5	40	52.5	62.5	87.5
110	32.5	42.5	55	65	90
125	32.5	45	57.5	67.5	95
145	35	47.5	60	70	97.5
145+	35	50	62.5	72.5	100
Over 60 years old					
52	15	20	22.5	30	35
56	15	20	25	30	37.5
60	17.5	22.5	27.5	32.5	40
67	17.5	25	32.5	35	45
75	20	25	35	40	50
82	20	30	37.5	42.5	57.5
90	22.5	30	40	45	60
100	22.5	32.5	40	47.5	65
110	25	32.5	40	50	67.5
125	25	35	42.5	50	70
145	27.5	37.5	42.5	52.5	72.5
145+	27.5	37.5	45	55	75

Women

Body Weight	Untrained	Novice	Intermediate	Advanced	Elite
44	15	17.5	22.5	30	40
48	15	20	25	32.5	42.5
52	17.5	22.5	27.5	35	45
56	17.5	22.5	27.5	37.5	47.5
60	17.5	25	30	40	50
67	20	27.5	32.5	42.5	55
75	22.5	30	35	47.5	62.5
82	22.5	32.5	37.5	50	65
90	25	35	40	52.5	67.5
90+	27.5	37.5	42.5	57.5	72.5
Over 40 years old					
44	12.5	15	20	25	35
48	15	17.5	22.5	27.5	37.5
52	15	20	25	30	40
56	15	20	25	32.5	40
60	17.5	22.5	27.5	35	42.5
67	17.5	25	27.5	40	47.5
75	20	25	30	40	55
82	20	27.5	32.5	42.5	57.5
90	22.5	30	35	45	60
90+	25	32.5	40	50	65
Over 50 years old					
44	10	15	17.5	22.5	30
48	12.5	15	17.5	25	32.5
52	12.5	17.5	20	25	35
56	15	17.5	20	27.5	37.5
60	15	20	22.5	30	40
67	15	20	25	35	42.5
75	17.5	22.5	27.5	37.5	47.5
82	17.5	25	27.5	40	50
90	20	27.5	30	42.5	52.5
90+	20	30	35	45	57.5
Over 60 years old					
44	7.5	10	15	18	22.5
48	10	12.5	15	20	25
52	10	15	17.5	22.5	25
56	12.5	15	17.5	22.5	27.5
60	12.5	15	17.5	25	30
67	12.5	17.5	20	25	32.5
75	15	17.5	20	27.5	32.5
82	15	17.5	22.5	30	35
90	15	20	25	30	40
90+	17.5	20	25	32.5	42.5

POWER SNATCH STANDARDS - POUNDS

Men

Body Weight	Untrained	Novice	Intermediate	Advanced	Elite
114	45	80	95	135	160
123	50	85	105	145	175
132	55	95	115	155	185
148	60	105	130	175	205
165	65	115	140	190	225
181	70	125	150	205	240
198	75	130	160	220	250
220	80	135	170	230	265
242	85	140	175	235	275
275	90	145	180	245	285
319	95	150	185	250	290
320+	100	155	190	260	300
Over 40 years old					
114	40	70	80	115	140
123	45	75	90	125	150
132	45	85	100	135	160
148	50	90	110	150	180
165	55	100	120	135	195
181	60	110	130	175	205
198	65	115	140	190	215
220	70	120	145	200	230
242	75	125	150	205	240
275	80	130	155	210	245
319	85	135	160	215	250
320+	90	140	165	225	260
Over 50 years old					
114	35	60	70	105	125
123	40	65	80	110	135
132	40	70	85	120	140
148	45	80	100	135	155
165	50	85	105	145	170
181	55	95	115	155	180
198	55	100	125	165	190
220	60	105	130	175	200
242	65	110	135	180	210
275	70	115	140	185	215
319	75	120	145	190	220
320+	80	125	150	200	230
Over 60 years old					
114	25	45	55	80	95
123	30	50	60	85	105
132	30	55	70	90	110
148	35	60	75	100	120
165	40	65	80	110	130
181	40	70	90	120	140
198	45	75	95	130	145
220	45	80	100	135	155
242	50	85	105	140	160
275	55	90	110	145	165
319	60	95	115	150	170
320+	65	100	120	155	175

Women

Body Weight	Untrained	Novice	Intermediate	Advanced	Elite
97	25	50	55	75	95
105	30	55	60	80	100
114	35	55	65	85	110
123	35	60	70	90	115
132	35	65	75	95	120
148	40	70	80	110	135
165	40	75	90	115	150
181	45	80	95	125	155
198	50	90	100	135	165
199+	55	95	110	140	175
Over 40 years old					
97	20	45	45	65	80
105	25	50	50	70	85
114	30	50	55	75	95
123	30	55	60	80	100
132	30	55	65	85	105
148	35	60	70	95	115
165	35	65	75	100	130
181	40	70	80	110	135
198	45	75	85	115	140
199+	50	80	95	120	150
Over 50 years old					
97	20	40	40	55	70
105	20	45	45	60	75
114	25	45	50	65	85
123	25	45	55	70	90
132	25	50	60	75	95
148	30	55	65	85	105
165	30	55	70	90	115
181	35	60	70	95	120
198	40	70	75	105	125
199+	40	75	85	110	135
Over 60 years old					
97	15	30	30	45	55
105	15	30	35	45	60
114	20	30	40	50	65
123	20	35	40	50	70
132	20	40	45	55	75
148	25	40	45	65	80
165	25	45	50	70	85
181	25	45	55	75	90
198	30	50	60	80	95
199+	35	55	65	85	105

POWER SNATCH STANDARDS - KILOGRAMS

Men

Body Weight	Untrained	Novice	Intermediate	Advanced	Elite
52	20.0	37.5	42.5	62.5	72.5
56	22.5	40.0	47.5	65.0	80.0
60	25.0	42.5	52.5	70.0	85.0
67	27.5	47.5	60.0	80.0	92.5
75	30.0	52.5	62.5	87.5	102.5
82	32.5	55.0	67.5	92.5	110.0
90	35.0	57.5	72.5	100.0	115.0
100	37.5	60.0	77.5	105.0	120.0
110	40.0	62.5	80.0	107.5	125.0
125	42.5	65.0	82.5	112.5	130.0
145	42.5	67.5	85.0	115.0	132.5
145+	45.0	70.0	87.5	117.5	137.5
Over 40 years old					
52	17.5	32.5	37.5	52.5	65.0
56	20.0	35.0	40.0	57.5	67.5
60	20.0	37.5	45.0	62.5	72.5
67	22.5	40.0	50.0	67.5	82.5
75	25.0	45.0	55.0	75.0	87.5
82	27.5	50.0	60.0	80.0	92.5
90	30.0	52.5	62.5	87.5	97.5
100	32.5	55.0	65.0	90.0	105.0
110	35.0	57.5	67.5	92.5	110.0
125	37.5	60.0	70.0	95.0	112.5
145	40.0	62.5	72.5	97.5	115.0
145+	42.5	65.0	75.0	102.5	117.5
Over 50 years old					
52	15.0	27.5	32.5	47.5	57.5
56	17.5	30.0	37.5	50.0	62.5
60	17.5	32.5	40.0	55.0	65.0
67	20.0	35.0	45.0	60.0	70.0
75	22.5	40.0	47.5	65.0	77.5
82	25.0	42.5	52.5	70.0	82.5
90	25.0	45.0	55.0	75.0	87.5
100	27.5	47.5	57.5	80.0	90.0
110	30.0	50.0	60.0	82.5	95.0
125	32.5	52.5	62.5	85.0	97.5
145	35.0	55.0	65.0	87.5	100.0
145+	37.5	57.5	67.5	90.0	105.0
Over 60 years old					
52	10.0	20.0	25.0	35.0	42.5
56	12.5	22.5	27.5	37.5	47.5
60	12.5	25.0	32.5	40.0	50.0
67	15.0	27.5	35.0	45.0	55.0
75	17.5	30.0	37.5	50.0	60.0
82	17.5	32.5	40.0	55.0	62.5
90	20.0	35.0	42.5	60.0	65.0
100	20.0	35.0	45.0	62.5	70.0
110	22.5	37.5	47.5	62.5	72.5
125	25.0	40.0	50.0	65.0	75.0
145	27.5	42.5	52.5	67.5	77.5
145+	30.0	45.0	55.0	70.0	80.0

Women

Body Weight	Untrained	Novice	Intermediate	Advanced	Elite
44	10.0	22.5	25.0	35.0	42.5
48	12.5	25.0	27.5	37.5	45.0
52	15.0	25.0	30.0	37.5	50.0
56	15.0	27.5	32.5	40.0	52.5
60	15.0	30.0	35.0	42.5	55.0
67	17.5	32.5	37.5	50.0	62.5
75	17.5	35.0	40.0	52.5	67.5
82	20.0	37.5	42.5	57.5	70.0
90	22.5	40.0	45.0	60.0	75.0
90+	25.0	42.5	50.0	62.5	80.0
Over 40 years old					
44	10.0	20.0	22.5	30.0	37.5
48	12.5	22.5	25.0	32.5	40.0
52	15.0	22.5	25.0	35.0	42.5
56	15.0	25.0	27.5	37.5	45.0
60	15.0	25.0	30.0	40.0	47.5
67	15.0	27.5	32.5	42.5	52.5
75	15.0	30.0	35.0	45.0	60.0
82	17.5	32.5	37.5	50.0	62.5
90	20.0	35.0	40.0	52.5	65.0
90+	22.5	37.5	42.5	55.0	67.5
Over 50 years old					
44	10.0	17.5	17.5	25.0	32.5
48	10.0	20.0	20.0	27.5	35.0
52	12.5	20.0	22.5	30.0	37.5
56	12.5	20.0	25.0	32.5	40.0
60	12.5	22.5	27.5	35.0	42.5
67	12.5	25.0	30.0	37.5	47.5
75	12.5	25.0	32.5	40.0	52.5
82	15.0	27.5	32.5	42.5	55.0
90	17.5	32.5	35.0	47.5	57.5
90+	17.5	35.0	37.5	50.0	62.5
Over 60 years old					
44	7.5	12.5	15.0	20.0	25.0
48	7.5	12.5	15.0	20.0	27.5
52	10.0	12.5	17.5	22.5	30.0
56	10.0	15.0	17.5	22.5	32.5
60	10.0	17.5	20.0	25.0	35.0
67	10.0	17.5	20.0	30.0	37.5
75	10.0	20.0	22.5	32.5	40.0
82	12.5	20.0	25.0	35.0	42.5
90	15.0	22.5	27.5	37.5	45.0
90+	15.0	25.0	30.0	40.0	47.5

BACK SQUAT STANDARDS - POUNDS

Men

Body Weight	Untrained	Novice	Intermediate	Advanced	Elite
114	80	145	175	240	320
123	85	155	190	260	345
132	90	170	205	280	370
148	100	190	230	315	410
165	110	205	250	340	445
181	120	220	270	370	480
198	125	230	285	390	505
220	130	245	300	410	530
242	135	255	310	425	550
275	140	260	320	435	570
319	145	270	325	445	580
320+	150	275	330	455	595
Over 40 years old					
114	70	125	150	205	275
123	75	135	165	225	300
132	80	145	175	240	320
148	85	165	200	270	355
165	95	175	215	290	385
181	100	190	230	320	415
198	105	200	245	335	435
220	110	210	260	355	455
242	115	220	265	365	475
275	120	225	275	375	490
319	125	230	280	385	500
320+	130	240	285	390	510
Over 50 years old					
114	60	110	135	180	245
123	65	120	145	200	260
132	70	130	155	215	280
148	75	145	175	240	310
165	85	155	190	260	340
181	90	165	205	280	365
198	95	175	215	295	385
220	100	185	230	310	405
242	105	195	235	325	420
275	110	200	240	330	435
319	115	205	245	340	440
320+	120	210	250	345	450
Over 60 years old					
114	45	85	100	135	180
123	50	90	105	150	195
132	50	95	115	160	210
148	55	105	130	175	230
165	60	115	145	195	250
181	65	120	155	210	270
198	70	130	160	220	285
220	75	140	165	230	300
242	80	145	175	240	310
275	80	150	180	245	320
319	85	155	185	250	325
320+	85	155	190	255	335

Women

Body Weight	Untrained	Novice	Intermediate	Advanced	Elite
97	45	85	100	130	165
105	50	90	105	140	175
114	55	100	115	150	190
123	55	105	120	160	200
132	60	110	130	170	210
148	65	120	140	185	230
165	70	130	150	200	255
181	75	140	165	215	270
198	80	150	175	230	290
199+	85	160	185	240	305
Over 40 years old					
97	40	75	85	110	140
105	45	80	90	120	150
114	45	85	100	130	165
123	50	90	105	140	170
132	50	95	110	145	180
148	55	105	120	160	200
165	60	110	130	170	220
181	65	120	140	185	230
198	70	130	150	200	250
199+	75	140	160	205	260
Over 50 years old					
97	35	65	75	100	125
105	40	70	80	105	135
114	40	75	85	115	145
123	45	80	90	120	150
132	45	85	100	130	160
148	50	90	105	140	175
165	55	100	115	150	195
181	55	105	125	165	205
198	60	115	135	175	220
199+	65	120	140	180	230
Over 60 years old					
97	30	50	55	75	100
105	30	50	60	80	105
114	35	55	65	85	115
123	35	60	70	90	125
132	35	65	75	95	135
148	40	70	80	105	150
165	40	75	85	110	165
181	45	80	95	115	180
198	45	85	100	125	195
199+	50	90	105	130	200

BACK SQUAT STANDARDS - KILOGRAM

Men

Body Weight	Untrained	Novice	Intermediate	Advanced	Elite
52	35.0	65.0	80.0	107.5	145.0
56	37.5	70.0	87.5	117.5	157.5
60	40.0	77.5	92.5	127.5	167.5
67	45.0	85.0	105.0	142.5	185.0
75	50.0	92.5	112.5	155.0	202.5
82	55.0	100.0	122.5	167.5	217.5
90	57.5	105.0	130.0	177.5	230.0
100	60.0	110.0	135.0	185.0	240.0
110	62.5	115.0	140.0	192.5	250.0
125	65.0	117.5	145.0	197.5	257.5
145	67.5	122.5	147.5	202.5	262.5
145+	70.0	125.0	150.0	207.5	270.0
Over 40 years old					
52	32.5	57.5	67.5	92.5	125.0
56	35.0	62.5	75.0	102.5	137.5
60	37.5	65.0	80.0	110.0	145.0
67	40.0	75.0	90.0	122.5	160.0
75	42.5	80.0	97.5	130.0	175.0
82	45.0	85.0	105.0	145.2	187.5
90	47.5	90.0	110.0	152.5	197.5
100	50.0	95.0	117.5	160.0	207.5
110	52.5	100.0	120.0	165.0	215.0
125	55.0	102.5	125.0	170.0	222.5
145	57.5	105.0	127.5	175.0	227.5
145+	60.0	110.0	130.0	177.5	232.5
Over 50 years old					
52	27.5	50.0	62.5	82.5	112.5
56	30.0	55.0	65.0	90.0	117.5
60	32.5	60.0	70.0	97.5	127.5
67	35.0	65.0	80.0	110.0	140.0
75	37.5	70.0	85.0	117.5	155.0
82	40.0	75.0	92.5	127.5	165.0
90	42.5	80.0	97.5	132.5	175.0
100	45.0	85.0	105.0	140.0	182.5
110	47.5	87.5	107.5	147.5	190.0
125	50.0	90.0	110.0	150.0	197.5
145	52.5	92.5	112.5	155.0	200.0
145+	55.0	95.0	115.0	157.5	205.0
Over 60 years old					
52	20.0	37.5	45.0	60.0	82.5
56	22.5	40.0	47.5	67.5	87.5
60	22.5	42.5	52.5	72.5	95.0
67	25.0	47.5	60.0	80.0	105.0
75	27.5	52.5	65.0	87.5	112.5
82	30.0	55.0	70.0	95.0	122.5
90	32.5	60.0	72.5	100.0	130.0
100	35.0	62.5	75.0	105.0	135.0
110	37.5	65.0	80.0	107.5	140.0
125	37.5	67.5	82.5	110.0	145.0
145	40.0	70.0	85.0	112.5	147.5
145+	40.0	70.0	87.5	115.0	152.5

Women

Body Weight	Untrained	Novice	Intermediate	Advanced	Elite
44	20.0	37.5	45.0	60.0	75.0
48	22.5	40.0	47.5	65.0	80.0
52	25.0	45.0	52.5	67.5	87.5
56	25.0	47.5	55.0	72.5	90.0
60	27.5	50.0	60.0	77.5	95.0
67	30.0	55.0	62.5	85.0	105.0
75	32.5	57.5	67.5	90.0	115.0
82	35.0	62.5	75.0	97.5	122.5
90	37.5	67.5	80.0	105.0	132.5
90+	40.0	72.5	85.0	110.0	137.5
Over 40 years old					
44	17.5	35.0	40.0	50.0	62.5
48	20.0	37.5	42.5	55.0	67.5
52	20.0	37.5	45.0	60.0	75.0
56	22.5	40.0	47.5	62.5	77.5
60	22.5	42.5	50.0	65.0	82.5
67	25.0	47.5	55.0	72.5	90.0
75	27.5	50.0	60.0	77.5	100.0
82	30.0	55.0	62.5	85.0	105.0
90	32.5	60.0	67.5	90.0	112.5
90+	35.0	62.5	72.5	92.5	117.5
Over 50 years old					
44	15.0	30.0	35.0	45.0	57.5
48	17.5	32.5	37.5	47.5	62.5
52	17.5	35.0	40.0	52.5	65.0
56	20.0	37.5	42.5	55.0	67.5
60	20.0	40.0	45.0	60.0	72.5
67	22.5	42.5	47.5	65.0	80.0
75	25.0	45.0	52.5	67.5	87.5
82	25.0	47.5	57.5	75.0	92.5
90	27.5	52.5	62.5	80.0	100.0
90+	30.0	55.0	65.0	82.5	105.0
Over 60 years old					
44	12.5	22.5	25.0	35.0	45.0
48	12.5	22.5	27.5	37.5	47.5
52	15.0	25.0	30.0	37.5	52.5
56	15.0	27.5	32.5	40.0	57.5
60	15.0	30.0	35.0	42.5	62.5
67	17.5	32.5	37.5	47.5	67.5
75	17.5	35.0	40.0	50.0	75.0
82	20.0	37.5	42.5	52.5	82.5
90	20.0	40.0	45.0	57.5	87.5
90+	22.5	40.0	47.5	60.0	90.0

PUSH-UP STANDARDS

Men

Age	Untrained	Novice	Intermediate	Advanced	Elite
Adult	20	35	43	61	76
Over 40 years old	14	24	34	58	70
Over 50 years old	10	16	25	46	60
Over 60 years old	5	10	18	40	55

Women

Age	Untrained	Novice	Intermediate	Advanced	Elite
Adult	4	13	18	35	46
Over 40 years old	2	5	13	30	40
Over 50 years old	0	2	10	25	34
Over 60 years old	0	1	8	21	28

PULL-UP STANDARDS

Men

Age	Untrained	Novice	Intermediate	Advanced	Elite
Adult	4	8	12	16	22
Over 40 years old	2	5	9	14	17
Over 50 years old	1	3	7	11	15
Over 60 years old	0	1	2	8	11

Women

Age	Untrained	Novice	Intermediate	Advanced	Elite
Adult	1	3	5	8	10
Over 40 years old	0	2	3	5	8
Over 50 years old	0	1	2	3	5
Over 60 years old	0	0	1	2	3

SIT-UP STANDARDS

Men

Age	Untrained	Novice	Intermediate	Advanced	Elite
Adult	27	43	50	69	80
Over 40 years old	18	29	38	62	76
Over 50 years old	13	25	30	53	68
Over 60 years old	9	18	27	50	64

Women

Age	Untrained	Novice	Intermediate	Advanced	Elite
Adult	27	43	50	69	80
Over 40 years old	18	29	38	62	76
Over 50 years old	13	25	30	53	68
Over 60 years old	9	18	27	50	64

ONE MILE RUN STANDARDS

Men

Age	Untrained	Novice	Intermediate	Advanced	Elite
Adult	7:45	7:15	6:45	6:00	4:30
Over 40 years old	9:15	8:00	7:30	6:45	5:15
Over 50 years old	9:45	8:30	8:00	7:15	5:45
Over 60 years old	10:00	8:45	8:15	7:45	6:30

Women

Age	Untrained	Novice	Intermediate	Advanced	Elite
Adult	9:00	8:30	8:00	7:30	5:15
Over 40 years old	10:45	10:00	9:15	8:30	6:45
Over 50 years old	11:15	10:30	9:45	8:45	7:15
Over 60 years old	11:45	11:00	10:15	9:30	8:15

1000 METER ROW STANDARDS

Men

Age	Untrained	Novice	Intermediate	Advanced	Elite
Adult	4:15	3:45	3:30	3:15	3:00
Over 40 years old	4:30	4:00	3:45	3:30	3:15
Over 50 years old	4:45	4:15	4:00	3:45	3:30
Over 60 years old	5:00	4:30	4:15	4:00	3:45

Women

Age	Untrained	Novice	Intermediate	Advanced	Elite
Adult	5:00	4:30	4:15	4:00	3:45
Over 40 years old	5:15	4:45	4:30	4:15	4:00
Over 50 years old	5:30	5:00	4:45	4:30	4:15
Over 60 years old	5:45	5:15	5:00	4:45	4:30

Made in the USA
Lexington, KY
27 November 2014